Medicine in the Mining Industries

Medicine in the Mining Industries

Edited by John M. Rogan M.D., F.R.C.P.Ed., D.P.H.

Chief Medical Officer, National Coal Board.
Director, Institute of Occupational Medicine, Edinburgh.

William Heinemann Medical Books Ltd
London

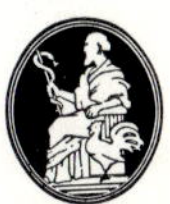

First published 1972

© John M. Rogan 1972

ISBN 0 433 28200 2

Text set in 10/11 pt. Monotype Times New Roman, printed by letterpress, and bound in Great Britain at The Pitman Press, Bath

Preface

This book is intended for those who are concerned with the health of
the miner. Its aim is to present a concise and accurate account of the
dangers inherent in mining and of the means to minimize them. They
include the dust-borne diseases, radio-activity, skin disease, extremes of
temperature, noise, noxious gases and accidents. The related topic,
absence from work, is discussed. As the efficiency of medical services
for mines is dependent on good administration in a business setting,
there is also a chapter on this subject.

Mining transcends national boundaries and it is therefore appropriate
that the contributors come from most of the major mining countries.
I am grateful to them for their painstaking work.

This is the first book of its kind, a fact surprising in the light of the
great expansion of mining in recent years.

January 1972.   J. M. R.

Contents

Contributors

R. McL. Archibald, M.B., Ch.B., D.I.H.
Assistant Chief Medical Officer, National Coal Board, London.

M. Bundy, M.D.
Director—Industrial Medicine, United States Steel Corporation, Pittsburgh.

R. B. Buzzard, B.M., B.Ch.
Director, National Institute of Industrial Psychology, London.

P. R. Davis, M.B., B.S., Ph.D.
Professor of Human Biology, University of Surrey.

P. E. Enterline, Ph.D.
Professor of Biostatistics, University of Pittsburgh.

M. Glick, M.B., Ch.B., F.R.C.S. F.R.A.C.S.
Chief Medical Officer, Joint Coal Board, New South Wales.

O. G. Griffin, M.Sc., A. Inst. P.
Principal Scientific Officer, Safety in Mines Research Establishment, Sheffield.

R. J. Hamilton, B.Sc., F. Inst. P.
Head of Dust Group, Mining Research and Development Establishment, Bretby, England.

M. Jacobsen, B.A.
Head of Statistics Branch, Institute of Occupational Medicine, Edinburgh.

J. J. Jarry, Docteur-en-Médecine
lately Chief Medical Officer, Charbonnages de France, Paris.

H. Jorgensen, M.D.
Chief Medical Officer, Luossavaara-Kiirunavaara AB, Kiruna, Sweden.

A. A. Knight, M.Sc., Ph.D.
Senior Ergonomist, Institute of Occupational Medicine, Edinburgh.

F. Lavenne, M.D.
Professor of Medicine, University of Louvain.

A. Lawrence, D. Comm., B.Econ.
Head, Personnel Research Division, Human Sciences Laboratory, Chamber of Mines of South Africa, Johannesburg.

P. J. Lawther, M.B., B.S., F.R.C.P.
Professor of Environmental Medicine, London University.

G. L. Leathart, M.D., F.R.C.P.
Senior Lecturer, Department of Industrial Health, University of Newcastle.

J. S. McLintock, M.B., Ch.B., D.P.H.
Deputy Chief Medical Officer, National Coal Board, London.

D. C. F. Muir, M.B., B.S., Ph.D., M.R.C.P., M.R.C.P.Ed.
Head of Physiology Branch, Institute of Occupational Medicine, Edinburgh.

S. Rae, M.B., Ch.B., F.R.C.P.Ed.
Head of Medical Branch, Institute of Occupational Medicine, Edinburgh.

Lynne Reid, M.D., F.R.C.P., F.R.A.C.P., F.R.C. Path.
Professor of Experimental Pathology, Institute of Diseases of the Chest, Brompton Hospital, London.

W. B. Roantree, M.A., M.D., F.R.C.S.Ed.
Medical Officer, Kent, National Coal Board, formerly Chief Medical Officer, Kolar Goldfields, India.

T. D. Spencer, M.D., D.P.H.
Assistant Chief Medical Officer, National Coal Board, London.

R. A. Steele, M.B., Ch.B., Ph.D., F.R.C.P.A.
Senior Lecturer in Morbid Anatomy and Experimental Pathology, University of Southampton.

H. R. Vickers, V.R.D., M.A., M.D., F.R.C.P.
Consultant Dermatologist, United Oxford Hospitals.

W. H. Walton, M.Sc., F. Inst. P.
Head of Environmental Branch, Institute of Occupational Medicine, Edinburgh.

I. Webster, M.B., B.Ch., B.Sc., F.R.C. Path.
Director, National Research Institute for Occupational Diseases, South Africa.

J. S. Weiner, M.Sc., M.A., Ph.D. M.R.C.S., L.R.C.P.
Professor of Environmental Physiology, University of London.

Norman Williams, M.D.
Professor of Preventive Medicine, Jefferson Medical College of Philadelphia, Pennsylvania. Formerly: Director of Occupational Health, Saskatchewan Department of Public Health, Canada.

Donald M. Williamson, M.D., M.R.C.G.P., D.I.H.
Consultant Dermatologist, Pontefract General Infirmary and Honorary Consultant Dermatologist, United Leeds Hospitals.

C. H. Wyndham, M.B., D.Sc., M.R.C.P., F.R.S.(S.A.)
Director, Human Sciences Laboratory, Chamber of Mines of South Africa.

Chapter 1
The Pathology of Coal Pneumoconiosis

Introduction

Coal workers' pneumoconiosis has recently been defined as "the response to prolonged retention in the lungs of abnormal amounts of dust derived from coal mining operations" (Rogan, 1970). The response of the lung tissue to such dust is here analysed, but in general it can be said that in "simple" pneumoconiosis the tissue response is unimportant; it is in the small group of miners in whom the condition has become "complicated" by progressive massive fibrosis and is associated with severe disability that the nature of the tissue response is paramount.

Even simple pneumoconiosis has become inextricably mixed with two other conditions, chronic bronchitis and emphysema, not to mention progressive massive fibrosis and cor pulmonale, to produce a veritable Gordian knot: the only way to "cut" the knot is first to consider each of these diseases separately and then in relation to simple pneumoconiosis.

The different forms of coal pneumoconiosis are described in the last section of the chapter which ends with a note on pathological examination of the lungs.

Chronic Bronchitis

Chronic bronchitis includes all chronic inflammatory conditions of the airways; it has also become a term of art to describe the hypersecretion of mucus which is not associated with any other identifiable pulmonary or cardiac condition (Medical Research Council, 1960). It is this condition to which Laennec (1827) applied the term "bronchial catarrh". Mucus is secreted in the normal bronchial tree from the goblet cells of the surface epithelium and from the secretory tubules of the bronchial glands deep in the bronchial wall. Although it is widely accepted that chronic bronchitis should be defined in clinical terms, a pathological basis for the hypersecretion of mucus can be recognized in hypertrophy of the mucous glands (Fig. 1), in increased numbers of goblet cells and in their extension to the peripheral part of the airways where they are normally sparse (Reid, 1954, 1960). The changes in the large airways are more uniform than those at the periphery and thus examination of one large airway will usually suffice to make the diagnosis of chronic bronchitis.

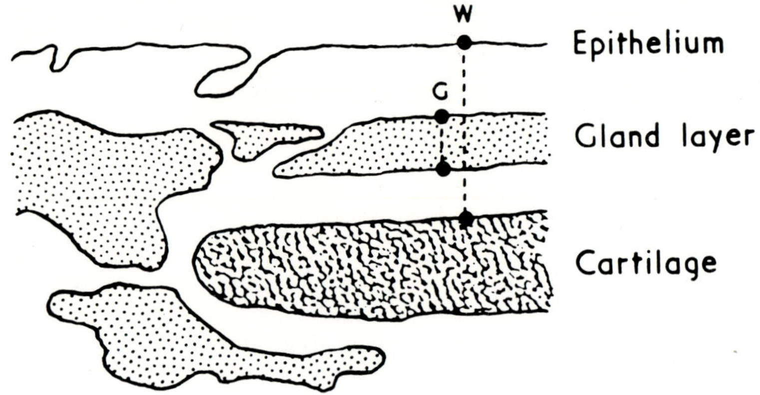

FIG. 1. Gland/wall ratio. At a site where epithelium is roughly parallel to cartilage, gland G and wall thickness W are measured. Increase in gland size is detected by rise in ratio.

Diagnosis of Chronic Bronchitis—Gland to Wall Ratio

Gland depth and the distance between the epithelium and the cartilage can be measured on the same radius of the bronchus, choosing a point in the bronchial wall where the epithelium is roughly parallel to the cartilage (Reid, 1960) as shown in Fig. 1. The mean of several readings may be expressed as a gland/wall ratio. For this purpose, the main or lobar bronchi offer the most convenient airways as glands are abundant between the epithelium and cartilage. In the trachea, cartilage rings are usually just under the epithelium with the glands bunched mainly in the spaces between them. In the enlarged glands the tubules are also enlarged and since gland hypertrophy can be assessed from this feature it can be diagnosed even on a surgical biopsy.

In patients whose condition fulfils the Medical Research Council definition (1960) of simple bronchitis, gland enlargement is uniform throughout the large airways (Reid, 1960).

The changes in the peripheral small airways are the more important in terms of respiratory disability. A relatively small amount of secretion in airways of a millimetre or so in diameter will produce much greater functional effect than the same amount lying on the surface of a large airway.

Cause and Pathogenesis

Epidemiological studies have shown that often the most important single factor associated with sputum production and hence with hypertrophy of mucus-secreting tissue is tobacco smoking (Oswald and Medvei, 1955), so much so that no other factor can be satisfactorily analysed unless allowance is made for smoking habits. It has thus been difficult to show whether any other factor has a significant effect in producing cough with sputum, but other conditions, such as climate and industrial exposure seem also to contribute.

Experimental studies on the effects of irritants on the respiratory system have established that in the airways increase in gland size and in goblet cells occurs without associated infection (Reid, 1963). A count of goblet cells and of the cells in mitosis (Lamb and Reid, 1968, 1969) offers a satisfactory way of assessing the effect of a given substance on the airway epithelium. Irritants may not necessarily have the same rating by each test. For example, cigarette and cigar tobacco score similarly on a goblet cell count; but the increase in mitotic cell activity was very much greater after exposure to cigarette smoke, cigar tobacco smoke producing a similar effect to that of sulphur dioxide exposure (Lamb and Reid, 1968). Humidity cannot be shown to produce an effect on goblet cells (Jones, Baetjer and Reid, 1971).

Chronic Bronchitis in Coal Miners

Recently, in Australia, McKenzie, Glick and Outhred (1969) investigated the gland size of the larger airways within the lungs of coal miners. They were able to show that the glands at this level were enlarged and encroached significantly on the bronchial lumen, a fact with important implications in the functioning of airways.

Recent epidemiological studies by Rae, Walker and Attfield (1971) have, for the first time, shown that over the years dust may contribute to the development of chronic bronchitis. It was only with the environmental information obtained over more than 10 years that a correlation between long-term dust exposure and the symptoms of chronic bronchitis emerged. Similar studies may well be necessary to show the effect of other environmental conditions such as atmospheric pollution and humidity, since short term experiments over a number of weeks have not, to date, sufficed to show that dust exposure or exposure to extremes of temperature or humidity will produce any detectable effect on mucus-secreting tissue.

Emphysema

It is now accepted that emphysema is best defined in structural terms. The following is the definition of emphysema recommended here (Reid, 1967):

> "Emphysema is a condition of the lung characterised by increase beyond the normal of the air spaces distal to the terminal bronchiolus, that is, within the acinus."

Anatomical Types

The enlarged air spaces of emphysema may affect the whole acinus or show a characteristic distribution within it. In Figure 2 are illustrated

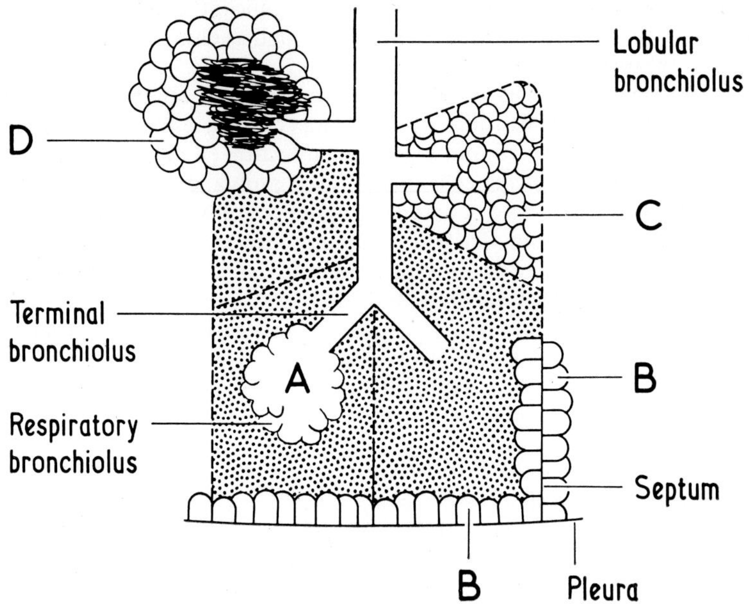

FIG. 2. Diagrammatic representation of the four anatomical types of emphysema.

the various types that are widely recognized—in centriacinar (or centri-lobular) emphysema* (A) the enlarged air spaces are found in the central part of the acinus and represent a dilatation or increase in size of the air spaces opening into the respiratory bronchioli; in periacinar, or paraseptal (B) emphysema the enlarged air spaces are found at the edge of an acinus but only where this is bounded by connective tissue, that is, the periacinar alveoli are only susceptible to this type of emphysema where they are also paraseptal; in panacinar emphysema (C) the enlargement of air spaces occurs throughout the acinus, although not

* A cluster of several acini make up the lobule; when this lesion was first described it was called centrilobular in that the large air spaces were centrally placed in the lobule rather than peripherally.

all acini are affected evenly—the enlargement may be so great that an acinus completely disappears; in scar emphysema (D) the enlarged alveoli are distributed irregularly within the acinus; it occurs around scars into which lung is often condensed, such as scars of progressive massive fibrosis or silicosis.

Emphysema under the pleura may elevate it and change the normal contour of the lung, such bulging of the pleura being described as a "bulla". If large enough, a bulla may be detected in the radiograph. It may be an isolated example of emphysema in an otherwise normal lung or bullae may develop as part of widespread emphysema. Within a bulla the emphysema is always panacinar in type.

The word "focal" has not been used here as it has been so variously applied that it has become a source of confusion.

Centriacinar Emphysema

A number of studies have shown that centriacinar emphysema is a common finding even in people without exposure to industrial dust. Snider and his co-workers in Chicago (1962), and Heard and Izukawa (1964) in London, have shown that this condition is common in subjects who, during life, were known to have a normal chest radiograph and had had no pulmonary symptoms. Centriacinar emphysema can be found in lungs in which there is no evidence of bronchiolitis. It is reported to be more common in the male than the female (Thurlbeck, 1963), which might suggest that the increase in size of centriacinar spaces is associated with an increase in overall lung volume. Since no increase in alveolar or acinar number has been reported in large as compared with small lungs, the male acinus must be larger on average than the female (Weibel, 1963).

Miners' lungs take up coal as particulate matter into macrophages which may be cleared along the ciliary escalator or incorporated into the alveolar and small airway walls and eventually reach lymph nodes from either the peribronchial or perivascular lymphatics. Within the acinus, dust-filled macrophages may concentrate (i) in the alveoli around the accessory bronchiolo-alveolar communications of Lambert (1955), (ii) within the alveoli opening into respiratory bronchioli, or (iii) in alveoli lying at the periphery of the acinus. Perhaps one of the most striking demonstrations of this pattern of deposition is seen in the lung after haemorrhage or after the experimental flooding of the alveolar spaces with blood which, at first, is throughout the acinus (Magarey, 1951) but within a few days the macrophages are concentrated in the regions described above.

Dust storage in the central part of the acinus occurs whether or not centriacinar emphysema is present (Figs. 3 and 4). Within any lung more dust will be found toward the apex than toward the base and the centriacinar lesions are predominantly found in the upper two thirds

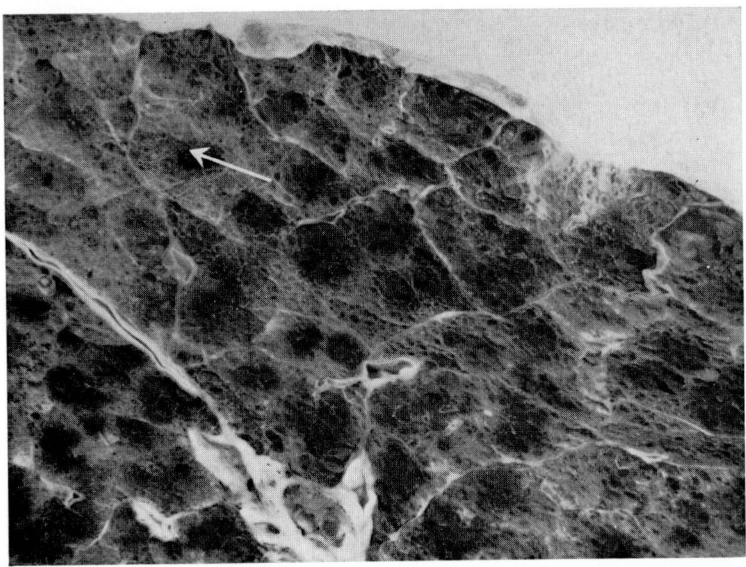

Fig. 3. Slice of lung showing macroscopically mild panacinar emphysema throughout with localized accumulation of dust in the centre of acinus (arrowed); centriacinar emphysema absent.

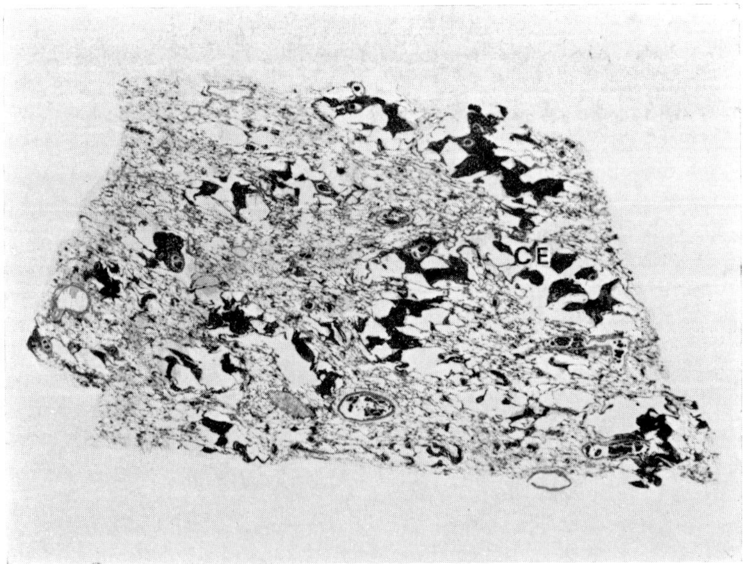

Fig. 4. Microscopic section of lung showing centriacinar emphysema (CE) etched by dust. ($\times 5$.)

of the lung with individual lesions tending to be larger nearer to the apex (Snider, Brody and Doctor, 1962; Thurlbeck, 1963). This, at first sight, might suggest a relationship between dust and centriacinar emphysema but, in many lungs, it is possible to show that at any given level centriacinar lesions are present and of the same size irrespective of the presence of dust. Several studies have failed to show a correlation between the presence of emphysema assessed pathologically and the amount of dust accumulated within the lung.

Over the years, it is the centriacinar type of emphysema that has come to be associated with the accumulation of industrial dust, particularly coal (Gough, 1940; Gough, James and Wentworth, 1949; Heppleston, 1954). It would seem best, at present, to regard it as an anatomical variant whose cause is not known. West (1971) has recently demonstrated that the tensions within the lung are greater toward the apex. It is not necessary to invoke infection as a cause of this type.

Periacinar Emphysema

Spontaneous pneumothorax may arise from rupture of periacinar subpleural lesions, which may be detected on the radiograph if they enlarge. Periacinar emphysema does not give rise to airways obstruction (Edge, Simon and Reid, 1966).

Panacinar Emphysema

(a) *Of Age*

Although the lung of an old person may be indistinguishable from that of a young one, even in those who during life had no respiratory symptoms and are known to have had a normal chest radiograph, with age a mild degree of panacinar emphysema, as in Fig. 3, may develop with air spaces up to 1 or 2 mm in diameter (Edge, Millard, Reid and Simon, 1964).

(b) *Primary Emphysema* (syn. Essential, Idiopathic or Cryptogenic)

A more severe form of panacinar emphysema may develop spontaneously. Sometimes it shows a familial incidence in patients who are deficient in α_1 antitrypsin (Hutchinson, Cook, Barter, Harris and Hugh-Jones, 1971). Many acini may completely disappear leaving large ragged spaces in the lung. In about a quarter of the patients who die from chronic bronchitis, this type of emphysema is sufficiently severe and widespread to be detected on the radiograph (Simon, 1964; Reid, 1967). In such cases the relative importance of the various mechanisms that may cause emphysema is not known.

Scar Emphysema

Scar emphysema may develop around lesions of progressive massive fibrosis or silicosis. Post-infective scarring also commonly shows a halo of this type of emphysema. The enlarged air spaces probably arise from previous inflammatory damage—with perhaps some compensatory over-inflation.

Difficulties in Diagnosis of type of Emphysema

Although there would be wide agreement among pathologists on the foregoing description of emphysema it is in their application to diagnosis that confusion has given rise to a seeming disagreement between pathologists.

In the aged lung, panacinar emphysema may be surprisingly uniform throughout and, for this reason, some authorities have restricted the use of the word "panacinar" to this subgroup.

It has also been suggested that centriacinar emphysema is diagnosed by a region of severe emphysema surrounded by a less affected zone. On occasions this has given rise to the diagnosis of centriacinar emphysema when a sub-segment was affected with panacinar and the rest of the lung was normal. Periacinar emphysema may cause a hole deep in the lung surrounded by normal alveoli.

A region of panacinar emphysema with a large amount of dust spread through it has given rise to the diagnosis of centriacinar on the ground that dust causes centriacinar, therefore the panacinar emphysema with a large amount of dust must have started as centriacinar. These examples show how confusion may arise.

The types of emphysema described above are anatomical and descriptive and should be applied to the anatomical lesion without any pathogenetic implication.

Disability from Emphysema

Any critical assessment of disability in patients with emphysema makes it clear that only one type of emphysema *per se* gives rise to airways obstruction; this is the widespread panacinar emphysema found in primary, essential, idiopathic or cryptogenic emphysema. In this condition there is no hypertrophy of the mucous glands, no increase in goblet cells and no airway fibrosis. The airway obstruction is due to secondary functional disturbance arising from reduction in elastic recoil of the lung on expiration which produces premature closure or collapse of airways (Dayman, 1951). This type of emphysema is capable of producing severe airways obstruction. It may, of course, co-exist with chronic bronchitis.

Chronic bronchitis may be associated with severe disability even if no emphysema is present. In some cases dying with severe airways obstruction, the types of emphysema found are similar to those in the "normal population"; these types include the panacinar type seen in the aged lung and centriacinar emphysema. Certainly these types may be present in the absence of disability but it is not known whether they contribute to disability if airways obstruction from chronic bronchitis is also present.

Confusion is still being caused by the assumption (Thurlbeck, Henderson, Fraser and Bates, 1970; Lancet, 1971) that centrilobular emphysema always causes disability.

Correlation between Radiographic Features of Emphysema and Pathological Findings

It has been shown that it is possible to detect, reliably, on the radiograph severe panacinar emphysema if it is widely enough distributed (Simon, 1964; Reid and Millard, 1964). Centriacinar emphysema is not apparent on the chest radiograph nor are mild degrees of panacinar, such as are found in the aged lung. The radiographic evidence of emphysema is found if either a localized region of lung is totally affected or a lung is affected through about two thirds of its volume by panacinar emphysema of Grade III severity (air spaces are larger than 2 mm in diameter). The radiographic features on which the diagnosis of severe panacinar emphysema can be reliably made, have recently been analysed in detail by Simon (1971). The main features can be summarized, thus:

(i) Excess of air in the lung shown by a low and flat diaphragm below the sixth intercostal space anteriorly;

(ii) Cardiovascular changes—a narrow vertical heart, 11·5 cm or less, with normal or prominent hilar and small intrapulmonary vessels;

(iii) A region of local vessel loss suggesting a bulla.

Only the first two signs are essential to the diagnosis.

The presence of right heart failure or of severe polycythaemia may mask the presence of emphysema since engorgement of vessels and elevation of the diaphragm then occurs.

Coal Pneumoconiosis

Changes in the Alveolar Wall associated with the Storage of Coal

The accumulation of macrophages within respiratory bronchioli may give the appearance of a small nodule of carbon with a halo of dilated spaces. Dust is not always as focal; it may occur diffusely through the lung and this would seem to be particularly so in cases of panacinar emphysema but the distribution of dust throughout the lung may also be diffuse with focal accentuation. Although in some miners the distribution of dust can be regarded as principally centriacinar, in others it is panacinar (Figs. 3 and 4).

Microscopic examination of accumulations of coal in the alveoli show that there is a slight increase in reticulin fibres and, to a lesser extent, of collagen within the alveolar wall (Heppleston, 1954; Duguid and Lambert, 1964). The importance of these changes has sometimes been exaggerated to the point at which simple coal miners' lung is regarded as a form of fibrosis. There is no evidence that the small increase in collagen or reticulin resulting from coal accumulation within alveoli, whose overall architecture is still intact, contributes to disability.

Even with more extreme degrees of fibrosis, as in patients who are known to have had sarcoid or tuberculosis, it is apparent that airways obstruction does not result from scar type emphysema, nor even from compensatory emphysema (Reid, 1967). The suggestion of Duguid and Lambert (1964) that condensation of alveoli associated with such lesions produces compensatory emphysema, does not explain therefore how these would give rise to airways obstruction—the reason for the shortness of breath complained of by the disabled miner.

Small Dust Lesions

The International Labour Organization Radiographic Classification (1970) recognizes three types of opacity—the pinhead, macular and nodular. The dust accumulations that give rise to these shadows range from about 1 mm to 10 mm or so in diameter and, on pathological examination, are usually found to be (i) coal and inert mineral (Rivers, Wise, King and Nagelschmidt, 1960), or rarely (ii) the above with silica also, or (iii) a necrobiotic nodule of the rheumatoid or "Caplan" type (Lindars and Davies, 1967). In the first type there is an accumulation of dust in which there is condensation of alveoli with increase in reticulin and collagen (Figs. 5 and 6). In the second, the appearance is that of a mixed lesion, part inert dust focus and part silicotic nodule as described in Chapter 2.

Progressive Massive Fibrosis (syn. "Complicated" Pneumoconiosis)

Sometimes the lung of a miner shows a large, solid, black mass (Fig. 7) which represents an accumulation of coal both within macrophages and between reticulin and collagen fibres. Analysis shows that this dust carries no higher content of silica than that in the lung of simple coal pneumoconiosis. These lesions are commonly found in the upper lobe against the fissure and, as they enlarge, may transgress the fissure so that the central part of the lung is converted into a dense, black mass. Occasionally such lesions are seen in the lower lobe and James (1954) has suggested that any black mass above 3 cm in diameter should be regarded as progressive massive fibrosis.

The lesions of progressive massive fibrosis may be quite large but their edge not show any dilatation of air spaces (Figs. 7 and 8), that is to say that even such extreme condensation of lung is not necessarily associated with emphysema. Chemical analysis of the dust suggests that silica is not the main cause of the fibrosis. Kilpatrick, Heppleston and

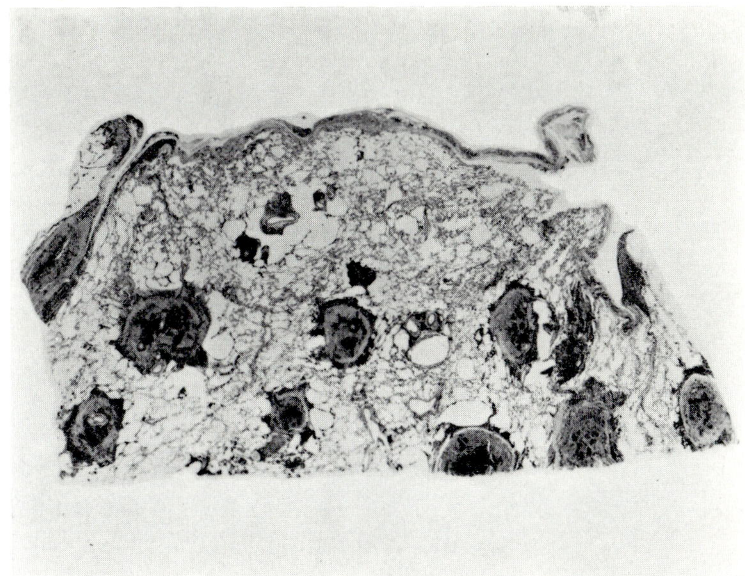

FIG. 5. Low power photomicrograph of lung section showing several dust nodules. (×5.)

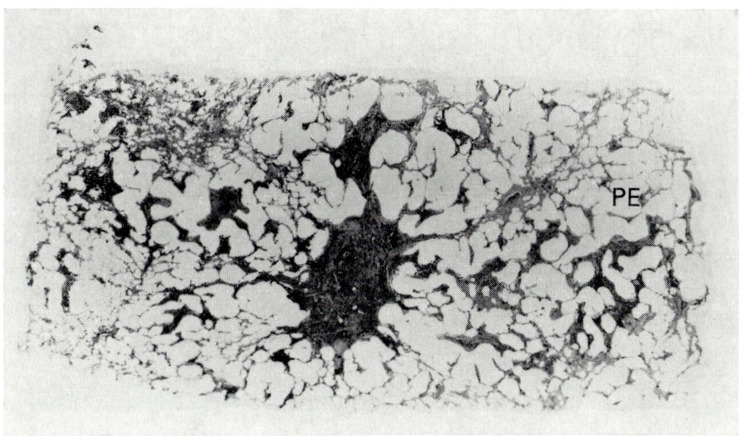

FIG. 6. Low power photomicrograph of dust nodule surrounded by panacinar emphysema (PE). (×5.)

Fletcher (1954) in their investigation of patients found that 27 of 104 with massive fibrosis had tubercle bacilli in their sputum and they regarded the condition as a modified form of tuberculosis. Attygalle, Harrison, King and Mohanty (1954) produced lesions resembling

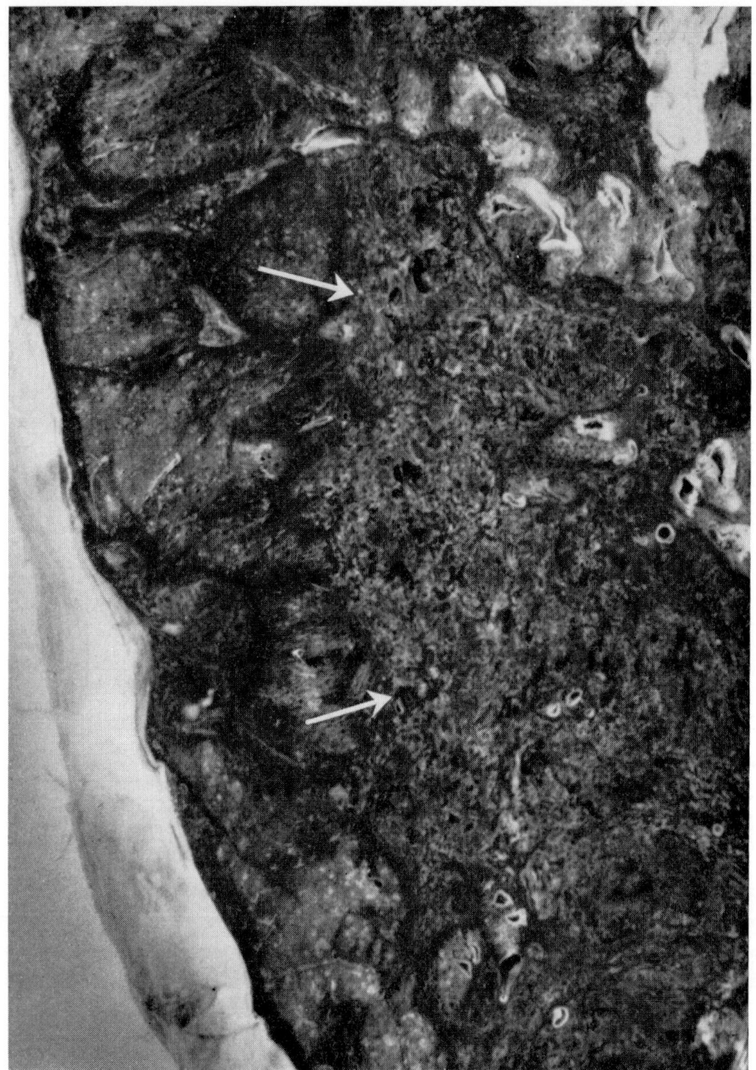

FIG. 7. Progressive massive fibrosis (PMF); the edge is shown by tip
of arrows and is free of emphysema.

massive fibrosis by intra-tracheal injection of coal dust and mycobacteria. Nevertheless, it is now considered that tuberculous infection
is likely to be a late sequel to massive fibrosis rather than its cause,
not least because of its failure to respond to tuberculosis chemotherapy
(Ball, Berry, Clarke, Gilson and Thomas, 1969). An immunological

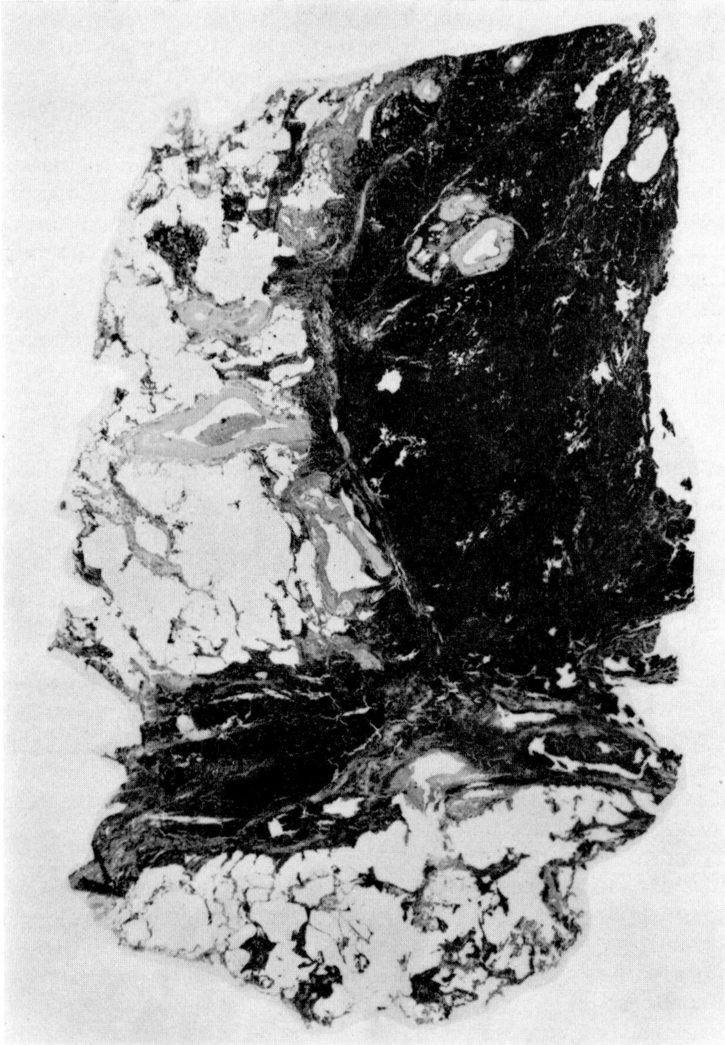

FIG. 8. Low power photomicrograph of edge of lesion of PMF showing severe panacinar emphysema (PE) in adjacent lung. (×5.)

theory of the aetiology of massive fibrosis has been advanced by Vigliani and Pernis (1958), but the immunological phenomena described may well be coincidental rather than causative. Despite much speculation and experiment the cause of progressive massive fibrosis remains unknown.

Caplan's Syndrome

In patients with rheumatoid arthritis, Caplan (1953) reported some, who were also coal miners, with multiple rounded shadows in their chest radiograph. These were basal as often as apical in contrast to progressive massive fibrosis, which is more usually apical. It emerged that these masses were necrobiotic nodules typical of rheumatoid arthritis. Necrobiotic nodules giving the characteristic radiographic appearance have now been reported in other industrial conditions. It seems possible that the presence of an increased amount of reticulin or collagen in the lung predisposes patients suffering from rheumatoid arthritis to this particular tissue response. Microscopically the lesions have a pale centre that is necrotic and may cavitate or occasionally calcify. The edge of the lesion is distinguished microscopically by the "palisaded" appearance of granulation tissue.

Correlation between the Radiograph and the Dust Content of the Lung

The amount of dust present in the lung correlates closely with the category of pneumoconiosis evident on the chest radiograph (I.L.O. Classification, 1958).

The progression from one radiographic category to another has recently been related to dust exposure in a 10 year period of observation (Jacobsen, Rae, Walton and Rogan, 1970).

In a series of coal miners applying for compensation the radiographic category of pneumoconiosis was related to the incidence of radiological evidence of emphysema (Caplan, Reid and Simon, 1966). The incidence of radiographic emphysema was low in all categories, but highest in O and of roughly the same severity in each of the other categories. Thus there was no evidence that the severity of pneumoconiosis influenced the incidence of emphysema.

It is easy to see how the idea of a relationship between dust and disability grew up. Close correlation between the radiographic appearance and the amount of dust retained in the lung meant that the radiograph was a reliable way to estimate the patient's dust exposure. The presence of emphysema is obviously more striking when the centriacinar holes are etched in dust. Without the support of quantitative studies, it was assumed that it was centriacinar emphysema that was responsible for the disability of the coal miner and, as a result, exposure to dust, then emphysema with disability because of shortness of breath became the accepted sequence. In fact, Category 3 pneumoconiosis on the radiograph can be present without any emphysema at all and emphysema may be present but not necessarily associated with disability. At present, the evidence suggests that disability in patients with simple pneumoconiosis arises from chronic bronchitis (Rogan, Chapman, Fay, Ashford, Duffield and Rae, 1961).

The Heart in Coal Miners' Pneumoconiosis and Airways Obstruction

Lung disease may affect the heart by causing right ventricular hypertrophy or right heart failure; the two may or may not be associated. Recognition of heart failure in certain cases of lung disease can be difficult because peripheral oedema may be associated with the blood gas disturbance found in obstructive airways disease although with no rise in jugular venous pressure. This means that, in analysing the effect of lung disease on the heart, peripheral oedema and a rise in jugular venous pressure should be separately recorded.

The World Health Organization (1961) has recently suggested that "cor pulmonale" should be defined as "right ventricular hypertrophy". This could lead to greater uniformity in the use of the term "cor pulmonale" but in studying any one case the other features of the effect on the right heart should also be separately noted.

At autopsy the diagnosis of right ventricular hypertrophy is best made by Fulton, Hutchinson and Jones' method (1952) in which the two ventricles are weighed separately. Fulton and his colleagues showed that the septum of the heart enlarged as part of the left ventricle, which means that the left ventricular and septal weight can be taken together and the right ventricular weight then expressed in relation to it. The normal weight of the right ventricle is less than 60 grammes. The criteria for right ventricular hypertrophy have been given as follows:

(*a*) mild, the ratio LV/RV being less than 2 even if the weight is not above 80 grammes.
(Weights between 65 and 80 grammes were regarded as normal if the ratio was within normal limits.)
(*b*) moderate, the weight being between 80 and 100 grammes.
(*c*) severe, the weight being above 100 grammes.

A right ventricular wall exceeding 5 mm in thickness will, of course, mean that hypertrophy is present, but dilatation may completely mask hypertrophy and prevent the wall thickness being used as a reliable guide to the degree of hypertrophy.

Using heart weight as the basis of the diagnosis of right ventricular hypertrophy, Millard (1967) was able to show that in the absence of disease of the left ventricle, the electrocardiogram during life offers a reliable way of diagnosing right ventricular hypertrophy in about 85 per cent of subjects. The criterion he used was of a right axis deviation (as shown on vectorcardiography) falling between over $+90°$ and $±180°$.

Right ventricular hypertrophy cannot be diagnosed from the radiograph since the heart with right ventricular hypertrophy may even appear narrow and vertical on the radiograph as described above for severe panacinar emphysema.

Simple pneumoconiosis would seem not to cause ventricular hypertrophy (Thomas, 1951; Wells, 1954) although ventricular hypertrophy may not uncommonly be found with massive fibrosis (James and Thomas, 1956). Airways obstruction causing hypoxia seems the strongest stimulus both to polycythaemia and to right ventricular hypertrophy presumably by causing pulmonary vasoconstriction. For these secondary effects of airways obstruction to develop, it seems that the peripheral small pulmonary arteries must be intact. It is paradoxical that the presence of severe panacinar emphysema, in spite of the loss of the peripheral vascular bed, seems to "protect" from the development of right ventricular hypertrophy (Reid, 1968).

Chronic bronchitis with no emphysema or with centriacinar emphysema (since in this most of the acinus is normal) are the conditions associated with the development of right ventricular hypertrophy.

Pathological Examination of Lungs

There is considerable need for improvement in the general standard of examination of lung specimens for diagnostic or research purposes. The proper assessment of the lungs and heart calls for consideration of the diagnosis of (i) chronic bronchitis, (ii) emphysema, (iii) cor pulmonale and, of course, (iv) the amount of dust in the lung, which is best assessed from the radiograph.

The diagnosis "cor pulmonale" should not be made unless there is evidence of right ventricular hypertrophy. If the right ventricle is more than 5 mm thick, right ventricular hypertrophy can be diagnosed but a wall of normal thickness does not preclude hypertrophy since dilatation may mask hypertrophy. Dissection of the adult heart by the method of Fulton *et al.* (1952) takes 15–20 minutes.

To assess the presence and type of emphysema, it is essential for proper examination that the lung be fixed in the inflated position. If speedy examination is necessary, it is even possible for the lung to be removed early during necropsy, fixed in formalin and cut at the end of the necropsy.

Slicing the lung will show whether emphysema is present, will reveal its anatomical type and enable its distribution to be assessed. There is no evidence that any emphysema present is related to the presence of dust.

The paper mounted section is useful if it is desirable to circulate lung slices over distances. The "dry" methods of fixing lung by steam, vapours or gas are of little use in diseased lungs as they do not give adequate fixation.

Larger or confluent lesions may suggest a silicotic element and microscopically crystals of silica may be revealed by polarized light. Haematoxylin-eosin stains can be supplemented by special stains for elastin, collagen and reticulin fibres. The normal alveolar wall contains reticulin, collagen and elastic fibres so their presence is not abnormal. In 5 μm sections the reticulin usually appears as short fibres across the alveolar wall with the cut ends pointing toward the alveolar space. Short segments of collagen and elastic fibres are seen running within the alveolar wall parallel to the alveolar surface. On occasion, incineration of lung may be desirable to analyse any dust present. The presence of mucous gland hypertrophy can be detected by studying gland size in a section of a main or lobar bronchus.

References

Attygalle, D., Harrison, C. V., King, E. J. and Mohanty, G. P. (1954), "Infective pneumoconiosis. 1. The influence of dead tubercle bacilli (B.C.G.) on the dust lesions produced by anthracite, coal-mine dust, and kaolin in the lungs of rats and guinea-pigs." *British Journal of Industrial Medicine*, **11**, 245.

Ball, J. D., Berry, G., Clarke, W. G., Gilson, J. C. and Thomas, J. (1969), "A controlled trial of antituberculous chemotherapy in the early complicated pneumoconiosis of coalworkers." *Thorax*, **24**, 399.

Caplan, A. (1953), "Certain unusual radiological appearances in the chest of coal-miners suffering from rheumatoid arthritis." *Thorax* **8**, 29.

Caplan, A., Reid, L. and Simon, G. (1966), "The radiological diagnosis of widespread emphysema and categories of simple pneumoconiosis." *Clinical Radiology*, **17**, 68.

Dayman, H. (1951), "Mechanics of airflow in health and in emphysema." *Journal of Clinical Investigation*, **30**, 1175.

Duguid, J. B. and Lambert, M. D. (1964), "The pathogenesis of coal miner's pneumoconiosis." *Journal of Pathology and Bacteriology*, **88**, 389.

Edge, J. R., Millard, J. C., Reid, L. and Simon, G. (1964), "The radiographic appearances of the chest in persons of advanced age." *British Journal of Radiology*, **37**, 769.

Edge, J., Simon, G. and Reid, L. (1966), "Emphysema: its clinical, radiological and physiological features." *British Journal of Diseases of the Chest*, **60**, 10.

Fulton, R. M., Hutchinson, E. C. and Jones, A. M. (1952), "Ventricular weight in cardiac hypertrophy." *British Heart Journal*, **14**, 413.

Gough, J. (1940), "Pneumoconiosis in coal trimmers." *Journal of Pathology and Bacteriology*, **51**, 277.

Gough, J., James, W. R. L. and Wentworth, J. E. (1949), "A comparison of the radiological and pathological changes in coalworkers' pneumoconiosis." *Journal of the Faculty of Radiologists* (London), **1**, 28.

Heard, B. E. and Izukawa, T. (1964), "Pulmonary emphysema in fifty consecutive male necropsies in London." *Journal of Pathology and Bacteriology*, **88**, 423.

Heppleston, A. G. (1954), "The pathogenesis of simple pneumoconiosis in coalworkers." *Journal of Pathology and Bacteriology* **67**, 51.

Hutchinson, D. C. S., Cook, P. J. L., Barter, C. E., Harris, Harry, and Hugh-Jones, P. (1971), "Pulmonary emphysema and α_1 antitrypsin deficiency." *British Medical Journal*, **1**, 689.

International Labour Organisation (1970), International classification of radiographs of pneumoconioses (revised 1968). *Occupational Safety and Health Series, No. 22.* International Labour Office, Geneva.

Jacobsen, M., Rae, S., Walton, W. H. and Rogan, J. M. (1970), "New dust standards for British coalminers." *Nature*, **227**, 445.

James, W. R. L. (1954), "The relationship of tuberculosis to the development of massive pneumokoniosis in coalworkers." *British Journal of Tuberculosis*, **48**, 89.

James, W. R. L. and Thomas, A. J. (1956), "Cardiac hypertrophy in coalworkers' pneumoconiosis." *British Journal of Industrial Medicine*, **13**, 24.

Jones, R., Baetjer, A. M. and Reid, L. (1971), "The effect of extremes of temperature and humidity on the goblet cell count in the rat airway epithelium." *British Journal of Industrial Medicine.* (In press.)

Kilpatrick, G. S., Heppleston, A. G. and Fletcher, C. M. (1954), "Cavitation in the massive fibrosis of coalworkers' pneumoconiosis." *Thorax,* 9, 260.

Laennec, R. T. H. (1827), *A Treatise on the Diseases of the Chest and on Mediate Auscultation,* p. 148. Translated from the French by John Forbes, 2nd edit. T. and G. Underwood, London.

Lamb, D. and Reid, L. (1968), "Mitotic rates, goblet cell increase and histochemical changes in mucus in rat bronchial epithelium during exposure to sulphur dioxide." *Journal of Pathology and Bacteriology,* 96, 97.

Lamb, D. and Reid, L. (1969), "Goblet cell increase in rat bronchial epithelium after exposure to cigarette and cigar tobacco smoke." *British Medical Journal,* 1, 33.

Lambert, M. W. (1955), "Accessory bronchiole—alveolar communications." *Journal of Pathology and Bacteriology,* 70, 311.

Lancet: Annotation (1971), "Chronic obstructive lung diseases." *Lancet,* 1, 1172.

Lindars, D. C. and Davies, D. (1967), "Rheumatoid Pneumoconiosis." *Thorax,* 22, 525.

McKenzie, H. I., Glick, M. and Outhred, K. G. (1969), "Chronic bronchitis in coal miners: ante mortem/post mortem comparisons." *Thorax,* 24, 529.

Magarey, F. R. (1951), "Experimental pulmonary haemosiderosis." *Journal of Pathology and Bacteriology,* 70, 311.

Millard, F. J. C. (1967), "The electrocardiogram in chronic lung disease." *British Heart Journal,* 29, 43.

Medical Research Council (1960), "Standardized questionnaires on respiratory symptoms." *British Medical Journal,* 2, 1665.

Oswald, N. C. and Medvei, V. C. (1955), "Chronic bronchitis: the effect of cigarette smoking." *Lancet,* 2, 843.

Rae, S., Walker, D. D. and Attfield, M. D. (1971), "Chronic Bronchitis and Dust Exposure in British Coalminers." In *Inhaled Particles and Vapours, III,* ed. W. H. Walton. Unwin, London.

Reid, L. (1954), "Pathology of chronic bronchitis." *Lancet,* 1, 275.

Reid, L. (1960), "Measurement of the bronchial mucous gland layer: a diagnostic yardstick in chronic bronchitis." *Thorax,* 15, 132.

Reid, L. (1963), "An experimental study of hypersecretion of mucus in the bronchial tree." *British Journal of Experimental Pathology,* 44, 437.

Reid, L. (1967), *The Pathology of Emphysema.* Lloyd-Luke (Medical Books) London. Monograph.

Reid, L. (1968), *Form and Function in the Human Lung,* ed. Cumming, G. and Hunt, L. B., E. & S. Livingstone, Ltd. Edinburgh and London.

Reid, L. and Millard, F. J. C. (1964), "Correlation between radiological diagnosis and structural changes in emphysema." *Clinical Radiology,* 15, 307.

Rivers, D., Wise, M. E., King, E. J. and Nagelschmidt, G. (1960), "Dust content, radiology and pathology in simple pneumoconiosis of coalworkers." *British Journal of Industrial Medicine,* 17, 87.

Rogan, J. (1970), "Coalworkers' Pneumoconiosis. A Review." *Journal of Occupational Medicine,* 12, 321.

Rogan, J. M., Chapman, P. J., Fay, J. W., Ashford, J. R., Duffield, D. P., and Rae, S. (1961), "Pneumoconiosis and respiratory symptoms in miners at eight collieries." *British Medical Journal,* 1, 1337.

Simon, G. (1964), "Radiology and emphysema." *Clinical Radiology,* 15, 293.

Simon, G. (1971), *Principles of Chest X-ray Diagnosis.* Butterworths, London.

Snider, G. L., Brody, J. S. and Doctor, L. (1962), "Subclinical pulmonary emphysema. Incidence and anatomic patterns." *American Review of Respiratory Diseases,* **85,** 666.

Thomas, A. J. (1951), "Right ventricular hypertrophy in the pneumoconiosis of coalminers." *British Heart Journal,* **13,** 1.

Thurlbeck, W. M. (1963), "The incidence of pulmonary emphysema, with observations on the relative incidence and spatial distribution of various types of emphysema." *American Review of Respiratory Dieases,* **87,** 203.

Thurlbeck, W. M., Henderson, J. A., Fraser, R. G. and Bates, D. V. (1970), *Medicine,* **49,** 81.

Vigliani, E. C. and Pernis, B. (1958), "Immunological factors in the pathogenesis of the hyaline tissue of silicosis." *British Journal of Industrial Medicine,* **15,** 8.

Weibel, E. (1963), *Morphometry of the Human Lung.* Springer-Verlag. Berlin, Göttingen, Heidelberg.

Wells, A. L. (1954), "Cor pulmonale in coal-workers' pneumoconiosis." *British Heart Journal,* **16,** 74.

West, J. B. (1971), "Distribution of mechanical stress in the lung, a possible factor in localisation of pulmonary disease." *Lancet,* **1,** 839.

World Health Organization (1961), Report on an Expert Committee on chronic cor pulmonale, p. 15. World Health Organization Technical Respiratory Service No. 213.

Chapter 2

The Pathology of Silicosis: Morbid Anatomy and Histology

Unique Effect of Finely Divided Silica

The usual response of living tissues to the introduction of inanimate particulate material is the foreign body reaction. This consists essentially of an accumulation of phagocytic cells, called macrophages, which are the scavenger cells of the body and are derived from the circulating monocytes of the blood and form part of the reticulo-endothelial system (R.E.S.), the formation of multinucleated giant cells from the macrophages and sometimes a slowly developing fibrous encapsulation of strictly limited distribution. Large crystals of silica evoke this reaction in the same manner as most other foreign substances (Gardner, 1937a). However, finely divided silica, especially if the particle size is less than $5\,\mu$m in diameter, causes a progressive fibrosis of a very distinctive pattern. This results in nodular lesions in which the collagen fibres tend to be arranged concentrically and to undergo a form of hyaline degeneration (Fig. 1). As the only common route by which finely divided silica may accidentally enter and remain in the human body is the respiratory tract, it is in the lungs that the fibrogenic properties of silica manifest themselves as the disease silicosis.

The Silicotic Nodule

The essential lesion of silicosis is the silicotic nodule, which although seen almost exclusively in the lungs, will form in other tissues under experimental conditions and in rare cases of miliary silicosis. In this latter disorder so much silica accumulates in the lungs that it overflows into the circulation and the characteristic lesions form in the spleen. The nodules in the lung vary in size from 2–3 mm to several cm (Fig. 2), though the larger lesions are usually found to consist of confluent masses of smaller fibrous nodules (Fig. 3). In its simplest form the silicotic nodule consists of a central core of hyalinized fibres of reticulin which tend to be concentrically arranged towards the periphery where they blend with coarser fibres of collagen which form a distinct capsule (Figs. 4a and b). Reticulin fibres are more delicate and have greater affinity for silver than collagen fibres, though the latter are usually considered to develop from them. The whole lesion contains very few cells, is avascular, and looks deceptively inactive. It has been shown by Heppleston (1962) that in experimental silicosis of rats, haematite dust inhaled after the nodular response to silica was established, became incorporated in the centre of the older lesions. This suggests that there

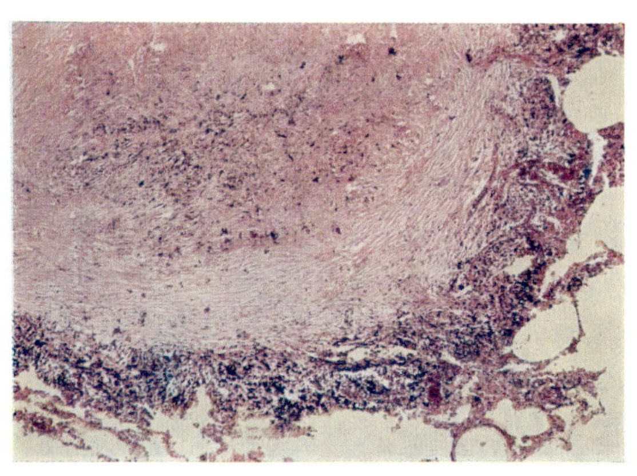

Fig. 1

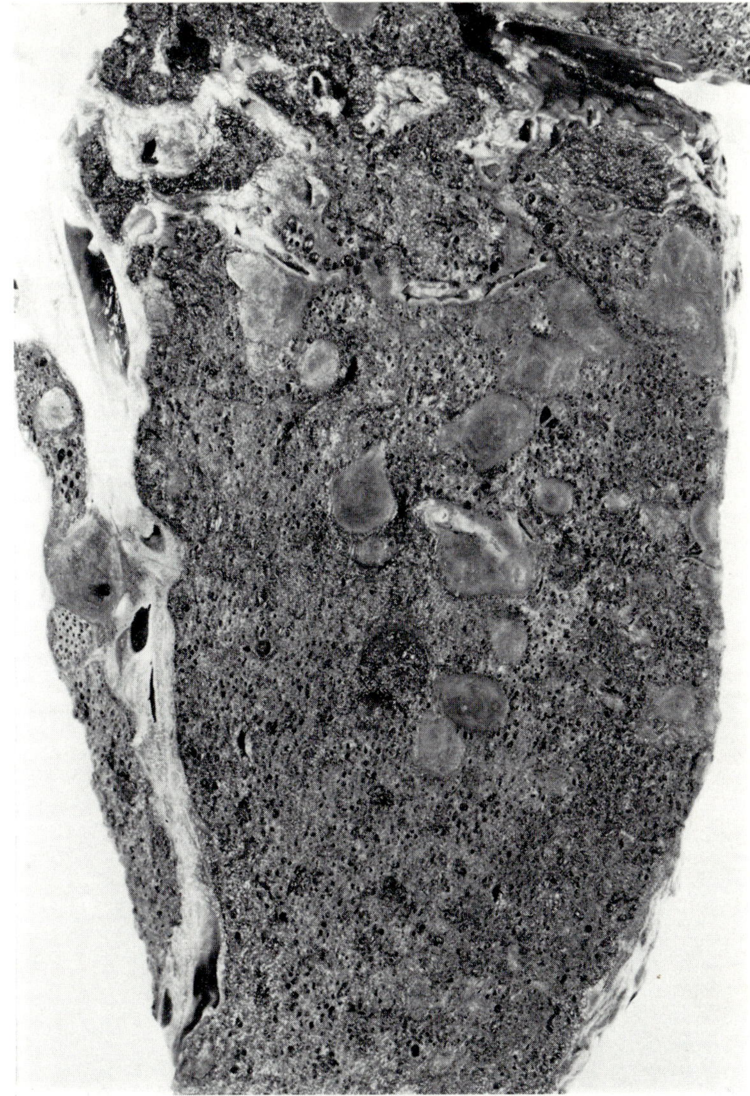

FIG. 2. A slice of human lung. Discrete fibrotic nodules of variable size can be seen.

(From the Museum of the Department of Pathology, University of Edinburgh.)

may be much more turnover of dust within the nodules than was once thought, and that silica in the centre is not inaccessible to macrophages at the periphery.

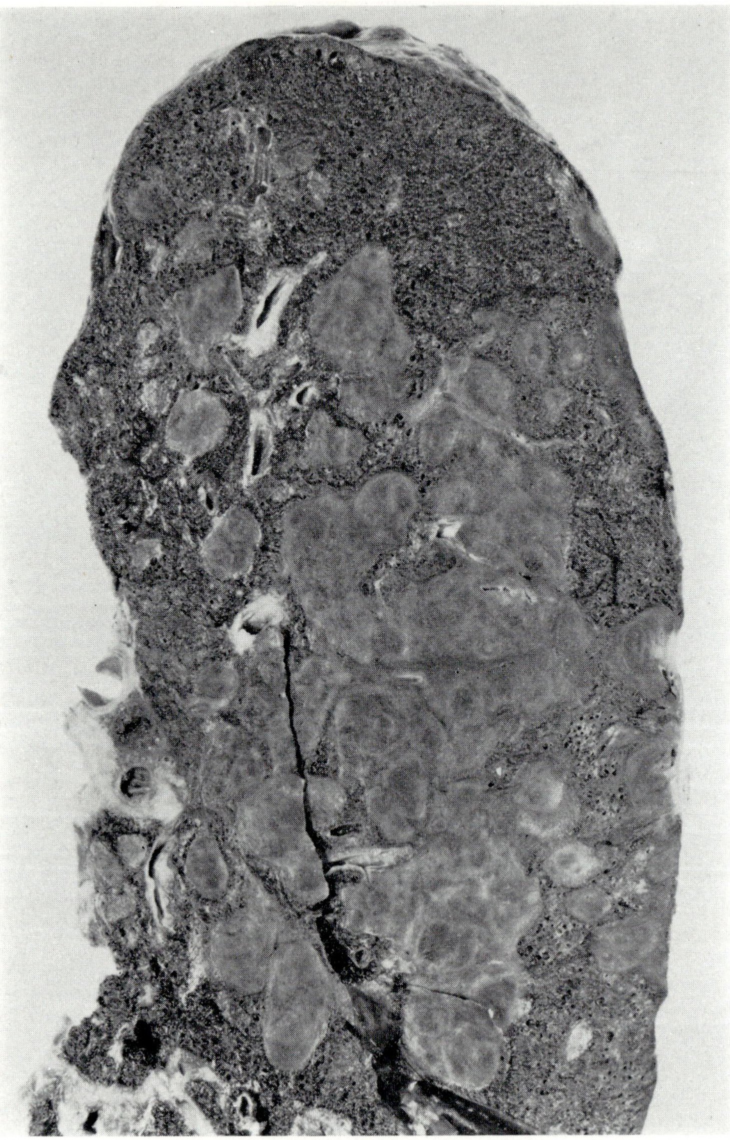

Fig. 3. A slice from the upper lobe of the left lung from the same case
as Fig. 2. Conglomerate nodular lesions replace most of the lung.

The silica particles responsible for the reaction are too small to be
seen in ordinary microscopic sections, and even under polarized light,
although birefringent, only particles of more than 1 μm in diameter can

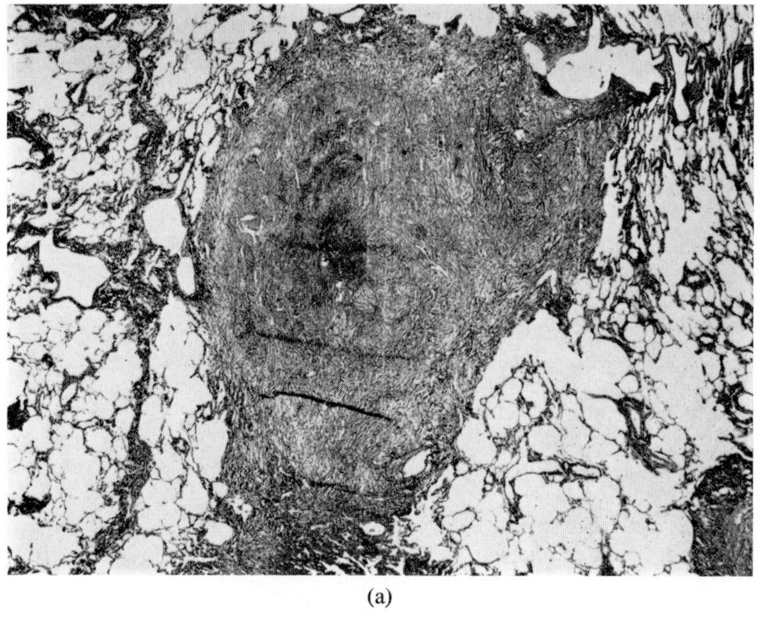

(a)

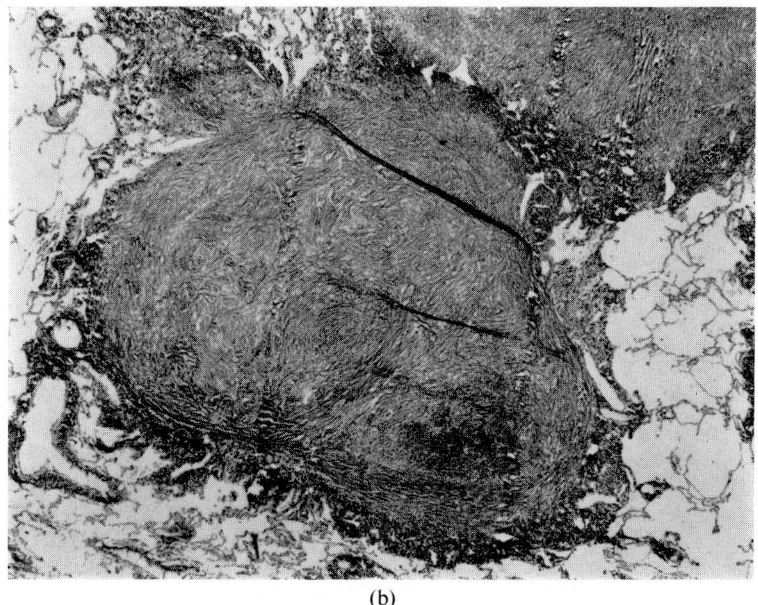

(b)

FIG. 4a and 4b. Silicotic nodules from a human lung stained for reticulin by Gordon and Sweet's method. (4a ×12; 4b ×17.)

be seen easily. Toluidine blue staining will sometimes reveal meta-
chromasia of the particles (Curran, 1953) but the most satisfactory
method of demonstrating their presence and distribution is by dark field
illumination after incinerating the section at 600°C and treating with
concentrated hydrochloric acid. Comparison of the pattern of dust left
on the slide with the next serial section enables the site of dust deposition
within the nodule to be visualized (Figs. 5 and 6). For details of the

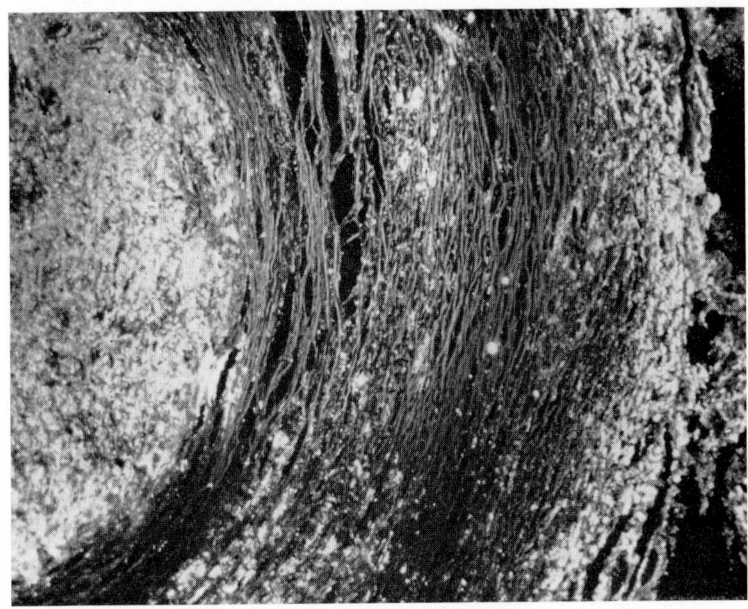

FIG. 5. A quadrant of a silicotic nodule from a human lung, stained
for reticulin (Gordon and Sweet) and photographed with dark field
illumination. The collagen fibres of the capsule can be clearly seen and
relatively little dust (white) is seen amongst them. (Original magnification ×60; Magnification of print ×210.)

technique Gross and Tolker (1966) should be consulted. By micro-
incineration it was found that the silica in human lesions had a very
characteristic distribution (Belt, 1939; Belt, Ferris and King, 1940).
There is a halo of silica particles around the outer margin of the nodule,
but little or none in the heavy collagenous capsule. In the centre is a
fine mist-like deposit of silica forming a skeleton of the tissue elements
as though they had been saturated in a solution of it. In contrast to
anthracosis, with its simpler type of reaction, the reaction to silica is
out of proportion to the amount of foreign material present, small
quantities of silica producing large amounts of fibrous tissue.

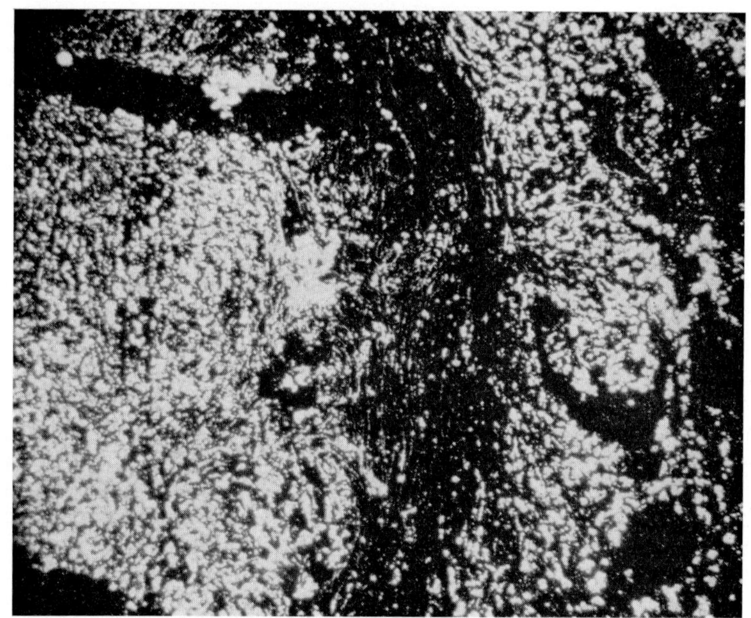

FIG. 6. The same field as Fig. 5 from a subsequent serial section treated by micro-incineration and concentrated hydrochloric acd. Also photographed with dark field illumination.

Experimental Silicosis

It is possible to produce a nodular variety of pulmonary fibrosis in rats and guinea pigs by injecting a suspension of silica and saline down the trachea (King and Harrison, 1960). A slower method, but one approaching more closely the conditions of human silicosis, is to expose mice to silica dust in special dust chambers for many hours a day for several weeks. Both techniques give a large number of positive results, but the lesions are not quite the same as those seen in human lungs. The concentric fibre pattern is not so clear, the distribution of dust into peripheral and central zones is not seen, and hyalinization, so typical of the human lesion, does not develop (Belt *et al.*, 1940). It is probable that these differences are merely the result of the relative immaturity of the experimental lesions, but when so much speculative theory is based on these experiments it is well to remember that they do not reproduce exactly the human disease.

Development of the Lesions

In both experimental animal lungs and human lungs the earliest lesions of silicosis occur in the walls of the respiratory bronchioles, which are the most proximal airways to bear alveoli. In animals, at least, these lesions form from aggregations of macrophages which engulf the dust particles within the alveolar spaces. There is good evidence that a similar mechanism operates in man (Duguid and Lambert, 1964). The little cluster of dust-laden macrophages becomes enmeshed in a reticulin framework and when the alveolar epithelium grows over the collection it becomes incorporated into the wall of the respiratory bronchiole at the cost of obliterating the original alveolus in which it was formed. Occasionally so much reticulin is formed that the bronchiole becomes obstructed (Gross, McNerney and Babyak, 1963; Gross and Brieger, 1966). That it should be the alveoli of the respiratory bronchiole that are affected is explained by Gross, Pfitzer and Hatch (1967) as being due to the great concentration of dust collecting at that point during the clearance of the more peripheral airways. The surface area of the respiratory bronchiole is only 1/500 of the surface area that is drained through it. Another factor that favours the local aggregation of dust laden macrophages and thus the formation of silicotic nodules, is the relative immobility of the tissues adjacent to fixed elements such as pulmonary arteries, interlobular septae and the pleura. Alveoli situated beside these structures are also likely to become filled with phagocytes. The subsequent development of the lesions is thought to be dependent on the death of the macrophages, the consequent release of the ingested particles, the accumulation of more macrophages and the progression of fibrosis in a manner which will be discussed later. It suffices here to point out that unlike most dusts, silica, in all those forms that provoke fibrosis, has a rapidly lethal effect on cells that ingest it.

Gross Appearances and Varieties

The lungs of a person dying from silicosis are typically dense and retain their shape on opening the chest. The pleural spaces are commonly obliterated by fibrous adhesions and the grey, mottled pleural surfaces studded with whitish mamillated nodules. The cut surface is marked by aggregates of dense, hard, grey-black nodules that may be so crowded as to leave practically no normal lung tissue at all (Middleton, 1936). The upper lobes and the hilar lymph nodes are frequently more severely affected than the bases of the lungs. The colour of the lungs depends to some extent on the nature of the industry in which the silicosis was contracted, but as silicotic lungs retain more dust of every type than do healthy lungs, they tend to be of a darker hue than normal.

In the early stages of the disease small isolated nodules are formed, and mild cases may never progress beyond this stage which is termed discrete nodular silicosis. In severe cases the numerous enlarging nodules may be so close together that they form a continuous mass of fibrous tissue, but close examination reveals that this is composed of many compressed nodules. This is the condition known as massive conglomerate nodular silicosis.

Progressive massive fibrosis of the lung is a form of the disease that should be distinguished from massive conglomerate nodular silicosis, for it probably has a different aetiology. In the former a single mass of fibrous tissue may eventually occupy the greater part of a lobe or even extend across an interlobar fissure, and its appearance is not that of a conglomeration of smaller discrete nodules but of a solitary lesion. Progressive massive fibrosis is seen in other forms of pneumoconiosis besides silicosis and is sometimes associated with infection, but the real nature of the condition is not known. Cavitation is not uncommon in the lesions of progressive massive fibrosis and may be either tuberculous or ischaemic in origin (Vorwald, 1941). However, haemorrhage, which is so common in cavitating non-silicotic tuberculosis, is unusual in progressive massive fibrosis because of the poor blood supply to the affected area (Spencer, 1968).

Association with Tuberculosis

The association between silicosis and tuberculosis is too frequent to be coincidental. There is experimental evidence that the presence of silica potentiates the growth of M. tuberculosis in macrophage cultures (Allison and D'Arcy Hart, 1968), and it has been known for years that non-pathogenic strains of mycobacteria will cause progressive lesions in guinea pigs if inoculated mixed with finely divided silica (Gardner, 1934). In days when tuberculosis was more common in the general community, as many as 65–75 per cent of fatal cases of silicosis had coexistent tuberculosis (Gardner, 1937b), while in Northern Rhodesia between 1950–1960 the incidence of tuberculosis in silicotic copper miners was thirty times greater than in non-silicotic miners (Paul, 1961). Even in the 1960's amongst white South African gold miners over 20 per cent of those with silicosis had active tuberculosis (Chatgidakis, 1963). Not only does silicosis encourage and modify unfavourably the progress of tuberculosis but also it may affect the morphology of the tuberculous lesions. The usual features of endothelioid cell proliferation, Langhans' giant cell formation and even the lymphocytic reaction may be suppressed and it may be impossible to identify organisms histologically or even by culture or guinea pig inoculation. Caseous necrosis in the centre of a silicotic nodule is sometimes the only indication of a coexistent tuberculous infection (Spencer, 1968).

Effects on the Heart and Pulmonary Blood Vessels

As well as reducing resistance to acid fast bacilli and replacing the spongy respiratory tissue of the normal lung with dense rounded masses of collagen, silicosis affects the pulmonary blood vessels and is one cause of cor pulmonale, that is heart disease brought on by a primary disorder of the lungs. In one autopsy series, 50 per cent of cases of silicosis had pathological enlargement of the right ventricle, though only 10 per cent died from right sided heart failure (Geever, 1947). The fact that many nodules form adjacent to blood vessels enables the developing fibrous tissue to produce obstruction of the lumen by compression of the wall of the artery or arteriole. The vessel wall may be more directly damaged by infiltration with dust laden macrophages and fibroblasts in the form of granulation tissue. Large vessels, over 1 mm in diameter, are involved only in massive conglomerate silicosis, but small arteries, 0·1–0·4 mm in diameter, and arterioles, under 0·1 mm in diameter, are often affected even in discrete nodular silicosis. All the layers of the vessel wall are sometimes involved by degenerative changes in muscle and elastic with replacement of these specialized tissues by fibrous tissue, which itself may undergo degeneration in much the same manner as in any ageing artery (Geever, 1947). It was long thought that pulmonary hypertension was simply a result of such mechanical obstruction and destruction of the vascular bed, but it seems likely that abnormal blood gas levels resulting in vasoconstriction are more important. This may explain why cor pulmonale is less common in silicosis, despite frequent gross mechanical distortion of the vessels, than it is in chronic bronchitis or emphysema. In the latter diseases gas exchange is often more seriously impaired than the apparent degree of lung damage would indicate and it is hypoxia, and to a lesser extent hypercapnia, that causes spasm of the pulmonary arterioles and produces the rise in pulmonary blood pressure that ultimately leads to right heart failure (Heard, 1969).

Association with Malignancy

There is no evidence that silica itself is carcinogenic and cases of silicosis amongst South African gold miners have no increased incidence of malignant disease (Chatgidakis, 1963). However, there is good evidence that haemitite miners in Cumberland (England) have 70 per cent more lung cancer than do male controls in the same area who do not work in the mines (Boyd, Doll, Faulds and Leiper, 1970). It is not suggested that this is due to silica itself. It may well be the result of some extraneous factor such as radioactivity in the mines, but in view of the carcinogenic properties of asbestos, which is also an iron-silica combination, it is possible that under some circumstances silica can act as a co-carcinogen with iron.

The Pathogenesis of Silicosis

Effect of Silica on the Macrophage

The observations of Allison, Harington and Birbeck (1966) and Allison, Harington, Birbeck and Nash (1967) on the effects of feeding dust particles to phagocytes in tissue culture, have led to a reorientation of ideas on the processes involved in the silicotic reaction. They found that silica, amorphous carbon and diamond dusts of similar particle size were all taken up by the cultured cells. However, cells fed on carbon or diamond dust continued to thrive, while those which ingested silica rounded up, stopped moving and died within 24 hours. Combining this technique with electron microscopy they were able to demonstrate that the particles were initially taken into phagosomes, which are intracellular vacuoles bounded by a plasma membrane—the outer membrane of the cell—included by a process of invagination. Subsequently the lysosomes, which are small bodies located in the cytoplasm capable of secreting potent lytic enzymes, came to lie adjacent to the phagosome and poured their enzymes into it, turning it into a secondary lysosome. With the inert dusts this was all that happened, but if silica was present in the phagosome then the membrane lining it appeared to break down, for the silica particles were seen to lie free in the cytoplasm, and enzymes normally confined to the lysosome were released into the culture medium where they could be detected by various methods (Comolli, 1967; Nadler and Goldfischer, 1970). By this time the macrophages containing the silica were dead.

Protective Substances and their Aetiological Significance

Further observations which have led to a better understanding of the way in which silica acts, are those concerning various protective substances which modify or inhibit the toxic and fibrogenic effects of silica. One of the first of these to be discovered was metallic aluminium. Denny, Robson and Irwin (1937; 1939) showed that less than 1 per cent of grease free finely divided aluminium dust, uniformly mixed with powdered quartz, prevented any fibrosis developing in the lungs of rabbits made to inhale the mixture, while rabbits given quartz dust alone all developed silicotic lesions. They found that the silica particles became coated with an impermeable layer of hydrated alumina. This was held to support the theory that silica exerted its effects by dissolving slowly in the tissues, releasing silicic acid which caused the fibrosis. This so-called solubility theory lost favour when it was found that the fibrogenic properties of different forms of silica did not parallel their solubility (King, Mohanty, Harrison and Nagelschmidt, 1952) and that silica placed in diffusion chambers in the tissues did not provoke any fibrosis (Curran and Rowsell, 1958; Curran and Ager, 1962). It has been pointed out, however, that such experiments are not decisive, as the particles dissolve too slowly for the polymerization of silicic acid into its toxic form to take place (Heppleston, Ahlquist and Williams, 1961).

When cortisone became available, its ability to lessen the fibrous reaction in such diseases as rheumatoid arthritis soon led to its being tried in silicosis. In experimental conditions it reduced the fibrosis in rats, though it did not affect the maturation of collagen (Harrison,

King, Dale and Sichel, 1952); it also reduced the amount of collagen formed and lessened hyaline degeneration (Marenghi and Rota, 1954) and varied in its effects on different species (Magarey and Gough, 1952), a fact that should be remembered when interpreting human disease in the light of experimental results. Though its effect is probably multi-factorial one of its actions is to stabilize biological membranes.

Studying the toxic effect of silica on cultured phagocytes Marks (1957) discovered that the histamine liberator compound 48/80 had a powerful protective action. Later Marks, James and Morris (1958) found that it was also effective *in vivo* in preventing fibrosis of the liver and fatal silica shock in mice given intravenous tridymite. Its mode of action is unknown but 48/80 reduces the solubility of silica.

The most powerful protective agent against silica yet discovered is the polymer polyvinyl pyridine-N-oxide (PNO). This substance was discovered by Schlipkoter and Brockhaus (1961) and has the formula

$$CH_2—CH—CH_2—CH— \quad \text{the pyridine oxide group being}$$

with PyO groups attached below each CH, the oxygen atom at position N having a high negative charge and being capable of forming strong H-bonds. It protects macrophages completely against the toxic action of silica if either they or the silica are treated with it before they are brought into contact. An attractive explanation of its mode of action is given by Nash, Allison and Harington (1966), who point out that the silicic acid is an H-donor which polymerizes into the following form,

$$\begin{array}{cccc} OH & OH & OH & OH \\ | & | & | & | \\ Si—O—Si—O—Si—O—Si—OH \\ | & | & | & | \\ OH & OH & OH & OH \end{array}$$

Chains such as this cross link with the elimination of water to form colloidal silica the outer surface of which is covered by OH groups. They present evidence that polymeric silicic acid forms H-bonded complexes with quaternary and phosphate ester groups of phospholipids and to a less extent with peptide groups of proteins. By this mechanism it could disrupt the normal structure of the membrane lining the secondary lysosome. PNO, which gets into the same phagosome as the silica particle, may form preferential H-bonds with silicic acid preventing the permeability changes produced by the latter on biological membranes.

There are still some discrepancies which prevent complete acceptance of this theory of the action of silica within macrophages. The failure of

PNO to protect red blood cells against the haemolytic action of the asbestos chrysotile (Macnab and Harington, 1967), the finding that alkaline treated (etched) quartz ls toxic to macrophages but does not haemolyse red cells, while ground quartz haemolyses red cells but is harmless to macrophages (Sakabe, Koshi and Hayashi, 1971), both call for further explanation. However, it is not unlikely that the plasma membrane of a red cell differs significantly from the membrane of the secondary lysosome of a macrophage. There is electron microscopic evidence to suggest that the latter is not so simple as may have been supposed (von Bruch, 1971). More significant is the failure of a crystalline form of silica, stishovite, to harm macrophages or provoke fibrosis (Brieger and Gross, 1967). This type of silica only forms at very high pressures and temperatures and is found naturally in certain meteorite craters in Arizona. It has similar solubility to the other crystalline forms of silica, quartz, cristobolite, tridymite and coesite, all of which are fibrogenic, but unlike these, the atoms of stishovite are arranged in an octahedral configuration instead of in tetrahedrons. This suggests that some surface action on the particle of silica itself is important in determining its effects on the cell as well as the action of dissolved silica within the secondary lysosome. Further evidence that the spatial arrangement of the bonds may be important was provided by Holt, Lindsay and Beck (1970), who, while investigating the protective action of several derivatives of PNO, found that 2 stereo regular forms of poly (2-vinyl pyridine 1-oxide) differed in their effectiveness although only the spatial arrangements of their structural units were different. They also showed that the N-oxide group was not essential for protective powers and that some polymers actually increased the cytotoxicity of quartz when it was pretreated with them.

A further fact which does not readily fit the theory of Allison and Harington is the protective action of reduced glutathione when macrophages are incubated with cytotoxic forms of silica (Nutt and Harington, 1964). This substance is thought to exert its effect by maintaining an equilibrium between the sulphur containing groups SH—SS which are important in maintaining the integrity of biological membranes. Poisons such as arsenite, cadmium and selenite are known to interfere with these sulphur containing groups and produce remarkable changes in vascular permeability (Steele and Wilhelm, 1967), but silica had not been thought to act in such a manner.

Basic Processes in the Development of Silicosis

Heppleston (1969) has emphasized that the death of macrophages with the consequent reliberation of silica into the tissues is only the first of four basic processes in the development of the lesions of silicosis. The others are the continuous production of phagocytes to reingest the silica and be killed in their turn, the formation of collagen, and the hyalinization of the collagen formed. Any theory of pathogenesis must explain all these phenomena or be found wanting. He has summarized his own hypothesis of silicotic fibrogenesis in diagrammatic form (Fig. 7), and further reference will be made to this below.

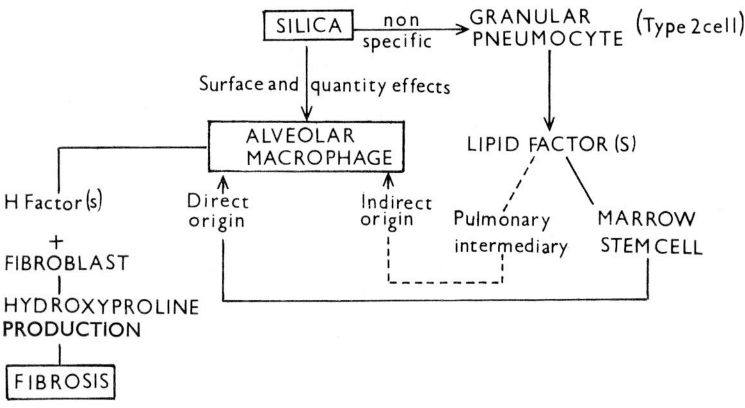

Fig. 7. A hypothesis to account for silicotic fibrogenesis. (Redrawn from Heppleston, 1971, with the permission of Professor A. G. Heppleston.)

The Supply of Macrophages

The initial stimulus to the appearance of sufficient macrophages in the lung may be the presence of the dust itself. There is evidence that the number of macrophages produced in the first 24 hours is proportional to the number of particles introduced into the lung (Brain, 1971), but the initial reaction, to intratracheal coesite at least, is polymorpho-nuclear (Gross and Brieger, 1966), and this could mean that a prior polymorph response is necessary for subsequent monocyte emigration (Page and Good, 1958). There is now good reason to believe that lung macrophages are derived from the blood monocytes, though they may require a period of maturation and division in the interstitial tissue of the lung to develop the distinctive characteristics of the alveolar macrophage (Bowden, Davies and Wyatt, 1968; Bowden, Adamson, Grantham and Wyatt, 1969). The stimulus to their continuous replacement may come from the dying macrophage itself. Conning and Heppleston (1966) have demonstrated that silica enhances the activity of the reticulo-endothelial system, a property shared by triolein, tricaprin, oestradiol and B.C.G. Heppleston (1971) comments that there are several leads pointing to a link between a lipid component released from macrophages by silica and the stimulus to further macrophage production, emigration and perhaps maturation in the tissues of the lung (Fig. 7). There is also some evidence that the monocyte count is increased in the early stages of human silicosis (Velican, Latis, Popa, Popa and Steinbach, 1959; Warraki, Gammal and Awny, 1965).

The Stimulus of Collagen Formation

An explanation is next required for the manner in which the death of macrophages leads to the overproduction of collagen. For many years the pioneer work of Fallon (1937) was taken to provide the answer. He had shown that phospholipid extracted from early silicotic lesions in rabbit lungs produced fibrosis when injected into the peritoneum, which was very similar to the effect of finely divided quartz itself. Unfortunately Fallon omitted to perform the control experiment of injecting extracts of non-silicotic rabbit lungs which are also rich in phospholipid. The work of Heppleston and Styles (1967) strongly supports the theory that macrophages which have ingested silica release a substance which stimulates fibroblasts to produce increased amounts of fibrous tissue (Fig. 7). They incubated macrophages with silica, inert dust, silica plus PNO, PNO alone, and without any additive. They subsequently disrupted the macrophages by repeated freeze-thawing and deposited the cell debris and silica by centrifugation. The supernatant was then used as a culture medium for fibroblasts. They found that the supernatant from macrophages which had ingested silica alone caused a significant increase in hydroxyproline (HOP) production by the fibroblasts. None of the other macrophage preparations yielded potent supernatant fluids and in particular PNO completely blocked the effect of silica, no increase in HOP production resulting from the incubation of fibroblasts in the fluid from disrupted macrophages previously cultured with both silica and PNO. They also showed that addition of silica directly to the fibroblast culture had no effect on HOP production. Heppleston (1969) has pointed out that evidence is accumulating that it is the non-lipid fraction of macrophage disintegration products that has the power to stimulate fibrosis. In particular he notes the work of Webster, Henderson, Marasas and Keegan (1967) who found that the lipid free fraction of silica dusted macrophages provoked subcutaneous granuloma formation in guinea pigs, while the lipid fraction did not. Webster *et al.* (1967) themselves suggest that the active substance may be a kinin, possibly bradykinin, which they have demonstrated in increased amounts in the serum of rabbits following the injection of intravenous silica suspension. They also cite a unique case of human silicosis reported from Finland (Halonen, Koskelo, Frick and Merenmies, 1962) of a woman who developed typical nodular lung lesions in association with a metastasising carcinoid tumour, a type of tumour known to produce both serotonin and bradykinin (Oates, Melmon, Sjoerdsma, Gillespie and Mason, 1964).

Hyalinization of the Collagen

The final stage in the development of human silicotic lesions is the hyalinization of collagen. By this process the fibres of connective tissue become embedded in an eosinophilic acellular glassy matrix. This silicotic hyaline has been shown by Vigliani and Pernis (1958) to have a similar composition to amyloid, which is sometimes laid down around cells and fibres in conditions of abnormal activity of the reticulo-endothelial system. Like amyloid, silicotic hyaline is rich in globulins, particularly gamma globulins, which include the antibodies produced by the R.E.S. in response to foreign materials. In the last decade much work was done in an attempt to explain the entire silicotic reaction in terms of an abnormal immunological response. However the more recent findings of Allison, Heppleston, Webster and others have tended to direct attention away from a purely immunological theory towards the hypothesis outlined above. Stimulation of the R.E.S. is an essential feature of silicosis, and it is not only phagocytosis that is increased but also plasma cell and gamma globulin production (Englebrecht and Thiart, 1966). Abnormalities in the response may be caused by other disorders involving the immunological system such as rheumatoid arthritis (Caplan, Cowen and Gough, 1958) and hypersensitivity states (Powell and Gough, 1958). But although these may alter the pattern of the silicotic process, and immunological phenomena may be responsible for the hyalinization of collagen, they are not the direct cause of the basic reaction of the tissues to the presence of finely divided silica.

A Possible Role for Type II Cells and a Field for Speculation

Lest it should be thought that the response of the lungs to silica is now completely understood and further research unnecessary, some consideration will be given to recent work indicating a possible role in the reaction to dust played by the granular pneumocyte. This cell, also known as the type II epithelial cell, is the larger and normally less numerous of the two varieties of epithelial cell that line the alveoli. These cells are thought to be the source of surfactant which is the substance that reduces surface tension and forms a very thin film between the air and the cells of the alveolar wall (Bensch, Schaefer and Avery, 1964). Three recent reports hint that a failure in the normal functions of these cells may prevent the usual silicotic reaction from taking place. Gross, de Villiers and de Treville (1967) found that the Syrian hamster reacted peculiarly to injection of intratracheal quartz. Very few nodules formed and the quartz remained diffusely distributed in the lungs. Later Gross and de Treville (1968) discovered that typical silicotic nodules also failed to develop if very large amounts of dust were inhaled by rats, guinea pigs or hamsters. Instead of a nodular fibrosis a diffuse consolidation of the lungs was produced which in places resembled the human disease known as alveolar proteinosis. The authors suggested that the quartz was rendered non-wettable by finely divided lipid that was present in such lungs. The third report (Heppleston, 1967) stated that specific pathogen-free rats reacted differently to inhaled silica from standard rats. They developed an irregular intraalveolar fibrosis and an accumulation of foamy histiocytes containing P.A.S. positive granules as well as a large amount of eosinophilic granular material which also stained with the periodic acid Schiff (P.A.S.) technique, and it was amongst this material, which was sometimes rich in lipid, that the silica particles were found. Heppleston also noted the similarity between this atypical reaction to silica and alveolar proteinosis. In this latter condition P.A.S. positive granules also appear, but in the type II pneumocytes, which then degenerate and liberate lipid rich material. It has been suggested that alveolar proteinosis is caused by an inhibition of lipolytic enzymes in the alveolar wall (Spencer, 1968).

Heppleston (1971) claims that early in the atypical reaction to silica there is an increase in the number and activity of the type II cells and that the alveoli subsequently become filled by a lattice derived from lipoprotein containing lamellar bodies excreted by the type II cells. This lattice appears to prevent macrophages from reaching the silica particles enmeshed in it, and thus breaks the chain of events the continuity of which is essential for the development of the typical silicotic reaction.

The significance of these, as yet unconfirmed, observations is still not fully appreciated, whether in regard to the normal functions of type II cells, the aetiology of alveolar proteinosis or the development of human silicosis. It may be that some simple explanation will be found and the atypical reaction to silica shown to be irrelevant to any human disease, or it may be the first clue to a hitherto unsuspected protective mechanism or to a further facet of the complex reaction of tissues to the presence of silica.

References

Allison, A. C. and D'Arcy Hart, P. (1968), "Potentiation by silica of the growth of mycobacterium tuberculosis in macrophage cultures." *British Journal of Experimental Pathology*, **49,** 465.

Allison, A. C., Harington, J. S. and Birbeck, M. (1966), "The examination of the cytotoxic effect of silica on macrophages." *Journal of Experimental Medicine*, **124,** 141.

Allison, A. C., Harington, J. S., Birbeck, M. and Nash, T. (1967), "Observations on the cytotoxic action of silica on macrophages." In *Inhaled Particles and Vapours, II*, ed. C. N. Davies, p. 121. Pergamon Press, Oxford.

Belt, T. H. (1939), "Silicosis of the spleen: a study of the silicotic nodule." *Journal of Pathology and Bacteriology*, **49,** 39.

Belt, T. H., Ferris, A. A. and King, E. J. (1940), "The silicotic nodule in human and experimental silicosis: a comparative study." *Journal of Pathology and Bacteriology,* **51,** 263.

Bensch, K., Schaefer, K. and Avery, M. E. (1964), "Granular pneumocytes: Electron microscopic evidence of their exocrine function." *Science,* **145,** 1318.

Bowden, D. H., Davies, E. and Wyatt, J. P. (1968), "Cytodynamics of pulmonary alveolar cells in the mouse." *Archives of Pathology,* **86,** 667.

Bowden, D. H., Adamson, I. Y. R., Grantham, G. and Wyatt, J. P. (1969), "Origin of the lung macrophage. Evidence derived from radiation injury." *Archives of Pathology,* **88,** 540.

Boyd, J. T., Doll, R., Faulds, J. S. and Leiper, J. (1970), "The report of the M.R.C. statistical unit on the incidence of lung cancer in haematite miners." *British Journal of Industrial Medicine,* **27,** 97.

Brain, J. D. (1971), "The effects of increased particles on the number of alveolar macrophages." In *Inhaled Particles, III,* ed. W. H. Walton, p. 209, Unwin, London.

Brieger, H. and Gross, P. (1967), "On the theory of silicosis. III Stishovite." *Archives of Environmental Health,* **15,** 751.

Bruch, von J. (1971), "Elektromikroskopische Beobachtungen zur Quartzstaub-phygozytose." In *Inhaled Particles, III,* ed. W. H. Walton, p. 447. Unwin, London.

Caplan, A., Cowen, E. D. H. and Gough, J. (1958), "Rheumatoid pneumoconiosis in a foundry worker." *Thorax,* **13,** 181.

Chatgidakis, C. B. (1963), "Silicosis in South African white gold miners. A comparative study of the disease in its different stages." *Medical Proceedings,* **9,** 383.

Comolli, R. (1967), "Cytotoxicity of silica and liberation of lysosomal enzymes." *Journal of Pathology and Bacteriology,* **93,** 241.

Conning, D. M. and Heppleston, A. G. (1966), "Reticulo-endothelial activity and local particle disposal. A comparison of the influence of modifying agents." *British Journal of Experimental Pathology,* **47,** 388.

Curran, R. C. (1953), "Observations on the formation of collagen in quartz lesions." *Journal of Pathology and Bacteriology,* **66,** 271.

Curran, R. C. and Ager, J. A. M. (1962), "The diffusion chamber in experimental silicosis." *Journal of Pathology and Bacteriology,* **83,** 1.

Curran, R. C. and Rowsell, E. V. (1958), "The application of the diffusion chamber technique to the study of silicosis." *Journal of Pathology and Bacteriology,* **76,** 561.

Denny, J. J., Robson, W. D. and Irwin, D. A. (1937), "The prevention of silicosis by metallic aluminium." *Canadian Medical Association Journal,* **37,** 1.

Denny, J. J., Robson, W. D. and Irwin, D. A. (1939), "The prevention of silicosis by metallic aluminium." *Canadian Medical Association Journal,* **40,** 213.

Duguid, J. B. and Lambert, M. W. (1964), "The pathogenesis of coal miners pneumoconiosis." *Journal of Pathology and Bacteriology,* **88,** 389.

Englebrecht, F. M. and Thiart, B. F. (1966), "Plasma cells in the pathogenesis of silicosis." *South African Medical Journal,* **40,** 121.

Fallon, J. T. (1937), "Specific tissue reaction to phospholipids: A suggested explanation for the similarity of the lesions of silicosis and pulmonary tuberculosis." *Canadian Medical Association Journal,* **36,** 223.

Gardner, L. U. (1934), In *First Symposium on Silicosis.* Trudeau School of Tuberculosis, Saranac Lake, New York.

Gardner, L. U. (1937a), "The similarity of the lesions produced by silica and by the tubercle bacillus." *American Journal of Pathology,* **13,** 13.

Gardner, L. U. (1937b), "The significance of the silicotic problem." In *Third Symposium on Silicosis.* Trudeau School of Tuberculosis, Saranac Lake, New York.

Geever, E. F. (1947), "Pulmonary vascular lesions in silicosis and related pathological changes." *American Journal of Medical Science,* **214,** 292.

Gross, P. and Brieger, H. (1966), "Silicotic bronchiolitis obliterans—a focal clearance failure." *Archives of Environmental Health*, **12**, 5.

Gross, P., McNerney, J. M. and Babyak, M. A. (1963), "Experimental silicosis: a model for the study of inflammatory pulmonary reticulin." *Diseases of the Chest*, **43**, 113.

Gross, P., Pfitzer, E. A. and Hatch, T. F. (1967), "Alveolar clearance: its relation to lesions of the respiratory bronchiole." In *Inhaled Particles and Vapours, II*, ed. C. N. Davies, p. 169. Pergamon Press, Oxford.

Gross, P. and Tolker, E. B. (1966), "Dust particles in lung sections. Some notes on methods of their visualisation." *Archives of Environmental Health*, **12**, 213.

Gross, P. and de Treville, R. T. P. (1968), "Experimental acute silicosis." *Archives of Experimental Health*, **17**, 720.

Gross, P., de Villiers, A. J. and de Treville, R. T. P. (1967), "Experimental silicosis. The 'atypical' reaction in the Syrian hamster." *Archives of Pathology*, **84**, 87.

Halonen, P. I., Koskelo, P., Frick, M. H. and Merenmies, L. (1962), "Metastatic carcinoid tumour associated with complicated silicosis." *Acta Medica Scandinavica*, **171**, 477.

Harrison, C. V., King, E. J., Dale, J. C. and Sichel, R. (1952), "The effect of cortisone on experimental silicosis." *British Journal of Industrial Medicine*, **9**, 165.

Heard, B. E. (1969), *Pathology of Chronic Bronchitis and Emphysema*, p. 96. J. and A. Churchill, London.

Heppleston, A. G. (1962), "The disposal of dust in the lungs of silicotic rats." *American Journal of Pathology*, **40**, 493.

Heppleston, A. G. (1967), "Atypical reaction to inhaled silica." *Nature* (London), **213**, 199.

Heppleston, A. G. (1969), "The fibrogenic action of silica." *British Medical Bulletin*, **25**, No. 3 (Mechanisms of Toxicity), 282.

Heppleston, A. G. (1971), "Observations on the mechanism of silicotic fibrogenesis." In *Inhaled Particles, III*, ed. W. H. Walton, p. 357. Unwin, London.

Heppleston, A. G., Ahlquist, K. A. and Williams, D. (1961), "Observations on the pathogenesis of silicosis by means of the diffusion chamber technique." *British Journal of Industrial Medicine*, **18**, 143.

Heppleston, A. G. and Styles, J. A. (1967), "Activity of a macrophage factor in collagen formation by silica." *Nature* (London), **214**, 521.

Holt, P. F., Lindsay, H. and Beck, E. G. (1970), "Some derivatives of polyvinyl-pyridine 1-oxides and their effect on the cytotoxicity of quartz in macrophage cultures." *British Journal of Pharmacology*, **38**, 192.

King, E. J. and Harrison, C. V. (1960), "Reaction of the lung to dust." In *Industrial Pulmonary Diseases*, eds. E. J. King and C. M. Fletcher, pp. 37–43. J. and A. Churchill, London.

King, E. J., Mohanty, G. P., Harrison, C. V. and Nagelschmidt, G. (1952), "The action of different forms of pure silica on the lungs of rats." *British Journal of Industrial Medicine*, **10**, 9.

Macnab, G. and Harington, J. S. (1967), "Haemolytic activity of asbestos and other mineral dusts." *Nature* (London), **214**, 522.

Magarey, F. R. and Gough, J. (1952), "The effect of cortisone on the reaction to quartz in the peritoneal cavity." *British Journal of Experimental Pathology*, **33**, 76.

Marenghi, B. and Rota, L. (1954), "Effect of cortisone on experimental silicosis in rats." *Archives of Industrial Hygiene and Occupational Medicine*, **9**, 315.

Marks, J. (1957), "The neutralization of silica toxicity *in vitro*." *British Journal of Industrial Medicine*, **14**, 81.

Marks, J., James, D. M. and Morris, T. S. (1958), "The treatment of experimental silicosis with 48/80." *British Journal of Industrial Medicine*, **15**, 1.

Middleton, E. L. (1936), "Industrial pulmonary disease due to the inhalation of dust with special reference to silicosis." *Lancet*, **2**, 1 and 59.

Nadler, S. and Goldfischer, S. (1970), "The intracellular release of lysosomal contents in macrophages that have ingested silica." *Journal of Histochemistry and Cytochemistry*, **18**, 368.

Nash, T., Allison, A. C. and Harington, J. S. (1966), "Physico-chemical properties of silica in relation to its toxicity." *Nature* (London), **210**, 259.

Nutt, A. and Harington, J. S. (1964), "The reaction of reduced glutathione with quartz powder and with associated iron and copper." *La Medicina del Lavoro*, **55**, 176.

Oates, J. A., Melmon, K., Sjoerdsma, A., Gillespie, L. and Mason, D. T. (1964), "Release of kinin peptide in the carcinoid syndrome." *Lancet*, **1**, 514.

Page, A. R. and Good, R. A. (1958), "A clinical and experimental study of the function of neutrophils in the inflammatory response." *American Journal of Pathology*, **34**, 645.

Paul, R. (1961), "Silicosis in Northern Rhodesia copper mines." *Archives of Environmental Health*, **2**, 96.

Powell, D. E. B. and Gough, J. (1958), "The effect on experimental silicosis of hypersensitivity induced by horse serum." *British Journal of Experimental Pathology*, **40**, 40.

Sakabe, H., Koshi, K. and Hayashi, H. (1971), "On the cell toxicity of mineral dusts." In *Inhaled Particles, III*, ed. W. H. Walton, p. 423. Unwin, London.

Schlipkoter, H. W. and Brockhaus, A. (1961), "Die Hemmung der experimentellen Silikose durch subcutane Verobreichung von Polyvinylpyridin-N-oxyd." *Klinische Wochenschrift*, **39**, 1182.

Spencer, H. (1968), *Pathology of the Lung*. 2nd Ed. Pergamon Press, Oxford.

Steele, R. H. and Wilhelm, D. L. (1967), "The inflammatory reaction in chemical injury II." *British Journal of Experimental Pathology*, **48**, 592.

Velican, C., Latis, G., Popa, M., Popa, Gr. and Steinbach, M. (1959), "Investigations concerning the pre-radiological stage of silicosis." *British Journal of Industrial Medicine*, **16**, 40.

Vigliani, E. C. and Pernis, B. (1958), "Immunological factors in the pathogenesis of the hyaline tissue of silicosis." *British Journal of Industrial Medicine*, **15**, 8.

Vorwald, A. J. (1941), "Cavities in the silicotic lung. A pathological study with clinical correlation." *American Journal of Pathology*, **17**, 709.

Warraki, S. E., Gammal, M. Y. and Awny, A. Y. (1965), "Bone marrow changes in silicosis." *British Journal of Industrial Medicine*, **22**, 279.

Webster, I., Henderson, C. I., Marasas, L. W. and Keegan, D. J. (1967), "Some biologically active substances produced by the action of silica and their possible significance." In *Inhaled Particles and Vapours, II*, ed. C. N. Davies, p. 111. Pergamon Press, Oxford.

Chapter 3

The Pathology of Asbestosis

Introduction

Although asbestosis may have been recognized before 1907, Murray (1907) is usually credited with the first description of the autopsy findings of the lungs in a patient who died after 10 years exposure to asbestos dust. Eighteen years later Cooke (1924) recorded another case of asbestosis in a young textile worker and drew attention to the coated asbestos fibres which he called "curious bodies". Between 1927 and 1931 a number of papers were published. Seiler (1928) produced convincing evidence of the relationship between pulmonary fibrosis and the inhalation of asbestos. McDonald (1927) described the histology of asbestosis in a case in Great Britain and Simson (1928) of cases in South Africa. Stewart (1930) called the "curious bodies" "asbestosis bodies" thereby implying that the presence of the bodies in the lung or sputum suggested that asbestotic fibrosis was present. Some three years later Gloyne (1929) suggested that the term "asbestos body" should be used. Gough (1965) considered that mineral particles of needle shape other than those of asbestos could give rise to structures which had the appearance of asbestos bodies. He referred to them as mineral fibre bodies. Gross, de Treville and Haller (1970) described such bodies in animals inoculated intratracheally with a fibre glass suspension and introduced the term, ferruginous body, with which Goldstein and Rendall (1970) concur as in their experiments other fibrous materials became coated with a ferruginous protein complex. Heppleston (1970) considers that the term "ferruginous body" lays undue emphasis on one feature of the envelope and prefers the descriptive but non-committal term—"coated fibre".

The definition of the exact pathogenesis and morbid anatomy of asbestosis presents many problems which are being investigated in different laboratories throughout the world. The particular parameter in an asbestos dust cloud which relates most closely to the fibrogenic effect of the dust, the sites in the lung at which fibrosis occurs, the mechanism through which fibrosis and calcified plaques develop and the relationship of asbestos exposure to the development of malignant conditions of the lung, pleura and other organs, are the subjects of intensive research.

The Fibrogenic Parameter of an Asbestos Dust Cloud

Using rabbits King, Clegg and Rae (1946) found that whereas asbestos fibres approximately 15 microns in length caused a nodular fibrosis, animals inoculated intratracheally with a suspension of fibres 2·5 microns long, developed a diffuse increase in the interstitial reticulin. In the writer's laboratory two groups of South African Vervet monkeys were exposed to crocidolite asbestos dust clouds, the one consisting of fibres up to 150 microns in length and the other of the same asbestos which had been so ground that the dust cloud consisted mainly of particles of 2 microns. On electron microscopy these small particles were shown to consist of fibres and by electron diffraction the unaltered crystalline structure of asbestos has been confirmed.

The monkeys exposed to the finely ground asbestos showed that the main lesion consisted of perivascular and intra-alveolar aggregations of dust-laden macrophages (Fig. 1) and even five years after exposure there was no evidence of any increase in reticulin fibres. In the animals

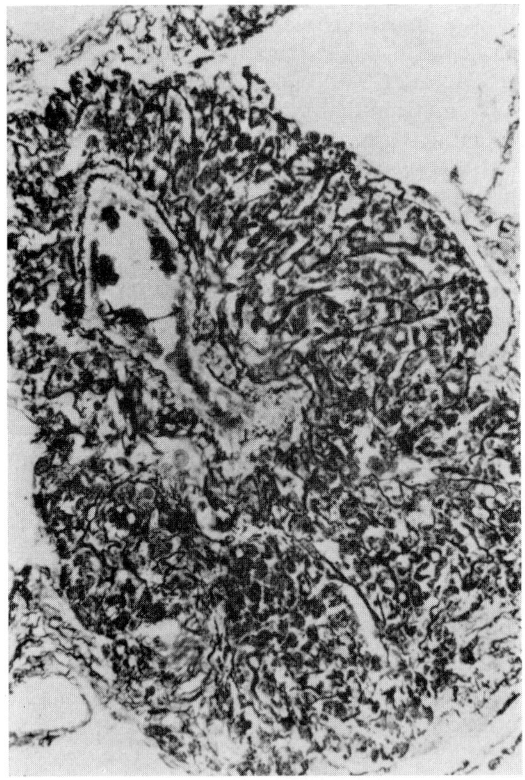

Fig. 1. Section from the lung of a monkey exposed to finely ground crocidolite approximately 3 years after commencement of exposure showing aggregations of dust laden macrophages in the perivascular tissues and adjacent alveoli.

exposed to the dust cloud consisting of long fibres asbestotic fibrosis developed (Fig. 2).

In both groups of animals there was evidence of a chronic fibrous pleurisy and in the animals exposed to the long fibre asbestos fibrous parietal and diaphragmatic plaques were present.

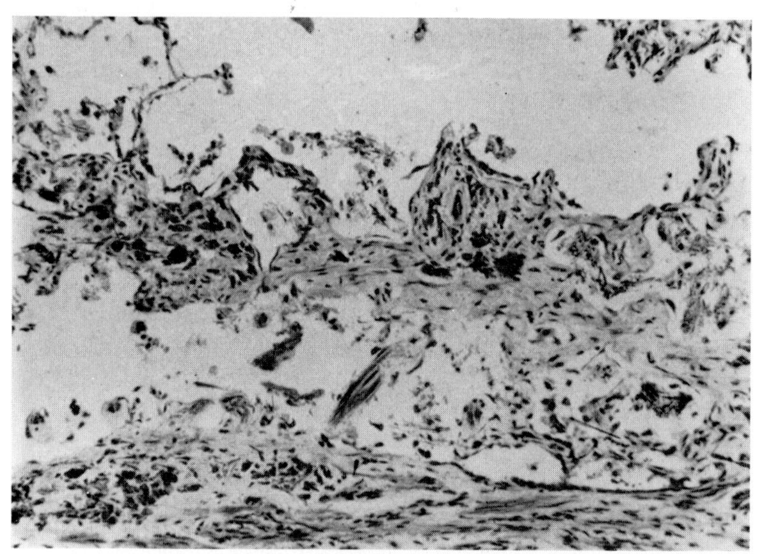

Fig. 2. Section from the lung of a monkey exposed to long fibre crocidolite showing fibrosis of the lung parenchyma in the region of the respiratory bronchiole.

Asbestotic Fibrosis

Asbestosis has been regarded as an interstitial fibrosis in which the walls of the lower respiratory tract were thickened. As in other diseases in which the pathological changes were originally classified in the general group of interstitial fibrosis, a more accurate definition of the part of the lower respiratory tract involved in asbestosis is now possible. The exact role of long and short fibres in the development of asbestotic parenchymal fibrosis has been established, but the relationship of these to the chronic pleurisy and pleural plaque formation has not yet been established.

One of the striking features of a focus of asbestotic fibrosis is that the bodies and fibres are in groups, both in the fibrous connective tissue and in spaces in the area of fibrosis (Fig. 3). Elastic staining shows the elastic network of an alveolus around the groups of bodies and needle and around the spaces in which asbestos can be seen, indicating that

the predominating fibrosis is intra-alveolar and not in the walls of the
air spaces (Webster, 1970).

Although fibrosis of the walls of the lower respiratory tract does occur,
the main component, and indeed the basic pathology of asbestotic

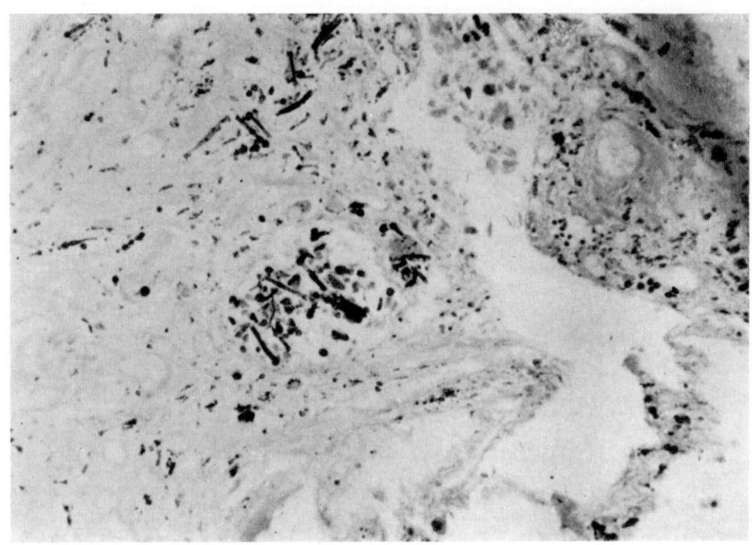

Fig. 3. Section from the lung of an asbestos miner showing an area
of fibrosis in which groups of asbestos needles and bodies can be seen.

fibrosis, is an organizing alveolitis (Fig. 4). The presence of asbestos in
the alveolar spaces causes swelling of the alveolar epithelial cells which
then desquamate giving the appearance of a desquamative alveolitis
which becomes organized by collagen fibrils probably originating from
the connective tissue of the alveolar walls. When this occurs in the
alveoli of a respiratory bronchiole, the appearance suggests thickening
of the walls of the bronchiole (Webster, 1970).

On occasion areas of fibrosis can be found in workers who have been
exposed to asbestos though no evidence of ferruginous body formation
can be seen even after digestion of the tissue using the method described
by Gross, de Treville and Haller (1969). When the extract is examined
under polarized light, numerous asbestos needles can be seen. This is
supportive evidence, in man, of the experimental investigation carried
out by Vorwald, Durkan and Pratt (1951) in which they found that the
coated fibres did not produce fibrosis in the guinea pig lung. Gough and
Heppleston (1960) suggested that the coating rendered the asbestos
fibre innocuous. Observations in South Africa therefore support the
view that the coating of the asbestos fibre appears to be a defence

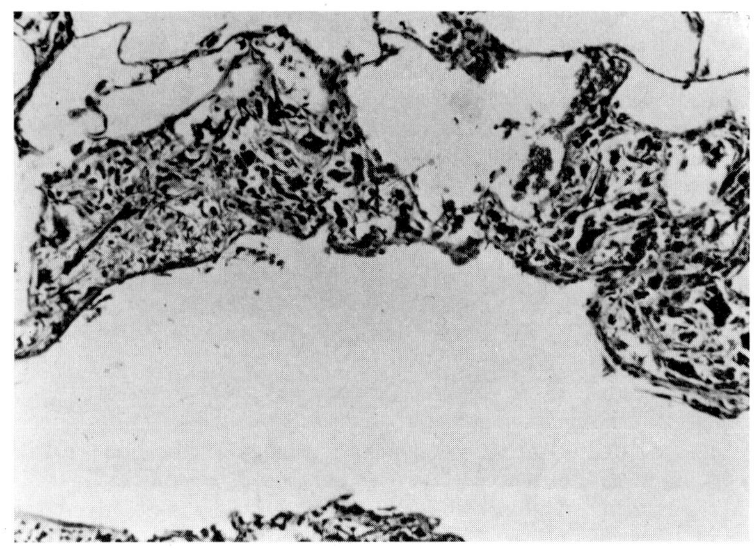

FIG. 4. Sections of a lung showing that the lesion of asbestosis is in the alveoli related to the respiratory bronchiole with almost no change in the wall of the bronchiole.

mechanism on the part of the body which renders the asbestos fibre non-fibrogenic.

It has been suggested that the segmental form of some bodies is indicative of degeneration but even after short exposure such forms can be found in the lungs of primates.

Areas of massive fibrosis have been found in the lungs of asbestos miners and although only a few such cases have been described, there does not appear to be any particular distribution of these areas in the lung. In the Vervet monkeys exposed to the long fibre asbestos, areas of pigmented fibrosis measuring up to 1·5 cms in diameter were found in both the upper and lower lobes.

Although there was evidence of a tuberculous infection in some of the cases of massive fibrosis in mineworkers, in the monkeys, however, there is no doubt that areas of massive fibrosis developed without an initiating tuberculous infection.

Histologically these areas show that the organizing alveolitis has affected a larger area of lung tissue, but that the basic pathological change is the same as in asbestosis without massive fibrosis.

Basal Asbestosis

According to Thomson, Kaschula and McDonald (1963) and Thomson (1965) in the person not exposed to asbestos dust in mines or in industry the inhalation of asbestos fibres can occur from polluted urban atmosphere. Asbestos needles move downwards into the lung bases before becoming coated with an iron protein complex. Thomson considers that once a fibre becomes an "asbestos body" it is unlikely to move further as it is too large to be phagocytosed. Over a lifetime a focal concentration of these bodies occurs at the lung bases and while the amount present, if dispersed thoughout the lung, would be in-effective, when concentrated it is fibrogenic.

It is indeed strange that this type of lesion is not encountered in the mining population of South Africa, where the pathological examinations of the lungs of miners are all carried out in one institution where the examination is designed to detect even the minimal changes due to the inhalation of mineral dust.

Basal asbestosis therefore tends to occur in people exposed to small amounts of asbestos dust in an urban environment. The lesions appear to be associated with pieural changes, usually calcification or with malignant disease of the pleura or peritoneum (Thomson, 1965).

More recently Whitwell and Rawcliffe (1971) have described this type of asbestosis in five cases of pleural mesothelioma.

Chronic Pleurisy

A chronic non-specific thickening of the pleura is a more frequent finding in the pathological examination of asbestos miners (75·8 per cent) than in gold miners (16·9 per cent) in South Africa. The pleurisy may be widespread but is usually more marked over the lateral basal and subapical bronchopulmonary segments of the lower lobe. The interlobar fissures are often obliterated and the pleurae of two adjoining obes are thickened.

The histological examination of the pleura shows that there is an increase of fibrous connective tissue outside the elastic membrane of the pleura together with a fibrosis between the elastic membrane and the subpleural alveoli. The underlying alveoli are obliterated by collagen bundles in the alveolar spaces. Although in the majority of specimens the fibrous connective tissue is without any cellular infiltrate, occasional lymphocytes and plasma cells may be present in the thickened pleura.

The subpleural lymphatics are usually dilated and in some specimens there may be congestion of the smaller blood vessels. The elastic membrane may not be broken but in foci there may be reduplication and increased size of the elastic fibres.

It is the exception to find ferruginous bodies in the fibrous tissue except that of the alveolar spaces, but in the monkeys exposed to an asbestos dust cloud consisting of particles of 2 microns and below, macrophages laden with the small asbestos particles were found in the loose connective tissue of a papillary type of pleurisy.

Classification of Asbestosis

It is the practice in South Africa and in some other countries to classify asbestosis into three grades—slight, moderate or marked. This classification depends on the degree of interstitial fibrosis, and the extent of parenchymal involvement.

It is considered that the presence of a chronic pleurisy may be associated with a degree of atelectasis of the lung parenchyma. As this will accentuate the appearance given by asbestotic fibrosis of the lung parenchyma, the grading of asbestosis into slight, moderate and marked categories is unreliable. There is some justification for indicating that the lesion is a minimal one especially when the fibrosis is focal and confined to the lower lobes as described by Thomson (1965). Similarly, in order to conform to the classification of the other pneumoconioses asbestosis with massive fibrosis might be considered as "marked" although the descriptive phrase "asbestosis with massive fibrosis" is preferred.

Asbestotic Plaques

According to Selikoff (1965) the earliest reports of pulmonary asbestosis do not mention pleural calcification and he considers that this was because workers died of asbestosis after a relatively short exposure at the time when these reports were written. Pleural calcification, if it is to occur, only becomes apparent approximately twenty years after the onset of exposure. In 1931, however, Sparks did describe calcification in the lower zones of the chest. Gloyne (1933) discussing the morbid anatomy of asbestosis described lesions which were probably pleural plaques.

Although Siegal, Smith and Greenberg (1943a, 1943b) described plaques in talc miners and millers it was only later that the significance of the tremolite nature of the talc was recognized. The association of calcified pleural plaques and anthophyllite asbestos was noted by Kiviluoto (1960). Sleggs (1960) noted plaque formation in cases of mesothelioma in people exposed to crocidolite asbestos and this was confirmed in the survey carried out in the North Western Cape Province of South Africa by the Pneumoconiosis Research Unit of the South African Council for Scientific and Industrial Research (1964).

More recently plaque formation has been found in workers from the amosite mine in the Transvaal Province of South Africa.

The pathology of these calcified pleural plaques was described by Meurman (1966) in his extensive monograph published in 1966 in which there is a complete description of the morbid anatomy, frequency and distribution of the plaques associated with anthophyllite asbestos in Finland.

The pathogenesis of these plaques has always been obscure but Thomson (1970) suggested that the plaque formation may be the result of a sensitivity reaction because of the small numbers of asbestos fibres found in relation to the fibrotic reaction and the cellular reaction in the deepest part of the plaque. He suggests that the gravitation of the asbestos fibres in the lung explains the siting of the plaques.

Fibrous plaques may develop on the parietal pleura, the diaphragm and the pericardium. Although the plaque formation of the parietal pleura is often associated with fibrous plaques on the visceral pleura, the extent of such plaque formation is far less on the visceral pleura. A chronic fibrous pleurisy of the visceral pleura usually accompanies plaque formation, and there is often thickening of the pleura of the interlobar fissures.

Plaque formation of the parietal pleura is most commonly found on the pleura adjacent to the ribs and extends along a line which is parallel to the ribs (Fig. 5).

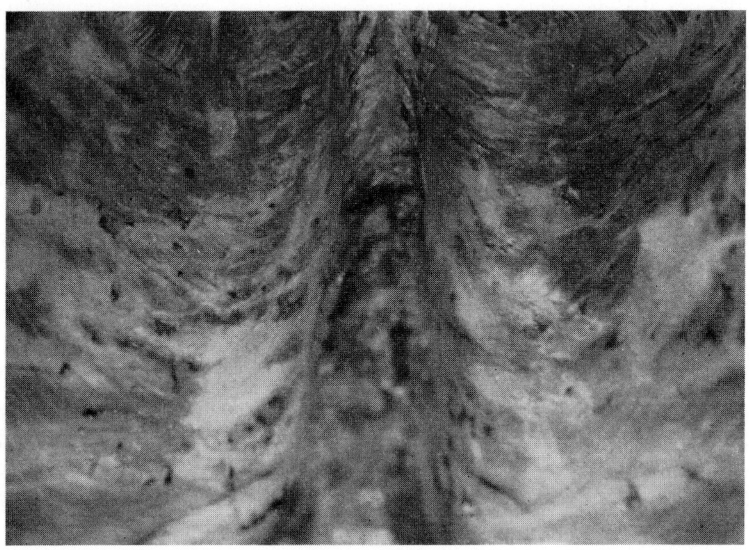

FIG. 5. The thoracic cage of a non-mining industrial worker in whom there was a history of asbestos exposure, showing plaque formation.

The diaphragmatic plaques are more obvious on the domes on both sides. There may, however, be extensive and multiple plaque formation involving almost the whole diaphragm (Fig. 6).

Pericardial plaque formation may be found when diaphragmatic plaque formation has occurred and is situated on that part of the pericardium which touches the diaphragm plaque during cardiac pulsation. This "kissing" feature is most obvious when the plaques are seen at thoracotomy.

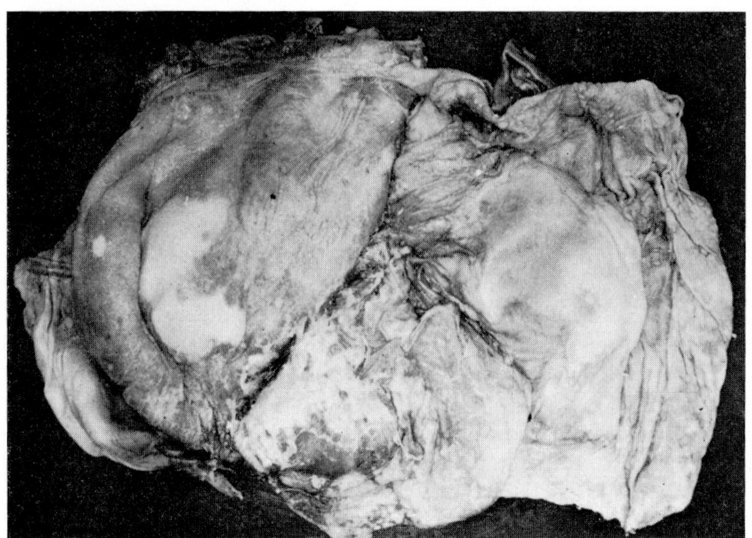

Fig. 6. The diaphragm of an asbestos miner showing calcified plaques.

The fibrous plaques tend to calcify and this change may lead to extensive focal calcification of the parietal pleura and diaphragm. When calcified the plaques on the diaphragm are usually visible at a radiological examination.

Malignant Tumours associated with Asbestos Exposure

Wood and Gloyne (1934) reported on 100 cases of asbestosis of whom 28 had died. Although it is recorded that two of the cases showed evidence of cancer of the lung and one showed the presence of malignant tumour nodules on the pleura, the possible association between asbestos and cancer of the lung was probably first recognized by Lynch and Smith (1935).

Buchanan (1965) reviewed the death certificates of 584 people who had died with asbestosis in the United Kingdom from 1924–1963 and found that 30·9 per cent of the males and 13 per cent of the females were reported as having a lung tumour. The exposure to asbestos was industrial in contrast to that of mining where, for example, in South Africa the incidence of bronchogenic carcinoma is only slightly above that expected in the unexposed population.

In the insulation workers of the United States, Hammond, Selikoff and Churg (1965) found 17·3 per cent of bronchogenic carcinoma in 307 consecutive deaths. In the same group 11·1 per cent of the deaths were attributed to cancer of the gastro-intestinal tract; however the authors refrained from drawing conclusions on the relationship between asbestos exposure and gastro-intestinal carcinoma.

Without doubt, the association which is of great interest and the subject of much research work is that of the group of mesotheliomatous tumours. This association was first suggested by Wagner (1960) who described 26 cases in which there was histological confirmation. Of these there was an association with the Northern part of the Cape Province of South Africa in twenty.

Since that time numerous studies have been reported from different parts of the world recording cases of mesothelioma. Gilson (1970) indicated that 550 cases had been diagnosed in the United Kingdom up to the end of 1968 but did not give the numbers exposed to asbestos, but such an association with exposure has been noted by Elmes and Wade (1965), Wagner (1965) and Newhouse (1970). Selikoff, Hammond and Churg (1970), found that of 380 deaths in insulation workers since 1943, 6 were from pleural mesothelioma and 16 peritoneal. In Canada where the exposure is to chrysotile, 165 cases of mesothelioma have been reported by McDonald, Harper, El Attar and McDonald (1970), but there has not been a case of mesothelioma reported from Rhodesia (Gelfand and Morton, 1970) where chrysotile is also mined. In Finland where anthophyllite asbestos has been mined since 1919 no case of mesothelioma has been described (Kiviluoto and Meurman, 1970). From other countries cases have been reported though the epidemiological studies are not complete (Vigliani, 1970; Avril and Champeix, 1970). There is then some evidence that at least one type of asbestos is not associated with the development of mesothelioma but it is probable that most information will be obtained from South Africa because it is in that country that three of the main types of asbestos are mined and milled. There it is possible for a mining employee to be exposed to only one of crocidolite, amosite or chrysotile. Unfortunately the proportion of people exposed to chrysotile asbestos is relatively small.

The great majority of the cases of mesothelioma found in South Africa have been exposed to crocidolite in the Northern Cape Province (Fig. 7) but no case has been described in the population exposed to a similar crocidolite mined and processed in the Northern Transvaal. Although three cases of mesothelioma have been found in the mining population of the amosite mine in the Transvaal Province, it is possible that in two of these cases there may have been exposure to other types of asbestos. No case of mesothelioma has yet been found in the population of the South African chrysotile mines.

At the end of 1969 the Asbestos Tumour Reference Panel in South Africa had registered 179 cases of pleural mesothelioma collected over the last 20 years. Those in which the environmental history is known or in which no history could be obtained are summarized in Table 1.

As can be seen from this Table, in 16 per cent of the cases an exposure

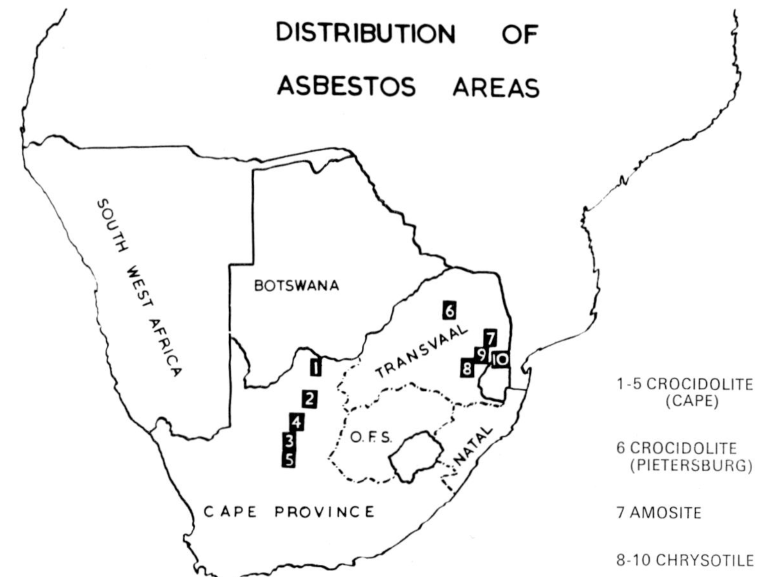

FIG. 7. Map of the asbestos areas of South Africa.

Table 1

Environmental and Occupational Exposure

(179 Cases—Definite Mesothelioma of Pleura)

Asbestos Mines		54
Crocidolite (Northern Cape)	51	
Amosite	3	
Asbestos + Manganese Mines		21
Manganese Mines only		2
Asbestos Mines and Other Industry		4
Asbestos Exposure—Other Industries		12
Possible Environmental Exposure (Northern Cape)		31
No Evidence of Asbestos Exposure		24
		148
Unknown		31
Total		179

to asbestos could not be elicited. In approximately one third of the
cases of mesothelioma a mining history was obtained and in a further
third it is possible that there was environmental exposure in the Cape
crocidolite asbestos fields either by domicile or by working there. In

the remaining third of the cases neither an occupational nor environmental history could be obtained. It must be stressed that together with asbestos there are deposits of other minerals such as iron and manganese in the Northern Cape area. It is possible, therefore, that environmental and mining exposure may well have been to manganese and iron as well as asbestos. In some cases there has only been exposure to manganese.

It is for the above reasons that it is considered that in addition to asbestos some other factor is necessary for the development of a mesothelioma.

Mesothelioma

It is probable that the mesothelioma of the pleura (Fig. 8) develops in a fibrous plaque but not in a plaque which has undergone calcification. The tumour may develop in a number of different foci and even when the tumour macroscopically appears to be localized to the costophrenic angle or the apex of the thoracic cage, microscopic foci can be found scattered in different parts of the pleura.

Although the histological pattern can vary in different parts of the tumour three main types have been identified:

(*a*) Mixed type;

(*b*) Spindle cell type, and

(*c*) "Epithelial Cell" type.

The mixed type of mesothelioma (Fig. 9) is the tumour which is most frequently found and characteristically it consists of bundles of mature collagen in which there are clefts lined by or filled with cells which are similar to those lining the pleura. Although there may be pleomorphism of the cells there is usually a uniform staining reaction and the usually folded nucleus is vesicular. In parts the mature collagen bundles are replaced by a more cellular connective tissue and in this desmoplastic reaction sarcomatous change may be evident.

The spindle cell type (Fig. 10) may be localized or diffuse. The localized form includes tumours previously classified as fibromata of the pleura. In the diffuse type the tumour may have the appearance of a spindle cell sarcoma but in other tumours of this group occasional foci can be seen in which there are clefts similar to those found in the mixed type of mesothelioma.

The "epithelial cell" type (Fig. 11) consists of masses of cells with the characteristics described in the mixed type. Throughout some tumours and in parts of others these cells are vacuolated. It is possible to demonstrate the presence of hyaluronic acid in the vacuolated cells in certain tumours of this group and also in cells of the mixed type of mesothelioma, but the lack of hyaluronic acid does not discount the diagnosis of a mesothelioma. Many patients with a mesothelioma present with a history of recurrent pleural effusions. In some instances hyaluronic acid can be found in the pleural fluid.

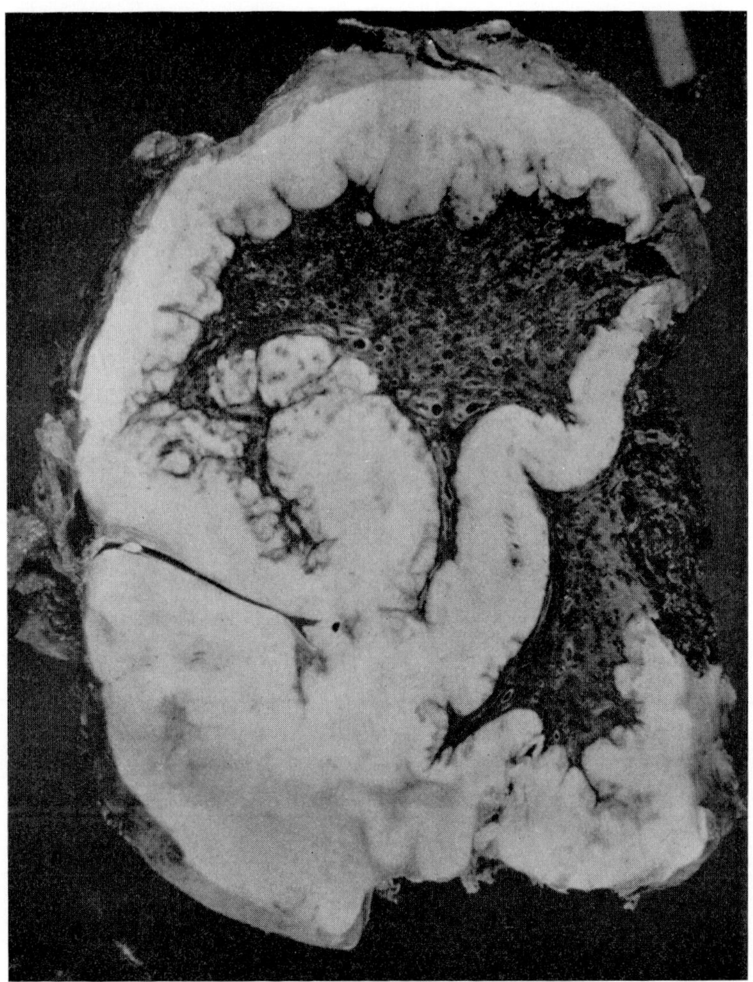

FIG. 8. Mesothelioma of the pleura showing the tumour extending
into the interlobar fissure and the lung parenchyma.

Mesothelioma of the pleura tends to spread by contiguity, for
example, through the diaphragm to the peritoneum. Not unusually it
may infiltrate any operation site in the chest wall, even along the track
of a needle biopsy. It may also spread into the lung parenchyma by
contiguity, though in this case it usually spreads in the perivascular and
peribronchiolar lymphatics. On occasion parenchymal involvement
may lead to confusion as it may be difficult to distinguish the "epithelial
cell" type of tumour from a peripheral bronchiolar carcinoma.

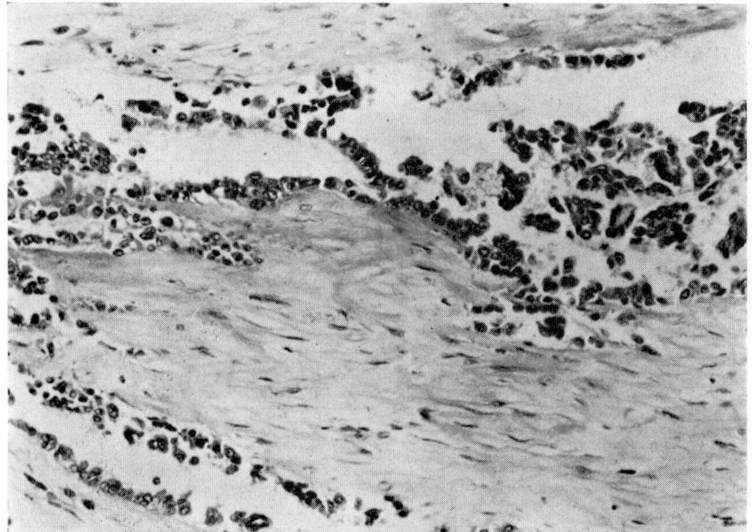

FIG. 9. Histological section of the mixed type of mesothelioma
showing the dense mature collagen in which clefts containing epithelial-
like cells can be seen.

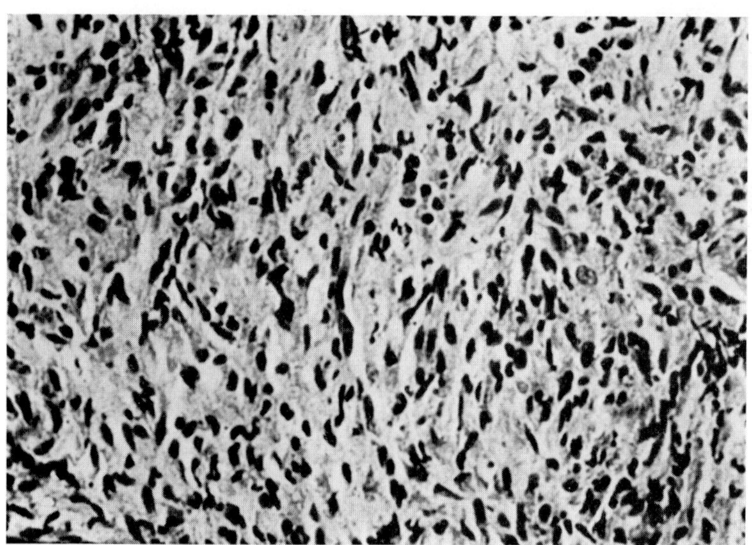

FIG. 10. Histological section of the spindle cell type of mesothelioma.

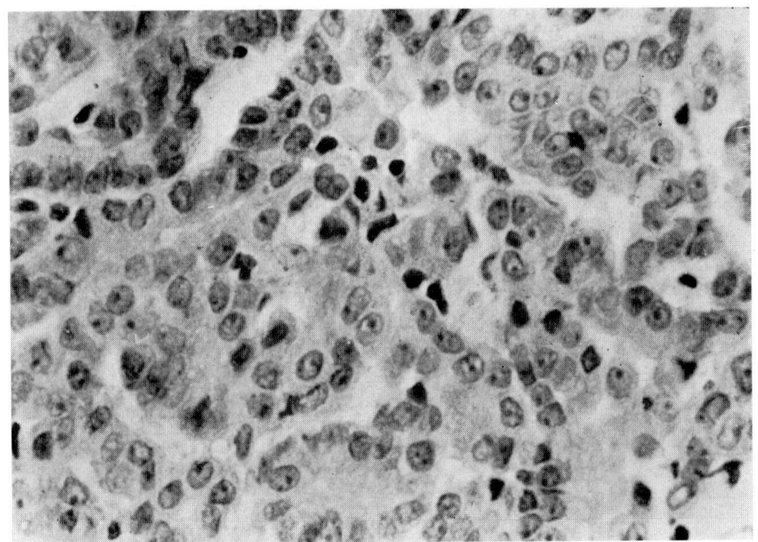

FIG. 11. Histological section of the epithelial type of mesothelioma.

References

Avril, J. and Champeix, J. (1970), "Results of asbestos exposure in France." *Pneumoconiosis: Proceedings of the International Conference, Johannesburg, 1969.* Ed. by H. A. Shapiro, p. 187. Oxford University Press, Cape Town.

Buchanan, W. D. (1965), *Asbestosis and Primary Intrathoracic Neoplasms. Annals of the New York Academy of Sciences,* **132,** 507. *Biological Effects of Asbestos.* New York, 1964, p. 507. New York Academy of Sciences, New York.

Cooke, W. E. (1924), "Fibrosis of the lungs due to the inhalation of asbestos dust." *British Medical Journal,* **2,** 147.

Elmes, P. C. and Wade, O. L. (1965), "Relationship between exposure to asbestos and pleural malignancy in Belfast." *Annals of the New York Academy of Sciences,* **132,** 549.

Gelfand, M. and Morton, S. A. (1970), "Asbestosis in Rhodesia." *Pneumoconiosis: Proceedings of the International Conference, Johannesburg, 1969.* Ed. by H. A. Shapiro, p. 204. Oxford University Press, Cape Town.

Gilson, J. C. (1970), "Asbestos health hazards; recent observations in the United Kingdom." *Pneumoconiosis: Proceedings of the International Conference, Johannesburg, 1969.* Ed. by H. A. Shapiro, p. 173. Oxford University Press, Cape Town.

Gloyne, S. R. (1929), "The presence of the asbestos fibre in the lesions of asbestos workers." *Tubercle,* **10,** 404.

Gloyne, S. R. (1933), "Morbid anatomy and histology of asbestosis." *Tubercle,* **14,** 445.

Goldstein, B. and Rendall, R. E. G. (1970), "Ferruginous bodies." *Pneumoconiosis: Proceedings of the International Conference, Johannesburg, 1969.* Ed. by H. A. Shapiro, p. 92. Oxford University Press, Cape Town.

Gough, J. (1965), "Differential diagnosis in the pathology of asbestosis." *Annals of the New York Academy of Sciences,* **132,** 368.

Gough, J. and Heppleston, A. G. (1960), "The pathology of the pneumoconiosis." *Symposium on Industrial Pulmonary Diseases, London*, 1958. Ed. by E. J. King and C. M. Fletcher, p. 23. J. & A. Churchill, London.

Gross, P., De Treville, R. T. P. and Haller, M. (1970), "Pulmonary ferruginous bodies studies on their origin." *Pneumoconiosis: Proceedings of the International Conference, Johannesburg, 1969*. Ed. by H. A. Shapiro, p. 86. Oxford University Press, Cape Town.

Gross, P., De Treville, R. T. P. and Haller, M. N. (1969), "Pulmonary ferruginous bodies in city dwellers; a study of their central fiber." *Archives of Environmental Health*, **19**, 186.

Hammond, E. C., Selikoff, J. J. and Churg, J. (1965), "Neoplasia among insulation workers in the United States with special reference to intra-abdominal neoplasia." *Annals of the New York Academy of Sciences*, **132**, 519.

Heppleston, A. G. (1970), Discussion: symposium on asbestosis. *Pneumoconiosis: Proceedings of the International Conference, Johannesburg, 1969*. Ed. by H. A. Shapiro, p. 107. Oxford University Press, Cape Town.

King, E. J., Clegg, J. W. and Rae, V. M. (1946), "The effect of asbestos, and of asbestos and aluminium, on the lungs of rabbits." *Thorax*, **1**, 188.

Kiviluoto, R. (1960), "Pleural calcification as a roentgenologic sign of non-occupational endemic anthophyllite-asbestosis." *Acta radiologica*, suppl. 194.

Kiviluoto, R. and Meurman, L. (1970), "Results of asbestos exposure in Finland." *Pneumoconiosis: Proceedings of the International Conference, Johannesburg, 1969*. Ed. by H. A. Shapiro, p. 190, Oxford University Press, Cape Town.

Lynch, K. M. and Smith, W. A. (1935), "Pulmonary asbestosis: carcinoma of lung in asbesto-silicosis." *American Journal of Cancer*, **24**, 56.

McDonald, A. D., Harper, A., El Attar, O. A. and McDonald, J. C. (1970), "Epidemiology of primary malignant mesothelial tumours in Canada." *Pneumoconiosis: Proceedings of the International Conference, Johannesburg, 1969*. Ed. by H. A. Shapiro, p. 197. Oxford University Press, Cape Town.

McDonald, S. (1927), "Histology of pulmonary asbestosis." *British Medical Journal*, **2**, 1025.

Meurman, L. (1966), "Asbestos bodies and pleural plaques in a Finnish series of autopsy cases." *Acta pathologica et microbiologica Scandinavica*, suppl. 181.

Murray, H. M. (1907), Report of the Departmental Committee on Compensation for Industrial Diseases. Minutes of evidence, appendices and index, p. 127. Wyman & Sons, London.

Newhouse, M. L. (1970), "The mortality of asbestos factory workers." *Pneumoconiosis: Proceedings of the International Conference, Johannesburg, 1969*. Ed. by H. A. Shapiro, p. 158. Oxford University Press, Cape Town.

Seiler, H. E. (1928), "A case of pneumoconiosis, result of the inhalation of asbestos dust." *British Medical Journal*, **2**, 982.

Selikoff, I. J. (1965), "The occurrence of pleural calcification among asbestos insulation workers." *Annals of the Academy of Sciences, New York*, **132**, 513.

Selikoff, I. J., Hammond, E. C. and Churg, J. (1970), "Mortality experiences of asbestos insulation workers, 1943–1968." *Pneumoconiosis: Proceedings of the International Conference, Johannesburg, 1969*. Ed. by H. A. Shapiro, p. 180. Oxford University Press, Cape Town.

Siegal, W., Smith, A. R. and Greenburg, L. (1943), "Study of talc miners and millers in St. Lawrence County." *Industrial Hygiene Bulletin*, **22**, 468.

Siegal, W., Smith, A. R. and Greenburg, L. (1943), "Dust hazard in tremolite talc mining, including roentgenological findings in talc workers." *American Journal of Roentgenology and Radium Therapy*, **49**, 11.

Simson, F. W. (1928), "Pulmonary asbestosis in South Africa." *British Medical Journal*, **1**, 885.

Sleggs, C. A. (1960), "Clinical aspects of asbestosis in the Northern Cape." p. 383, *Proceedings of the Pneumoconiosis Conference, Johannesburg, 1959.* Ed. by A. J. Orenstein. J. & A. Churchill, London.

South African Council for Scientific and Industrial Research. Pneumoconiosis Research Unit (1964), Field survey in the North Western Cape and at Penge in the Transvaal (Asbestosis and Mesothelioma). Report No. 1/1964. Johannesburg.

Sparks, J. V. (1931), "Pulmonary asbestosis." *Radiology*, **17,** 1249.

Stewart, M. J. (1930), "Asbestosis bodies in the lungs of guinea-pigs after three to five months exposure in an asbestos factory." *The Journal of Pathology and Bacteriology*, **33,** 848.

Thomson, J. G. (1965), "Asbestos and the urban dweller." *Annals of the New York Academy of Sciences*, **132,** 196.

Thomson, J. G. (1970), "The pathogenesis of pleural plaques." *Pneumoconiosis : Proceedings of the International Conference, Johannesburg, 1969.* Ed. by H. A. Shapiro, p. 138. Oxford University Press, Cape Town.

Thomson, J. G., Kaschula, R. O. C. and McDonald, R. R. (1963), "Asbestos as a modern urban hazard." *South African Medical Journal*, **37,** 77.

Vigliani, E. C. (1970), "Asbestos exposure and its results in Italy." *Pneumoconiosis: Proceedings of the International Conference, Johannesburg, 1969.* Ed. by H. A. Shapiro, p. 192, Oxford University Press, Cape Town.

Vorwald, A. J., Durkan, T. M. and Pratt, P. C. (1951), "Experimental studies of asbestosis." *A.M.A. Archives of Industrial Hygiene*, **3,** 1.

Wagner, J. C. (1960), "Some pathological aspects of asbestosis in the Union of South Africa," p. 373. *Proceedings of the Pneumoconiosis Conference, Johannesburg, 1959.* Ed. by A. J. Orenstein. J. & A. Churchill, London.

Wagner, J. C. (1965), "Epidemiology of diffuse mesothelial tumors: evidence of an association from studies in South Africa and the United Kingdom." *Annals of the New York Academy of Sciences*, **132,** 575.

Webster, I. (1970), "The pathogenesis of asbestosis." *Pneumoconiosis: Proceedings of the International Conference, Johannesburg, 1969.* Ed. by H. A. Shapiro, p. 117. Oxford University Press, Cape Town.

Whitwell, F. and Rawcliffe, R. M. (1971), "Diffuse malignant pleural mesothelioma and asbestos exposure." *Thorax*, **26,** 6.

Wood, W. B. and Gloyne, S. R. (1934), "Pulmonary asbestosis; a review of one hundred cases." *Lancet*, **227,** 1383.

Chapter 4

Dust Inhalation, Retention and Elimination

Introduction

The respiratory tract of man is adapted to facilitate gas exchange during breathing and also to resist damage by the external environment. In addition to protection against thermal injury and dehydration, the lungs are provided with a highly efficient system to eliminate any dust particles which may be inhaled. An understanding of the manner in which this airborne material is handled in the body is of great practical importance since it forms the basis of any assessment of the hazard presented by industrial dust.

The Functional Anatomy of the Lung

The main anatomical features of the lung are shown in diagrammatic form in Fig. 1. The nose and mouth are seen to form a common cavity

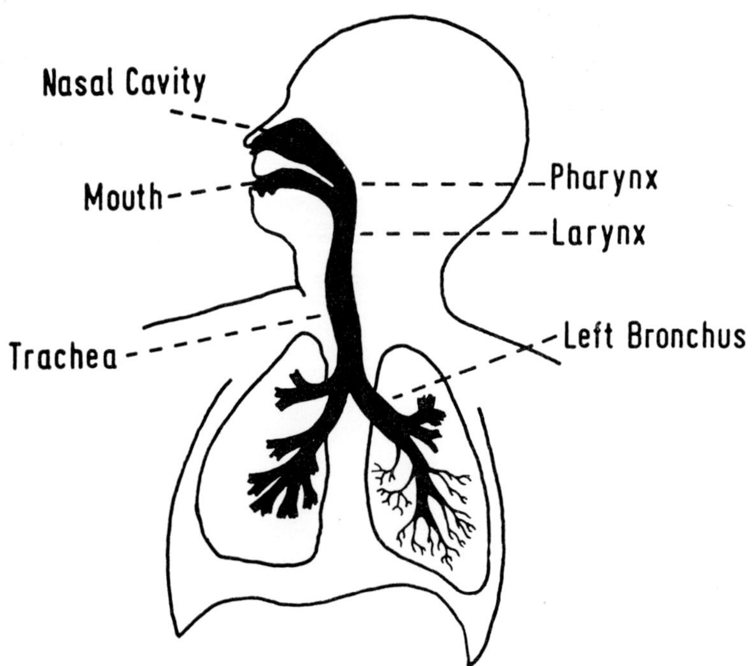

FIG. 1. Diagrammatic outline of the respiratory tract.

called the pharynx. This leads through the larynx ("Adam's Apple") to the trachea which is the main airway leading to the chest. It divides into a right and left bronchus which supply the two lungs. Each bronchus divides into two smaller airways which sub-divide in their turn. This branching is repeated some 23 times. The last seven divisions or generations have small sac-like openings in their walls called alveoli. There are about 300,000,000 alveoli in all and they give the cut surface of the lung its familiar sponge-like appearance. Each alveolus has a diameter of about 250 microns. The branching pattern was assumed to be symmetrical as a first approximation by Weibel (1963) who estimated the dimensions of the airways throughout the lung (Table 1). One of the fundamental features of the pulmonary anatomy can be seen from the values shown in Table 1. Although the calibre of the distal airways

Table 1

Dimensions of the Human Airways
(Model "A" from Weibel, 1963)

	Generation	Name	Number per generation	Length (cm)	Diameter (cm)	Total cross section (cm^2)
	0	Trachea	1	12·0	1·8	2·54
	1	Main bronchi	2	4·76	1·22	2·33
	2	Lobar bronchi	4	1·90	0·83	2·13
	3	Segmental bronchi	8	0·76	0·56	2·00
	4	Intrasegmental bronchi	16	1·27	0·45	2·48
	5	,,	32	1·07	0·35	3·11
	6	,,	64	0·90	0·28	3·96
Conducting zone (with cilia)	7	,,	128	0·76	0·23	5·10
	8	,,	256	0·64	0·186	6·95
	9	,,	512	0·54	0·154	9·56
	10	,,	1,024	0·46	0·130	13·4
	11	,,	2,048	0·39	0·109	19·6
	12	Bronchioles	4,096	0·33	0·095	28·8
	13	,,	8,192	0·27	0·082	44·5
	14	,,	16,384	0·23	0·074	69·4
	15	,,	32,768	0·20	0·066	113·0
	16	Terminal bronchioles	65,536	0·165	0·060	180·0
	17	Respiratory bronchioles	131,072	0·141	0·054	300·0
	18	,,	262,144	0·117	0·050	534·0
Respiratory zone (with alveoli)	19	,,	524,288	0·099	0·047	944·0
	20	Alveolar ducts	1,048,576	0·083	0·045	1,600·0
	21	,, ,,	2,097,152	0·070	0·043	3,222·0
	22	,, ,,	4,194,304	0·059	0·041	5,880·0
	23	Alveolar sacs	8,388,608	0·050	0·041	11,800·0

is minute their total cross sectional area is enormous. Since the velocity of airflow in any airway is inversely proportional to the total area of all the pathways in that generation the speed of airflow is very much slower in small airways in the depths of the lung than that measured in the trachea or major bronchi. The narrowest part of the respiratory tract is in fact in the nose and it is here that the highest rates of airflow are encountered.

Oxygen is absorbed into the blood and carbon dioxide eliminated within the alveoli. This region of the lung is therefore called the respiratory zone. The first sixteen generations of airways do not contain alveoli and this region, called the conducting zone, simply distributes inhaled air to the alveoli and returns exhaled air back to the environment. Both regions are equipped with highly efficient systems to get rid of dust particles which settle onto their surfaces. The non-respiratory conducting airways are lined with ciliated cells extending as far as the terminal bronchiole. The cilia consist of small hairs about 0·5 micron long, projecting into the lumen of the airway. They beat to and fro with a wave-like motion and propel the moist layer of mucus which covers them towards the pharynx. Any insoluble dust particles settling onto this moving surface are carried in the same direction and are removed eventually from the body after being swallowed. The ciliated epithelium is probably cleared of deposited material in less than twelve hours. Dust particles reaching the alveoli on the other hand, are cleared very much more slowly. After being engulfed by alveolar macrophages within a few hours of deposition they are also excreted eventually by the same mucus escalator which removes material trapped in the upper airways, but the whole process may take many months. Some dusts are retained permanently within the lung or hilar lymphatics and may cause tissue damage.

The effect of inhaled dust thus depends on the region of the lung within which it is deposited as well as on the toxicity of the individual particles.

That fraction of the dust which deposits in the upper airways may damage the mucosa and cause bronchitis. Particles which are able to penetrate beyond the terminal bronchiole tend to accumulate in the lung and may cause the group of diseases known as the Pneumoconioses. Very soluble substances are absorbed from all parts of the respiratory tract and the site of deposition is not usually important.

The site at which an individual airborne particle is deposited in the lung depends on the aerodynamic properties of the particle, on the dimensions of the airways and on the pattern of breathing. There is no direct evidence concerning the details of dust deposition within the lungs of man and much effort has, of necessity, been diverted to the problem of obtaining information by indirect means. There is general agreement on the broad outlines of the pattern but it cannot be assumed that important modifications will not be required in the light of future experimental work.

The Deposition of Airborne Particles in the Lung

All particles that remain airborne for a reasonable length of time and which can be inhaled are properly called aerosols. This generic name is applied to both liquid and solid particles whether they be of coal, iron or rock from industrial sources or dust of natural origin such as fungi or pollen grains and also includes therapeutic substances used in medicine. The inhaled particles closely follow the movement of the air in which they are suspended and are drawn into the lung with each inspiration. They possess a small independent movement of their own however, and this motion causes a certain proportion of them to touch the wall of the respiratory tract. Any particle which does touch the wall in this way cannot be resuspended in the airstream and is permanently deposited. It can only be removed from the lung by the macrophage and ciliary systems. Those particles which escape deposition are exhaled to the atmosphere once more. In the first instance it is convenient to consider the behaviour of single spherical particles and to discuss the behaviour of irregular aggregates and fibrous particles at a later stage.

There are several independent mechanisms that contribute to the movement of aerosol particles and which cause them to deposit on the surface of the respiratory tract.

Gravitational Sedimentation

All airborne particles sediment under the influence of gravity. Each individual particle falls at a constant speed. This speed, called the terminal velocity, is proportional to the density of the particle and to the square of its diameter. The larger and denser the particle the faster it falls. This mechanism causes aerosols to deposit in the lung during breathing. When an industrial process is associated with the production of dust containing a wide range of particle sizes the coarse material is removed preferentially by sedimentation and the remaining cloud contains an increasing proportion of fine particles.

Inertial Impaction

The momentum of a particle travelling in a moving airstream causes it to maintain its original direction of travel for a short distance despite a change in the direction of the airflow. As a result some of the aerosol is deposited at those points of the respiratory tract where sudden changes in the direction of airflow are encountered. The effect is related to the original velocity of the particle, to its density and to the square of its diameter. Impaction is an important cause of particle deposition in the nose and at the bifurcations of the larger airways.

Diffusion

All airborne particles are subject to bombardment by the surrounding
gas molecules. As a result they acquire a random motion of the type
known as Brownian movement, which may cause their deposition in
the lung. The degree of this movement, or coefficient of diffusion, is
independent of the density of the particles but is inversely proportional
to their diameter. Only particles smaller than about 0·1 micron in diameter have a high enough rate of diffusion to result in significant
intrapulmonary deposition as a result of this mechanism alone.

Findeisen (1935) was the first to consider the effects of these factors
on the behaviour of inhaled aerosols. He was able to calculate the speed
of airflow in each airway of the lung, and to estimate the probability
of particle deposition in the various regions. An analysis of this type
presents considerable difficulties. The lung is likened to a series of
filters through which the inhaled air must pass. The probability of
deposition due to sedimentation or diffusion in any one region during
inhalation and exhalation is related to the time which the particles
spend in that region, and to the calibre of the individual airway. In the
case of inertial impaction the probability of deposition at a branching
point depends on the speed of airflow and the angle of branching as
well as on the size and density of the particle. Each particle may be
considered as an independent unit and the concentration of an aerosol
does not affect the rate of its deposition.

Findeisen (1935) showed that both large and small particles are
completely deposited in the lung as a result of their high settling velocity
and diffusivity respectively. Their strong tendency to be deposited
prevents them from penetrating to the alveolar regions and they are all
trapped in the upper respiratory tract during inhalation. There is an
intermediate size range however where particles, having a low terminal
velocity and diffusivity, are able to penetrate to the alveoli. Because
of their low mobility many escape deposition altogether and are exhaled
once more. The rate of their overall deposition may therefore be low
but their importance lies in the fact that it is these particles alone which
can cause pneumoconiosis. This fraction of an airborne cloud is called
the "respirable dust" although it must not be forgotten that the
remaining particles are also important as a possible cause of bronchitis.

Findeisen's calculations have been modified by subsequent authors
(Landahl, 1950; Beeckmans, 1965) and a number of measurements of
the overall deposition of particles in the lung have been published
(Brown, 1931; Brown, Cook, Ney and Hatch, 1950; Dautrebande,
Beckmann and Walkenhorst, 1957; Altshuler, Yarmus, Palmes and
Nelson, 1957; Muir and Davies, 1967; Love, Muir and Sweetland,
1971; Dennis, 1971). Despite the very great importance of defining the
"respirable fraction" there is no direct experimental evidence of its
limits in men. Considerable use has been made of the results of Brown

et al. (1950) who examined the distribution of particles in the exhaled air of their subjects. The validity of this indirect approach to the measurement of the regional deposition of aerosols in the lungs is problematical. A more promising method has been used by Lippmann and Albert (1969) who used aerosols labelled with radioactive tracers. By assuming that particles cleared from the lungs of volunteer subjects within twenty-four hours of inhalation represented material initially deposited on the cilia, it was possible to calculate the fraction of the inhaled cloud which had penetrated to the alveoli. This work is still in progress and should give important information. The available evidence on the probable site of particle deposition in the lung has been summarized by a committee of the International Commission on Radiological Protection (1966) and the results for one pattern of breathing are shown in Fig. 2. The regional deposition of 3 micron diameter

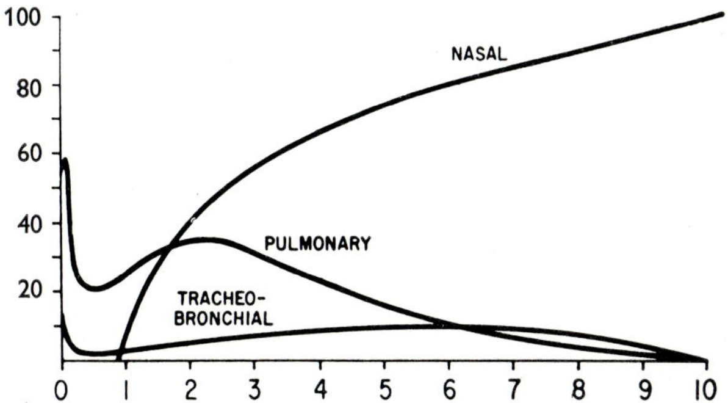

Fig. 2. Regional deposition of aerosols as a function of particle size (microns). Nasal breathing at 15 respirations/min, 750 cm³ tidal volume. The pulmonary compartment refers to the alveolated region and the tracheobronchial to the ciliated airways (From *Health Physics*, **12**, 179, 1966.)

particles will serve as an example. The curves in Fig. 2 show that about 58 per cent of such particles will be deposited in the nose, 35 per cent in the alveoli and 7 per cent on the ciliated airways.

The Effect of Particle Shape and Aggregation

The deposition of dust in the lungs depends on the terminal velocity and diffusion coefficient of the individual particles. The overall deposition pattern is most conveniently illustrated by diagrams of the type shown in Fig. 2, which refers to spherical aerosols with a specific gravity of 1 (i.e. equal to that of water). Most airborne dust in industry is of irregular shape however and may be aggregated into loose clumps. The behaviour of such dusts again depends entirely on the mobility of the individual particles and not on their apparent microscopic size. A

clump of coal dust may thus appear to be some 15 microns in diameter.
If its structure is very loose, however, it may only sediment with the
same speed as a 7-micron diameter sphere and, when inhaled into the
lung, it will be deposited in the same manner as a 7-micron diameter
sphere. The behaviour of a particle of this type is most easily described
by stating the size of sphere of unit density which has the same terminal
velocity and which will thus have an identical intrapulmonary deposition pattern. The diameter of the equivalent unit density sphere
(E.U.D.S.) of the 15-micron diameter coal dust particle mentioned
above is thus 7 micron.

It follows that microscopic sizing should not be used to estimate the
respirable fraction of an industrial dust. The terminal velocity of
individual particles cannot be determined outside the laboratory but it
is possible to design instruments which collect dust samples as a function
of the falling speed of each separate particle. These methods are
described in Chapter 9.

The Pattern of Breathing

The amount of dust inhaled each minute by a miner is determined by
the volume of air breathed during that time (the minute ventilation) and
by the ambient concentration of airborne particles. The minute ventilation of different miners while working underground was measured by
Hadden, Jones and Morgan (1965) and wide variations were noted. It
seems highly likely that consistent differences of this type will be
associated with different individual susceptibilities to the development
of pneumoconiosis. These may be related to the individual occupations
of the miners since some tasks demand much more physical effort than
others. They may also be related to differences in the volume of air
breathed by each man while performing the same task.

The pattern of breathing itself may affect the fraction of inhaled
particles which is deposited and the site of its deposition. Slow deep
breathing is associated with a greater overall deposition of dust within
the alveoli than rapid shallow breathing even though the total minute
ventilation may be identical in the two cases. This is because a greater
fraction of each breath penetrates to the alveoli and also because the
available time for sedimentation to take place is increased.

Nasal versus Mouth Breathing

Early calculations appear to have underestimated the true efficiency of
dust deposition in the nose. There is now increasing experimental
evidence (Wolfsdorf, Swift and Avery, 1969; Hounam, Black and
Walsh, 1971) that it is in fact a highly effective filter. Proctor and Swift
(1971) have pointed out that particles which escape deposition in the
nose are likely to escape deposition in the conducting airways altogether
and to be carried right through to the alveolus. A change from the

normal nasal manner of breathing to mouth breathing might thus increase the alveolar dust load and most certainly does increase the mass of particles depositing on the ciliated epithelium. Heavy exercise is normally accompanied by mouth, rather than nose breathing and the change occurs at a lower level of exercise in subjects who have nasal obstruction or who are breathless because of disease of the lungs.

Individual Variation in the Deposition of Inhaled Aerosols

Lehmann (1935) was the first to consider individual variations in the filtration efficiency of the airways as a causative factor in pneumoconiosis. He was unable to find such evidence from experimental work on the nasal filtration of particles. Altshuler *et al.* (1957) showed clear differences between the fractional deposition of inhaled particles in three normal subjects during mouth breathing. The rate of deposition appeared to be related to the amount of mixing of air in the lung and was evident when aerosols of various sizes were used. Love *et al.* (1971) carried out a detailed investigation of this problem. The fractional deposition of one micron diameter particles in the lungs was measured in eighteen coal workers with Category II simple pneumoconiosis and in forty control subjects whose chest X-rays were normal. The two groups were carefully matched for age and occupational history. The deposition characteristics of the two groups were compared after standardizing for the tidal volume and frequency of breathing. No significant differences were found. It was concluded that individual variations in the deposition pattern were unlikely to be an important factor in causing the development of simple pneumoconiosis in coal-workers and that the disease, at this stage, was not associated with an increased deposition pattern. This latter finding is important because Jacobsen, Rae, Walton and Rogan (1971) have shown that the X-ray changes of simple pneumoconiosis appear to progress at a faster rate once the initial pattern has developed. More serious disturbances of lung function are known to alter the behaviour of aerosols in the lung (Lipmann and Albert, 1969; Muir, 1970) but the effect of this on the pathogenesis of pulmonary disease is not known.

Clearance of Dust from the Lung

The ciliated epithelium is covered by a layer of mucus derived from secreting cells in the wall of the airway. The mucus is cleared by the cilia towards the oesophagus and carries with it any overlying insoluble particles. The rate at which a given particle is removed is related to the site of deposition. Dust deposited near the terminal bronchiole must traverse the entire mucosa and takes longer to reach the oesophagus than particles deposited near the major bronchi and trachea. Small particles penetrate further into the lung and are, therefore, cleared more slowly than large particles. The rate of clearance by the mucosa is not in itself sensitive to the particle size nor does it depend on the number of particles deposited unless they have some specific toxic action. The rate of clearance has been extensively studied in man by means of radioactive aerosols and by using external scintillation counters. The clearance of the mucosa appears to be essentially complete in less than twenty-four hours. The great majority of all particles trapped on the mucosa during a working shift are in fact cleared within a few hours and do not accumulate during regular daily work. The ciliary lining of the nose is also cleared within hours although much of the inhaled dust is trapped on the unciliated anterior portion where it remains until blown or wiped off.

Dust penetrating to the alveolus is engulfed by the alveolar macrophages within a few hours of being deposited. Non-toxic dusts are subsequently carried by the macrophages towards the ciliated epithelium where they are excreted by the mucus escalator. The initial phagocytic response appears to be a mechanism for the protection of the alvelor epithelium since this cannot be penetrated by the particles if they are within a phagocytic cell. The rate of this clearance process has been widely studied after brief exposure of human volunteers to low concentrations of dust labelled with radioactive tracers. There is uncertainty about the amount of dust which is cleared from the lung during daily exposure in industry. If the fractional deposition values shown in Fig. 2 are correct then a coalminer working under poor conditions may receive a total alveolar dust load of something like 1000 g during a life time of work. Despite this high figure it is unusual to find more than about 40 g of dust in the lungs of miners on post mortem examination. These figures suggest that the alveolar clearance mechanism is highly efficient. An alternative explanation is to suppose that the alveolar clearance is less efficient but that the initial rate of particle desposition within the alveolus is much lower than has previously been thought (Davies, 1967). There is certainly much experimental work to support the suggestion that alveolar clearance of dust following chronic exposure is a relatively slow process (Stöber, Einbrodt and Klosterkötter, 1967; Klosterkötter and Bünemann, 1961; Le Bouffant, 1961). Experimental work with animals has shown that the rate of clearance is proportional to the total amount of dust in the lungs provided that the initial burden is not too great. There is some evidence that this is also true in the case of human exposure. Dust does not appear to accumulate in the lungs of miners at a steady rate and the amount of dust in the lungs at any given time is not simply a function of the total number of days or years of exposure. Rather it tends to rise fairly rapidly during the first ten years or so and then level off or rise much more slowly (Stöber *et al.*, 1961).

These findings are based on post mortem examination of the lungs of miners and on their occupational exposure during life. Very little accurate information of long-term individual exposure is usually available and more studies of this type are required.

The rate of dust clearance is probably related to the availability of macrophages. Their number increases in response to an alveolar dust load (Brain, 1971) and the removal of the foreign matter is thus facilitated.

Individual Variations in the Clearance of Lung Dust

Le Bouffant (1961) noted wide variations in the rates of alveolar clearance in rats. Wright (1961) pointed out that these are not observed during long term exposure experiments. There is no information on variations in the clearance rate in man but this might be an important factor in determining individual susceptibility to occupational pulmonary disease. Wide variations in the rate of bronchial clearance have been found in human experiments (Lippmann and Albert, 1969) but the causes of this are not known at present.

Retention of Dust in the Lung

Some dust is always present in the lungs of city dwellers at post mortem examination.

Much greater amounts are seen in men with occupational exposure. In coal-workers the dust is found in depots round the respiratory bronchioles. These depots represent particles which are deposited in the first instance throughout the alveoli and are then transported by macrophages while still within the air space and packed into the alveoli opening off the respiratory bronchioles. These are eventually sealed off by the epithelium and are no longer in communication with the air space (Heppleston, 1961). Some dust penetrates the alveolar wall, is engulfed by macrophages and accumulates in the lymphatics and hilar lymph glands. Though it is usually contained within macrophages within lung tissue this does not imply that it penetrates the wall while within a macrophage (Schiller, 1961). Cytotoxic dusts such as quartz have a particularly marked tendency to penetrate the alveolar wall and to accumulate within the lung.

Lung dust is not a static accumulation of particles. Heppleston (1961) was able to demonstrate a progressive intermingling of particles in the lungs of rats exposed to two different non-fibrogenic dusts on different occasions separated by an interval of up to six months. This intermingling took place throughout the pulmonary dust foci and also within individual macrophages. The process is best explained by the repeated death of grossly laden cells with liberation of their dust and its subsequent ingestion by fresh generations of macrophages.

Size Distribution of Particles in Lung Dust

The first clue to our present knowledge of the behaviour of inhaled aerosols was obtained by McRae (1913) who noted that most of the particles in the lungs of miners were below one micron in diameter. The dust was very much finer than that in the inhaled air and it was correctly concluded that only fairly small particles could cause the pneumoconiosis. By comparing the size distribution of the lung dust and of the airborne dust, Davies (1964) has estimated the fractional deposition of inhaled particles. Unfortunately it is not possible to be certain of the terminal velocity of the aggregates in which most of the fine particles enter the respiratory tract. Without this information the deposition pattern of the aggregates cannot be determined. There is also evidence (Holma, 1967) that large particles are removed preferentially by the macrophage system and that the composition of the particles also determines the rate at which alveolar dust is taken up by macrophages. Holma (1967) found that carbon particles were ingested by macrophages much more avidly than polystyrene spheres of the same diameter. It is therefore highly likely that the size distribution and composition of alveolar dust changes with time and is not a reliable guide to the characteristics of the dust originally deposited in the lung.

The sensitivity of the macrophage system to the composition of the particles should also suggest some caution before it is assumed that industrial dusts are cleared from the lung at the same rate as experimental aerosols produced in the laboratory.

The Effects of Smoking and of Lung Disease

In addition to showing that there were wide individual variations in the regional deposition of inhaled aerosols, Lippmann, Albert and Peterson (1971) found that airway obstruction due to asthma or bronchitis increased the fraction of particles trapped in the larger airways. Sanchis, Dolovich, Chalmers and Newhouse (1971) also found that less aerosol was able to penetrate to the alveoli in smokers compared with non-smokers. They considered that this was due to small airway damage and was clearly not to the long term benefit of a miner despite the apparently reduced alveolar dust load. They also found that the rate of ciliary clearance was impaired in smokers although no difference was found by Thomson and Short (1969).

Although cigarette smoking may be associated with some change in the aerosol deposition pattern and in the rate of mucociliary clearance these are likely to be of minor importance in comparison with the known association with chronic bronchitis and its attendant disability.

Fibrous Dusts

The behaviour of a compact particle in the lung is determined by its aerodynamic properties.

Special consideration must be given to airborne fibres such as glass or asbestos. These may be over 100 microns in length but have a diameter of less than one micron. The settling velocity of a fibre is related to its diameter and density and not to its length. There is also a strong tendency for long fibres to be trapped, or intercepted, at the bifurcation of the smaller airways simply due to their size. A few long fibres are able to reach the alveoli because of their tendency to align themselves with the flow of air parallel to the axis of the airway. This may be more marked in the case of amphibole asbestos which is composed of straight thick fibres than in the case of chrysotile which has thin curved fibres (Timbrell and Skidmore, 1971).

Estimating the Hazard of Airborne Dust

Only certain portions of the total airborne dust in a mine can be regarded as representing a health hazard. The dust control engineer requires information from the physiologist concerning the identity of this fraction before a meaningful control programme can be instituted.

The dust which causes the pneumoconioses is the most important. A number of curves defining the probability of particles being deposited in, or having access to the alveoli have been derived. These are shown in Chapter 9 which also describes the various instruments which are used to measure the airborne dust. They are designed to accept a dust sample having the same size distribution as that of the "respirable" fraction. There is much discussion as to the preferred characteristics of such an instrument. That the samples collected in British coal mines represent a true measure of the hazard to man has now been amply confirmed by the findings of Jacobsen *et al.* (1971). Further information is required on the effect of the size distribution of the isolated particles within the respirable dust. Since there is some evidence that large particles are removed preferentially by the macrophages it may be that the small particles in the sample are particularly important in the causation of disease. Further experimental work on this point is required. A compositional factor must also be considered (see Chapter 9).

The coarser fraction of the total dust must also be measured since it may be a cause of chronic bronchitis. Much epidemiological work will be required before it is possible to indicate which fraction of the airborne cloud is of particular significance in this respect.

References

Altshuler, B., Yarmus, L., Palmes, E. D. and Nelson, N. (1957), "Aerosol deposition in the human respiratory tract." *American Medical Association Archives of Industrial Hygiene*, **15**, 293.
Beeckmans, J. M. (1965), "The deposition of aerosols in the respiratory tract." *Canadian Journal of Physiology and Pharmacology*, **43**, 157.

Brain, J. D. (1971), "The effects of inhaled particles on the numbers of alveolar macrophages." In *Inhaled Particles, III*, ed. W. H. Walton. Unwin, London.

Brown, C. E. (1931), "Quantitative measurements of the inhalation, retention and exhalation of dusts and fumes by man." *Journal of Industrial Hygiene and Toxicology*, **13**, 285.

Brown, J. H., Cook, K. M., Ney, F. G. and Hatch, T. (1950), "Influence of particle size upon the retention of particulate matter in the human lung." *American Journal of Public Health*, **40**, 450.

Dautrebande, L., Beckmann, H. and Walkenhorst, W. (1957), "Studies on deposition of submicronic dust particles in the respiratory tract." *American Medical Association Archives of Industrial Health*, **19**, 383.

Davies, C. N. (1964), "A comparison between inhaled dust and the dust recovered from human lungs." *Health Physics*, **10**, 1029.

Davies, C N. (1967), Editorial in *Inhaled Particles and Vapours, II*, p. xiii, ed. C. N. Davies. Pergamon Press, London.

Dennis, W. L. (1971), "The effects of breathing rate on the deposition of particles in the human respiratory system." In *Inhaled Particles, III*, ed. W. H. Walton. Unwin, London.

Findeisen, W. (1935), "Über das Absetzen Kleiner, in der Luft suspendierten Teilchen in der menschlichen Lunge bei der atmung." *Pflügers Archive für die gesamte Physiologie des Meschen und der Tiere*, **236**, 367.

Hadden, G. C., Jones, C. O. and Morgan, D. C. (1965), "A study of volumes of respired air in relation to dust exposures of coal miners. In *Inhaled Particles and Vapours, II*, p. 37, ed. C. N. Davies. Pergamon Press, London.

Heppleston, A. G. (1961), "Observations on the disposal of inhaled dust by means of the double exposure technique." In *Inhaled Particles and Vapours*, p. 320, ed. C. N. Davies. Pergamon Press, London.

Holma, B. (1967), "Lung clearance of mono- and di-disperse aerosols determined by profile scanning and whole-body counting." *Acta Medica Scandinavia*, Sup. No. 473.

Hounam, R. F., Black, A. and Walsh, H. (1971), "The deposition of aerosol particles in the nasopharyngeal region of the human respiratory tract." In *Inhaled Particles, III*, ed. W. H. Walton. Unwin, London.

International Commission on Radiological Protection (1966), "Deposition and retention models for internal dosimetry of the human respiratory tract." *Health Physics*, **12**, 173.

Jacobsen, M., Rae, S., Walton, W. H. and Rogan, J. M. (1971), "The relation between pneumoconiosis and dust exposure in British coal mines." In *Inhaled Particles, III*, ed. W. H. Walton. Unwin, London.

Klosterkötter, W. and Bunemann, G. (1961), "Animal experiments on the elimination of inhaled dust." In *Inhaled Particles and Vapours*, p. 327, ed. C. N. Davies. Pergamon Press, London.

Landahl, H. D. (1950), "On the removal of airborne droplets by the human respiratory tract. I. The Lung." *Bulletin of Mathematical Biophysics*, **12**, 43.

Le Bouffant, L. (1961), "Etude quantitative de l'epuration pulmonaire chez le rat; comparaison, entre poussières inertes et pousière nocives." In *Inhaled Particles and Vapours*, p. 369, ed. C. N. Davies. Pergamon Press, London.

Lehmann, G. (1935), "Dust filtering efficiency of human nose and its significance in causation of silicosis." *Journal of Industrial Hygiene*, **17**, 37.

Lippmann, M. and Albert, R. E. (1969), "The effect of particle size on the regional deposition of inhaled aerosols in the human respiratory tract." *American Industrial Hygiene Association Journal*, **30**, 257.

Lippmann, M., Albert, R. E. and Peterson, H. T. (1971), "The regional deposition of inhaled aerosols in man." In *Inhaled Particles, III*, ed. W. H. Walton. Unwin, London.

Love, R. G., Muir, D. C. F. and Sweetland, K. F. (1971), "Aerosol deposition in the lungs of coalworkers." In *Inhaled Particles, III*, ed. W. H. Walton. Unwin, London.

McRae, J. (1913), *The Ash of Silicotic Lungs.* South African Institute for Medical Research, Johannesburg.

Muir, D. C. F. and Davies, C. N. (1967), "The deposition of 0·5 micron diameter aerosols in the lungs of man." *Annals of Occupational Hygiene*, **10**, 161.

Muir, D. C. F. (1970), "The effect of airways obstruction on the single breath aerosol curve." In *Airway Dynamics*, ed. Arend Bouhuys. Charles C. Thomas, Springfield, U.S.A.

Proctor, D. F. and Swift, D. L. (1971), "The nose—a defence against the atmospheric environment." In *Inhaled Particles, III*, ed. W. H. Walton. Unwin, London.

Sanchis, J., Dolovich, M., Chalmers, R. and Newhouse, M. (1971), "Regional distribution and lung clearance mechanisms in smokers and non-smokers." In *Inhaled Particles, III*, ed. W. H. Walton. Unwin, London.

Schiller, E. (1961), "Inhalation, retention and elimination of dusts from dogs' and rats' lungs with special reference to the alveolar phagocytes and bronchial epithelium." In *Inhaled Particles and Vapours*, p. 342, ed. C. N. Davies. Pergamon Press, London.

Stober, W., Einbrodt, H. J. and Klosterkötter (1967), In *Inhaled Particles and Vapours, II*, p. 409, ed. C. N. Davies. Pergamon Press, London.

Thomson, M. L. and Short, M. D. (1969), "Mucociliary function in health, chronic obstructive airway diseases and asbestosis." *Journal of Applied Physiology*, **26**, 535.

Timbrell, V. and Skidmore, J. W. (1971), "The effect of shape on particle penetration and retention in animal lungs." In *Inhaled Particles, III*, ed. W. H. Walton. Unwin, London.

Weibel, E. R. (1963), *Morphometry of the Human Lung.* Springer, Berlin.

Wolfsdorf, J., Swift, D. L. and Avery, M. E. (1969), "Mist therapy reconsidered; an evaluation of the respiratory deposition of labelled water aerosols produced by jet and ultrasonic nebulisers." *Pediatrics*, **43**, 799.

Wright, B. M. (1961), Discussion in *Inhaled Particles and Vapours*, p. 398, ed. C. N. Davies. Pergamon Press, London.

Chapter 5

Physiological Aspects of Dust Disease

The functional effects of pneumoconiosis depend on the nature and extent of the pathological lesions. These in turn vary according to the type of inhaled dust. The effects of coalworkers' pneumoconiosis are thus very different from those found in asbestosis. On the other hand there is much variation within each type of pneumoconiosis according to the severity of the disease.

The problem is simplified by distinguishing two types of pulmonary dust disease:

(*a*) Classical Silicosis and Mixed Dust Pneumoconioses

These show a similar evolution from a micronodular stage towards one of massive fibrosis.

(*b*) Pneumoconioses such as Asbestosis

These are characterised by an initial stage of diffuse interstitial fibrosis with thickening of the interalveolar septum resulting from fibroblastic proliferation. Other types of pneumoconiosis in this group include those resulting from the inhalation of fibrous silicates such as talc, pneumoconiosis due to aluminium and hard metals, as well as acute silicosis which has occurred during the digging of tunnels and in the manufacture of abrasive materials.

The physiological tests which are of most value in the assessment of the effects of pneumoconiosis must also take account of the airway obstruction due to bronchitis and emphysema which is a common concurrent feature.

Screening Tests of Pulmonary Function in Pneumoconiosis and Obstructive Syndromes

1. Spirometry

The apparatus (spirometer) is simple and portable models are available. Its resistance should be as low as possible.

The vital capacity (VC) is obtained by asking the patient to inspire maximally and then to expire slowly and completely. The volume obtained represents the sum of the tidal volume and of the inspiratory and expiratory volumes. The forced vital capacity (FVC) is obtained by asking the patient to inspire maximally and then to exhale as rapidly and as forcefully as possible. During this manoeuvre the volume of air exhaled in a fixed interval of time can be measured by recording the movement of the spirometer on a paper chart but automatic timing devices are also available. Different expressions of the timed forced expiratory volume (FEV) are used: volume expired during the first second ($FEV_{1.0}$), volume expired in 0·75 of a second ($FEV_{0.75}$) and volume expired between 0·25 and 0·75 seconds after the beginning of expiration ($FEV_{0.25-0.75}$). The $FEV_{1.0}$ and $FEV_{0.75}$ have been found by Minette and Bruninx (1967) to be the most reproducible measurements.

All volumes are normally corrected for body temperature (37°C) and water vapour saturation at the ambient pressure (BTPS). Observed values are compared with the theoretical normal values taking account of the age and height of the subject using nomograms such as those of the European Coal and Steel Community (Jouasset, 1960).

The maximum rate of airflow during a forced exhalation is conveniently measured by means of Wright's peak flowmeter. The measurement, although closely related to the forced expiratory volume, is less reproducible. The extreme simplicity of the apparatus makes it very useful for epidemiological studies.

The vital capacity and forced expiratory volume both reflect the ventilatory capacity of the individual. Reduction in the ventilatory capacity as a result of narrowing of the lung airways, is called the obstructive syndrome and is typical of chronic bronchitis, asthma or widespread emphysema. The condition is characterised by a low value for the forced expiratory volume expressed as a percentage of the vital capacity (or of the forced vital capacity), i.e. the $FEV_{1.0}/VC$ per cent. This ratio is also known as Tiffeneau's ratio and its reduction below 70 per cent is accepted as a sign of obstructive pulmonary disease. The ratio decreases slowly with age and normal tables taking account of this decrease are available (Jouasset, 1960). The restrictive pulmonary syndrome is characterised by impairment of the ventilatory capacity due to a reduction in the vital capacity but without evidence of airway obstruction. The $FEV_{1.0}$ may be relatively normal and the Tiffeneau ratio or $FEV_{1.0}/VC$ per cent is normal or even increased. The syndrome is characteristic of conditions such as asbestosis where there is diffuse fibrosis of the alveolar tissue.

The vital capacity and forced expiratory volume may also be measured after the injection or inhalation of drugs. This is particularly useful in distinguishing the reversible bronchospasm of asthma from the fixed airway obstruction associated with bronchitis and emphysema. An increase of 10 per cent or more in the vital capacity and forced expiratory volume following the inhalation of a bronchodilator such as isoprenaline or orciprenaline is characteristic of asthma. In this condition there is also a marked fall in the vital capacity and forced expiratory volume following the inhalation of bronchoconstrictors such as acetylcholine and histamine.

2. Residual Volume and Total Lung Capacity

The residual volume (RV) is the volume of air which remains in the lungs at the end of a complete exhalation. Total lung capacity (TLC) is the sum of the residual volume and vital capacity. The residual volume is usually determined by a closed circuit method using helium as the tracer gas. The subject breathes through a spirometer circuit of constant volume for at least seven minutes to ensure that complete mixing of gas in the lungs takes place. The concentration of helium in the circuit is measured at the beginning and at the end of the test and the amount of its dilution enables the functional residual capacity (FRC) to be calculated. The residual volume is obtained by subtracting the expiratory volume from the functional residual capacity since the latter is the volume of air present in the lungs at the end of a normal expiration. The volume is normally corrected for BTPS conditions. It depends on the age and height of the subject but is less reproducible than the vital capacity and forced expiratory volumes. Theoretical normal values have been described by Jouasset (1960). An increase in the residual volume is characteristic of emphysema. The residual volume is often expressed as a percentage of the total lung capacity and this ratio is increased with emphysema. However the ratio may also be increased as a result of the reduction in the total lung capacity found in the restrictive pulmonary syndrome.

3. Ventilation, Respiratory Equivalents and Respiratory Quotient

Valuable information may be obtained by the measurement of the minute ventilation, oxygen consumption and carbon dioxide output during submaximal exercise. A number of closed circuit and open circuit methods are available. The latter are convenient, require less apparatus and enable oxygen uptake and carbon dioxide output to be measured with considerable accuracy.

The exercise may be performed either on a bicycle ergometer or on a treadmill. The standard method until recently has been to continue exercise at any given workload until the steady state condition has been established. This normally takes at least 3 minutes and measurements are made after the subject has been exercising for this period of time. Recent evidence however suggests that it may be advantageous to increase the workload in a step-wise fashion at intervals of as small as one minute. The procedure is quickly completed and does not impose the same amount of exercise on the subject as does the steady state method.

The results are usually expressed as the respiratory equivalent for oxygen which is the minute ventilation necessary for the consumption of a fixed volume of oxygen, either one litre or 1·5 litres. During submaximal exercise the minute ventilation is normally less than 30 litres for each litre of oxygen uptake.

Hyperventilation on exercise may be an index of pulmonary disease. It is particulary evident when there is diffuse alveolar disease but without airway obstruction, as in asbestosis or fibrosing alveolitis. It is also commonly noted in subjects with poor general physical fitness.

The respiratory quotient (R) is the ratio between the carbon dioxide output and the oxygen uptake each minute. During sub-maximal exercise a value greater than 1 indicates that the exercise is poorly tolerated, generally due to limitation of the cardiovascular system or of muscle metabolism. Hyperventilation due to emotional stress is not uncommon and is also associated with a respiratory quotient greater than unity.

4. Blood Gases at Rest and During Exercise

The oxygen and carbon dioxide content of the arterial blood are readily measured although arterial blood samples can normally only be taken in a fully equipped laboratory. The development of reliable electrodes has led to the wide-spread measurement of gas tensions. The measurement of the partial pressure (i.e. tension) of oxygen is also a more sensitive test of arterial blood oxygenation because of the S shaped dissociation curve of haemoglobin (Cotes, 1968).

The oxygen saturation of the arterial blood is normally greater than 95 per cent at rest and during exercise. The oxygen tension decreases with age but is normally about 90 mm Hg at the age of 40 (Raine and Bishop, 1963; Melemgaard, 1966). The partial pressure of carbon dioxide in the arterial blood normally varies between 36 and 47 mm Hg and does not exceed 47 mm Hg on exercise. The normal values of the arterial gases depend on the altitude at which the measurements are made since the partial pressure of oxygen in the inspired air falls with increasing altitude. Mining operations are carried out at high altitudes in some countries and low values for the arterial oxygen tensions are found in these situations. Compensatory hyperventilation may also cause a reduction in the arterial carbon dioxide tension.

Complex changes in the blood gas tensions may be found at rest and on exercise in association with different types of pulmonary disorder The uniformity of the blood flow and ventilation in each part of the lung (ventilation/perfusion ratio) is the dominant mechanism determining the degree and type of abnormality. In the early stages of classical silicosis and mixed dust pneumoconiosis only a minimal reduction in the arterial oxygen tension is present. When the disease has progressed to the stage of massive shadows there may be severe anoxia and hypercapnia. When diffuse interstitial fibrosis of the type associated with asbestosis is present the carbon dioxide tension in the arterial blood is normal or low but oxyhaemoglobin desaturation is an important early sign and there is often further desaturation on exercise. It may be evident on clinical examination and the degree of desaturation on exercise may be readily measured by ear oximetry.

5. Pulmonary Diffusing Capacity

Measurement of the oxygen transport capacity of the lungs is technically difficult and it is usually assessed by indirect methods using carbon monoxide. The test measures the transfer of molecules of carbon monoxide across the alveolar capillary membrane and their combination with haemoglobin in the pulmonary capillaries. It depends on the size and thickness of the alveolar membrane and on the effective area of the pulmonary capillaries which are in contact with ventilated alveoli. It is thus sensitive to the ventilation perfusion ratio in each region of the lung. For this reason Cotes has proposed that it should be called a measure of carbon monoxide transfer (TL_{CO}) rather than of diffusing capacity (DL_{CO}).

Two main techniques are available for the measurement of carbon monoxide transfer, the steady state and the single breath method. The steady state method requires little co-operation on the part of the subject but is particularly sensitive to inequalities of ventilation/perfusion ratios and probably gives a poor indication of the diffusing capacity of the alveolar membrane. Some methods of carrying out the steady state technique require arterial blood samples. Normal values for the steady state DL_{CO} are given by Dechoux, Pivoteau and Aubertin (1969). Their results are based on 200 normal male subjects in whom the DL_{CO} (ml of CO absorbed per minute per mm Hg difference between the partial pressure of CO in the alveoli and in the capillaries, i.e. ml per mm Hg) was found to be 16·75 (H) –0·17 (Y) –2·36 (± 4), where H is the height of the subject in metres and Y the age in years.

The single breath measurement of DL_{CO} is less influenced by abnormalities of the ventilation perfusion ratios and is a more specific test of the diffusing capacity of the alveolar capillary membrane. During the test the subject inhales a gas mixture containing a low concentration of carbon monoxide and of helium, holds his breath for approximately 10 seconds and then exhales. Each test takes approximately 10 to 15 minutes and no arterial puncture is necessary. Semi-automatic apparatus is now available which is particularly suitable for field survey work and the measurements can be carried out on a large scale without the necessity of maintaining a full research laboratory. Normal values for males are given by Cotes (1968) as DL_{CO} (ml per min per mm Hg) equals 30·4 (H) –0·28(A) –11·7 where H is the height of the subject in metres and A is age in years. In interpreting the results the total lung volume must also be taken into account since a low value for the DL_{CO} is not necessarily abnormal if it is associated with a low value for the total lung volume.

6. Other Tests

More complex tests of pulmonary function described below, are available for use in research laboratories. Further experience will be necessary before their place in the assessment of pneumoconiosis is established. It is convenient to divide these into tests of the mechanical properties of the lung, of pulmonary gas mixing and of pulmonary blood flow.

(*a*) Mechanics of Breathing

The airway resistance (expressed as centimetres of water per litre of air flow per minute) may be measured by means of a body plethysmograph. It is a major factor in determining the maximum rate of airflow that can be achieved by a subject during a forced exhalation and is closely related to spirometric airflow measurements, particularly the timed forced expiratory volume (Gary, Fessler and Ulmer, 1967). There are wide individual variations however, and maximal rates of airflow may be influenced by various additional factors such as pulmonary tissue compliance, chest wall elasticity and muscular expiratory forces (Pelzer and Thomson, 1969). The airway resistance is a sensitive test of airway obstruction and changes may be detected before there are abnormal clinical signs (Nolte and Ulmer, 1967) or before the $FEV_{1.0}$ is significantly reduced.

The compliance or distensibility of the lungs (expressed as millilitres per centimetre of water) may be represented by the change in intrathoracic volume per unit change in intrathoracic pressure. It is measured by means of an oesophageal catheter and balloon. The pressure change detected by the balloon is divided by the corresponding changes in the intrathoracic volume measured at the mouth with a spirometer as the subject inhales or exhales. A striking decrease in compliance may be found in asbestosis (Leathart, 1960) and in rare cases of acute silicosis (Buhlmann and Schuppli, 1960). Conflicting results in silicosis and coalworkers' pneumoconiosis have been reported by Muysers, Siehoff, Worth, Gasthaus and Smidt (1966) and Teculescu, Stanescu and Pilat (1967).

(*b*) Pulmonary Gas Mixing

A number of different methods are available for the investigation of the uniformity of gas distribution in the lungs during breathing. Both single breath and open circuit methods are available using various tracer gases such as helium, nitrogen and argon. Although abnormalities may be detected at an early stage in pneumoconiosis they may also be due to concurrent bronchitis and are sensitive to the smoking habits of the individual. There is a poor correlation between the unevenness of gas mixing and the extent of the pulmonary disease in pneumoconiosis and it is an unsatisfactory screening test for this condition.

(c) Pulmonary Haemodynamics

The pulmonary arterial pressure can be measured during right heart catheterisation. Investigations of this type can only be carried out in a fully equipped clinical research laboratory.

Summary of Functional Changes in Different Types of Pneumoconiosis Silicosis and Mixed Dust Pneumoconiosis

It is not always easy to distinguish functional changes from those due to chronic bronchitis with which they may be associated. In the early micronodular and nodular stages bronchitis may or may not be present while at the stage of massive shadows bronchitic and emphysematous changes are more common. In this discussion reference will be made to the International Radiological Classification of the ILO (Geneva, 1958) see Chapter 10.

(1) Micronodular and nodular stages

Conflicting spirometric results have been reported by different authors. Some have found a reduction in vital capacity at an early stage with a further decrease as the radiological shadows extend. Other workers have found no impairment of the vital capacity in simple pneumoconiosis. Gilson and Hugh-Jones (1955) found only small differences in vital capacity and ventilatory function in Welsh coalminers with Category 3 pneumoconiosis and those whose X-rays were normal, whatever the age range. However, their vital capacity measurements were below those of normal subjects who had not worked underground. This could be interpreted as indicating a wide-spread incidence of chronic bronchitis among the miners or that the mining population was a selected group who were unrepresentative of the general population.

Sartorelli and Magistretti (1958) did find a reduction in the vital capacity of their subjects who had silicosis. Those with nodular silicosis showed vital capacity values falling between those of subjects of micro-nodular pneumoconiosis and those with massive fibrosis. Brasseur (1963) compared 120 symptomless coalworkers aged between 35 and 45 years with 22 normal surface mineworkers. A moderate but statistically significant decrease in the vital capacity from Category 3 (p, m and n) onwards was found. At this stage the vital capacity measurements averaged only 87·7 per cent of the predicted normal values of Jouasset (1960).

As with the vital capacity measurements there are conflicting results on the timed forced expiratory volumes. Futher difficulties in interpretation arise because of different methods of carrying out the tests.

Part of the variability in these conflicting results is probably due to the method of selecting the subjects. Carpenter, Cochrane, Gilson and Higgins (1956) tried to allow for this difficulty by examining a random sample of miners who were still at work and others who were no longer working. There was no significant difference in the forced expiratory volumes of men with micronodular Category 3 pneumoconiosis and miners whose X-rays were normal. However, there was a significant reduction in these workers compared with non-mining subjects of the same age. As with vital capacity measurements the results could indicate a degree of bronchial irritation caused by smoke or dust underground or the fact that the mining population is a selected group within the general community.

A further difficulty in interpretation is the fact that self selection into dusty occupations underground must be common within the mining population itself.

In another study Cochrane and Higgins (1961) collected earlier data on miners and non-miners from various areas in Wales and England and found no obvious relationship between the extent of the X-ray opacities and the decrease in $FEV_{1.0}$ in simple pneumoconiosis. On the other hand, Lavenne, Brasseur, Oelbrandt and Belayew (1961), in a small group of miners aged between 35 and 45 years who were still at work underground, observed a significant decrease in the ratio $FEV_{1.0}/$ predicted $FEV_{1.0}$ at Category 3 simple pneumoconiosis.

A large scale British study of 9,758 subjects selected from eight different collieries showed a decrease in the $FEV_{1.0}$ from Category 3 simple pneumoconiosis onwards. Though the reduction in the $FEV_{1.0}$ was proportional to the extent of the X-ray opacities it was of little significance when compared with the progressive reduction in the $FEV_{1.0}$ due to age alone (Rogan, Ashford, Chapman, Duffield, Fay and Rae, 1961).

Brasseur (1963) examined 120 symptomless underground workers who had been exposed to dust at the coalface for at least 10 years. From Category 3 simple pneumoconiosis onwards he found a statistically significant reduction in the mean $FEV_{1.0}$. At this stage the $FEV_{1.0}$ averaged 81·4 per cent of the predicted normal value as against 91·3 per cent at Category 1 ($P < 0.05$). For a given category of pneumoconiosis Foubert, Nadiras and Batique (1954) as well as Sartorelli and Magistretti (1958) found a more frequent reduction in the timed forced expiratory volume in nodular than in micronodular pneumoconiosis.

In simple pneumoconiosis there is little or no change in the residual volume or in the total lung capacity.

On average the respiratory equivalent for oxygen is increased from Category 2 onwards but it is insufficient to be significant in any individual case (Brasseur, 1963). The arterial carbon dioxide is normal both at rest and on exercise but the arterial oxygen tension at rest is significantly lower from Category 2 (Brasseur, 1963) and even earlier onwards (Worth, Gasthaus, Muysers and Siehoff, 1961; Frans and Brasseur, 1970). In addition, from Category 2, the arterial oxygen tension does not return to normal during exercise as is the case in mild abnormalities of the ventilation/perfusion ratios. Among coal miners aged 35 to 45, still at work and having Category 3 pneumoconiosis, Brasseur found a mean arterial oxygen tension of 81·8 mm Hg during exercise at 120 watts whereas the value for surface workers of the same age was 93·8 mm Hg. Muysers, Siehoff, Worth and Gasthaus (1962) as well as Brasseur (1963) found a lower arterial oxygen tension in the pinhead forms than in the micronodular and nodular forms.

The steady state DL_{CO} is usually lower if there is associated obstructive airway syndrome (Dechoux, Pivoteau and Aubertin, 1969). Using the single breath method Billiet (1965) found only small reductions of DL_{CO}. The reductions were closely correlated with the total pulmonary capacity and were insufficient to account for any arterial desaturation. Exceptions to this rule were noted in cases with definite evidence of chronic bronchitis. For a given category of simple pneumoconiosis, Englert (1967) and Lyons, Clark, Hall and Cotes (1967) noticed a greater reduction in the DL_{CO} in the pinhead forms of the disease than in the micronodular and nodular types. Frans and Brasseur (1970) studying coalminers still at work, found occasional cases with a frankly pathological DL_{CO}, the correlation between the DL_{CO} and the arterial oxygen tension during exercise being better than previously believed.

The pulmonary artery pressure is significantly increased from Category 1 to Category 3. However, in the absence of obstructive airway disease, the increase is only occasionally important enough to be considered significant in an individual case (Kremer, 1969).

2. Pseudotumoral stage (progressive massive fibrosis)

The vital capacity and $FEV_{1.0}$ are characteristically abnormal. Associated bronchitis is accompanied by a reduction in the ratio $FEV_{1.0}/VC$ (Gilson and Hugh-Jones, 1955; Dechoux, 1956; Brasseur, 1963). The residual volume is increased but does not attain the values observed in cases of obstructive airway disease; the total lung volume is slightly reduced (Gilson and Hugh-Jones, 1955). Hyperventilation during exercise is, on average, slightly more marked than at the micronodular stage (Brasseur, 1963). The arterial oxygen tension, already reduced at rest, decreases further during exercise, initially without an increase in arterial carbon dioxide tension. Hypercapnia is only seen at the later stages of the disease (B and C) when there is severe impairment of the ventilatory capacity (Brasseur, 1963).

With both the steady state and single breath methods the DL_{CO} is more severely lowered than in the micronodular stage of the disease. This is chiefly due to imbalance in the ventilation perfusion ratios throughout the lung and the DL_{CO} is usually less reduced than in cases of diffuse interstitial fibrosis. In pseudotumoral pneumoconiosis it is unusual to find a fall in the arterial oxygen saturation during exercise despite hyperventilation sufficient to cause a reduction in the arterial carbon dioxide tension. The latter functional syndrome, found in pulmonary diffuse interstitial fibrosis, appears to be characteristic of alveolar capillary block (Lavenne, Meersseman and Brasseur, 1965). This term originally implied that the abnormality in gas transfer was caused by an inability of the molecules to diffuse across a thickened alveolar membrane. It is now recognised however, that part of the abnormality is caused by severe ventilation/perfusion inequalities and it is difficult to evaluate the role of diffusion impairment alone.

Even with minimal reduction of the spirometric values, pulmonary hypertension during exercise is common. At the stage where the arterial carbon dioxide levels are elevated pulmonary hypertension is present even at rest and carries a poor prognosis (Kremer, 1969).

Pulmonary Function in Asbestosis and Related Disorders

The functional findings in asbestosis are also found in talcosis (although usually to a minor degree), in pneumoconiosis due to aluminium and hard metals (cobalt, titanium, tungsten) and in chronic berylliosis. These conditions are all associated with thickening of the alveolar wall.

The vital capacity, initially well maintained (Bader, Bader, and Selikoff, 1957, 1961) may be greatly reduced in advanced cases. However, the FEV_1/VC ratio may remain normal and the ventilatory capacity may be preserved until a late stage (Austrian, McClement, Renzetti, Donald, Riley and Cournand, 1951). The residual volume, normal in the early stages (Wright, 1955; Bader, Bader and Selikoff, 1961) may be slighty increased as the disease advances (Bastenier, Denolin, De Coster, Cammaerts and Denolin-Reubens, 1952; Bader *et al.*, 1957, 1961; Wright, 1955). While breathlessness during exercise is due to a reduced ventilatory capacity in conditions such as silicosis, breathlessness in asbestosis is associated with a true hyperventilation on exercise.

In mild cases the arterial oxygen saturation and tension may be normal at rest. During exercise desaturation of the arterial blood may occur but without the development of hypercapnia (Williams and Hugh-Jones, 1960). Arterial desaturation during exercise was found by Wright (1955) even among asbestos workers who did not show a characteristic radiological picture.

Whatever the method used, all authors have observed a fall in the DL_{co}. Williams and Hugh-Jones (1960) found that this fall could occur before the appearance of radiological abnormalities and that there was a close relationship between the DL_{co} and the radiological grade of the disease as well as with the severity of dyspnoea and the degree of finger clubbing.

There has been much discussion about the cause of this abnormality in the carbon monoxide transfer capacity of the lung and of the increase in the alveolar-arterial oxygen gradient. Although there is no doubt that the alveolar capillary membrane is thickened and reduced in area, most of the findings are probably due to severe imbalance in the ventilation/perfusion ratios already noted.

There is little haemodynamic data concerning this group of conditions but they are probably associated with pulmonary hypertension caused by reduction in the pulmonary vascular bed.

References

Austrian, R., McClement, J. H., Renzetti, A. D., Donald, K. W., Riley, R. L. and Cournand, A. (1951), "Clinical and physiologic features of some types of pulmonary diseases with impairment of alveolar-capillary diffusion. The syndrome of 'alveolar capillary block'." *American Journal of Medicine*, **11**, 667.

Bader, M. E., Bader, R. A. and Selikoff, I. J. (1957), "Pulmonary function in asbestosis of the lungs; an 'alveolar capillary block' syndrome." *Journal of Clinical Investigation*, **36**, 871.

Bader, M. E., Bader, R. A., and Selikoff, I. J. (1961), "Pulmonary function in asbestosis of the lung: an alveolar-capillary block syndrome." *American Journal of Medicine*, **30**, 235.

Bastenier, H., Denolin, H., De Coster, A., Cammaerts, Ph. and Denolin-Reubens, E. (1952), "Etude clinique et physiopathologique d'un cas d'asbestose pulmonaire." *Archives belges de médecine sociale, hygiène, médecine du travail et médecine légale*, **10**, 61.

Billiet, L. (1965), *De bepaling van de pulmonaire diffusiecapaciteit door enkelvoudige inspiratie van koolstofmonoxyde en de toepassing ervan by longtuberculose en silicose*. p. 421, Arscia, Bruxelles.

Brasseur, L. (1963), *L'exploration fontionnelle pulmonaire dans la pneumoconiose des houilleurs*. p. 343, Arscia, Bruxelles and Maloine, Paris.

Buhlmann, A. and Schuppli, M. (1960): "Atemmechanische Untersuchungen bei Silikose." *Deutsche medizinische Wochenschrift*, **85**, 1745.

Carpenter, R. G., Cochrane, A. L., Gilson, J. C. and Higgins, I. T. T. (1956), "The relationship between ventilatory capacity and simple pneumoconiosis in coal-workers: the effect of population selection." *British Journal of Industrial Medicine*, **13**, 166.

Cochrane, A. L. and Higgins, I. T. T. (1961), "Pulmonary ventilatory functions of coalminers in various areas in relation to the X-ray category of pneumoconiosis." *British Journal of Preventive and Social Medicine*, **15**, 1.

Cotes, J. E. (1968), *Lung Function: Assessment and Application of Medicine*. p. 227, 2nd edition. Blackwell Scientific Publications, Oxford.

Dechoux, J. (1956), "Le retentissement fonctionnel des formes dites pseudotumorales dans les pneumoconioses des mineurs des charbonnages," p. 205. *Compte-rendu des Journées Françaises de Pathologie Minière*. Charbonnages de France, Paris.

Dechoux, J., Pivoteau, C. and Aubertin, X. (1969), "Analyse des troubles fonctionnels des pneumoconiotiques par la spirographie et le transfert du CO en régime stable et en inspiration unique." *Bulletin de Physio-pathologie respiratoire*, **5**, 179.

Englert, M. (1967), *Le réseau capillaire pulmonaire chez l'homme: Etude Physiopathologique*, p. 253, Masson, Paris.

Foubert, P., Nadiras, P. and Batique, L. (1954), "La spirographie au repos dans la silicose: Sa valeur et ses limites." *Revue médicale minière*, **25**, 3.

Frans, A. and Brasseur, L. (1970), "Capacité de diffusion par le CO, mesurée par la méthode en apnée chez des sujets normaux et chez des houilleurs pneumoconiotiques." Symposium Physiopathologie et clinique des affections respiratoires chroniques, Wiesbaden, 2–4 juin. *Communauté Européenne du Charbon et de l'Acier* (Luxembourg) (in press).

Gary, K., Fessler, Ch. and Ulmer, W. T. (1967), "Intrapleurale Druckschwankungen bei der Messung des 1—Sekundenwertes und beikörperlicher Arbeit (Zur problematik des 1—Sekundenwertes)." *Beiträge zur klinik des Tuberkulose und spezifischen Tuberkulose Forschung*, **134**, 295.

Gilson, J. C. and Hugh-Jones, P. (1955), "Lung function in coalworkers' pneumoconiosis." *Medical Research Council: Special Report Series*. No. 290, p. 266, London.

Jouasset, D. (1960), "Normalisation des épreuves fonctionnelles respiratoires dans les pays de la Communauté Européenne du Charbon et de l'Acier." *Poumon*, **16**, 1145.

Kremer, R.(1969), "Apport de l'hémodynamique pulmonaire à l'étude de la pneumoconiose des houilleurs." *Revue de l'Institut d'Hygiène des Mines*. **24**, 77. (Hasselt).

Lavenne, F., Brasseur, L., Oelbrandt, L. and Belayew, D. (1961), "Volumes pulmonaires et volume expiratoire maximum par seconde des pneumoconiotiques encore au travail." *Revue de l'Institut d'Hygiène des Mines*, **16**, 3.

Lavenne, F., Meersseman, F. and Brasseur, L. (1965), "Fibrose interstitielle diffuse et pneumoconiose des houilleurs." *Poumon*, **21**, 691.

Leathart, G. L. (1960), "Clinical, bronchographic, radiological and physiological observations in ten cases of asbestosis." *British Journal of Industrial Medicine*, **17**, 213.

Lyons, J. P., Clarke, W. G., Hall, A. M. and Cotes, J. E. (1967), "Transfer factor (diffusing capacity) for the lung in simple pneumoconiosis of coal workers." *British Medical Journal*, **4**, 772.

Mellemgaard, K. (1966), "The alveolar-arterial oxygen difference: its size and components in normal man." *Acta physiologica Scandinavica*, **67**, 10.

Minette, A. and Bruninx, M. (1967), "Etude de l'action bronchodilatatrice d'un dérivé hydroxyphényl de l'orciprénaline" (Th 1165). *Revue de l'Institut d'Hygiène des Mines*, **22**, 63.

Muysers, K., Siehoff, F., Worth, G. and Gasthaus, L. (1962), "Neuere Ergebnisse atemphysiologischer Untersuchungen von Kohlenbergarbeitern unter Berücksichtigung von Silikose, Bronchitis und Emphysem. V. Mitteilung: Endexpiratorisch-arterielle Sauerstoff und Kohlensauredruckdifferenzen in Ruhe und bei Körperbelastung." *Archiv für Gewerbepathologie und Gewerbehygiene*, **19**, 589.

Muysers, K., Siehoff, F., Worth, G., Gasthaus, L. and Smidt, U. (1966), "Neuere Ergebnisse atemphysiologischer Untersuchungen von Kohlenbergarbeitern unter Berücksichtigung von Silikose, Bronchitis und Emphysem." *Archiv für Gewerbepathologie und Gewerbehygine*, **22**, 215.

Nolte, D. and Ulmer, W. T. (1967), "Die Strömungswiderstände im normalen tracheobronchialbaum und bei obstruktiven Atemvegserkrankungen." *Beiträge zur Klinik der Tuberkulose und spezifischen Tuberkulose-Forschung*, **236**, 320.

Pelzer, A. M. and Thomson, M. L. (1969), "Body plethysmographic measurements of airway conductance in obstructive pulmonary disease." *American Review of Respiratory Diseases*, **99**, 194.

Raine, J. M. and Bishop, J. M. (1963), "A–a difference in O_2 tension and physiological dead space in normal man." *Journal of Applied Physiology*, **18**, 284.

Rogan, J. M., Ashford, J. R., Chapman, P. J., Duffield, D. P., Fay, J. W. J. and Rae, S. (1961), "Pneumoconiosis and respiratory symptoms in miners at eight collieries." *British Medical Journal*, **1**, 1337.

Sartorelli, E. and Magistretti, M. (1958), *Fisiopatologia respiratoria e cardiocircolatoria della silicosi*, p. 120, Unione tipografica, Milano.

Teculescu, D. B., Stanescu, D. C. and Pilat, L. (1967), "Pulmonary mechanics in silicosis." *Archives of Environmental Health*, **14**, 161.

Williams, R. and Hugh-Jones, P. (1960), "The significance of lung function changes in asbestosis." *Thorax*, **15**, 109.

Worth, G., Gasthaus, L., Muysers, K. and Siehoff, F. (1961), "Neuere Ergebnisse atemphysiologischer Untersuchungen von Kohlenbergarbeitern unter Berücksichtigung von Silikose, Bronchitis und Emphysem. III Mitteilung: alveolo-arterielle sauer-stoff und kohlensauredruckdifferenzen." *Archive fur Gewerbepathologie und Gewerbehygiene*, **18**, 581.
Wright, G. W. (1955), "Functional abnormalities of industrial pulmonary fibrosis." *Archives of Industrial Health*, **11**, 196.

Chapter 6

Clinical Aspects of Respiratory Disease due to Mining

Introduction

Inhaled dusts damage the lungs in two ways, (1) by a non-specific effect on the airways, common to all types of dust, and (2) by a specific action, peculiar to each type of mineral, exerted mainly on the respiratory surface and the interstitial tissues of the lung. This chapter will describe the non-specific effects of dust, and the clinical presentation, course and management of the specific disease due to the dusts commonly met with in the mining industry, viz.—coal, silica and asbestos.

Non-specific Effects of Dust

Dust inhalation tends to cause bronchospasm which can be alleviated or prevented by inhalation of a sympathomimetic drug (DuBois and Dautrebande, 1958) and which is more pronounced in those who smoke cigarettes, who are subject to allergic asthma, or have chronic obstruction of the airways. There is evidence that dust also increases the secretion of mucus (Rae, Walker and Attfield, 1971). Although these changes are usually too mild to attract attention they may occasionally present a picture resembling asthma, with wheeziness, productive cough and shortness of breath, brought on by working in a dusty atmosphere and relieved by a few hours away from work. It is probable that many years of this minor illness can cause changes in the bronchi which are indistinguishable from early stages of chronic bronchitis. Since those subjects who already have a productive cough (or smoke cigarettes) tend to show an exaggerated form of this response to dust it is indeed difficult to decide whether or not chronic bronchitis can be regarded as a result of dust exposure (Gilson, 1971). At present one must keep an open mind on this point, but the industrial medical officer should be aware of the possibility and should regard persistent complaints of shortness of breath, productive cough, or wheezing, towards the end of each shift as possible indicators of an unrecognized dust hazard—a view discussed in more detail by Gandevia and Ritchie (1966, 1968). In fact reduction of the forced expiratory volume in the course of a shift has not been demonstrable in coal miners (Duffield and Ashford, 1960) despite the development of increased airways' resistance following coal-dust inhalation in normal subjects (McDermott, 1962). On the other hand, a bronchial effect of silica has been reported (Šarić and Štritof, 1969). There are reasons for supposing that the dust particles producing this effect are outside the range commonly associated with silicosis, i.e. they are both smaller and larger in size.

Dust Disease in Coal Miners

In radiographs of coal miners (Chapter 10) two types of disease, (*a*) simple pneumoconiosis and (*b*) progressive massive fibrosis (P.M.F.) or complicated pneumoconiosis may be distinguished. These two types present contrasting clinical pictures. Simple pneumoconiosis (anthracosis) seldom causes either symptoms or signs; progressive massive fibrosis is not uncommonly associated eventually with respiratory failure and premature death.

Simple Pneumoconiosis

World-wide experience confirms what Stratton wrote in 1838: "Anthracosis may exist without any chest symptoms whatever". So nearly universal is this experience that one should beware of attributing a coal miner's symptoms to simple pneumoconiosis alone. If symptoms are present the coal miner probably has some other disease, even though the chest radiograph is typical. The same considerations apply to physical signs in the chest and probably also to abnormalities of function (see Chapter 5); if examination reveals material abnormalities these suggest that the pneumoconiosis, if present, is accompanied by some other disease, and that further investigation is needed.

Differential Diagnosis

What other diseases can masquerade as radiological pneumoconiosis or be concealed by it? The most important of these is miliary tuberculosis, especially in countries where the population has little natural immunity, and the doctor alert to this possibility is unlikely to miss it. Other fairly common conditions with a radiological picture indistinguishable from simple pneumoconiosis are sarcoidosis and extrinsic allergic alveolitis. The first of these presents particular difficulties because there are often no accompanying symptoms or signs in the chest, but gas transfer factor is diminished and help may be obtained by uncovering a history of erythema nodosum or by finding enlarged lymphatic glands and spleen, and an increase of plasma globulin, none of which occur in pneumoconiosis. Extrinsic allergic alveolitis may be encountered among miners in Britain because pigeon breeding is one of their common hobbies. It is distinguished from pneumoconiosis by the severe dyspnoea and by the finding of moist sounds (crepitations) at the lung bases, clubbing of the fingers, and specific precipitins in the serum. Less common conditions include histiocytosis X, histoplasmosis, and lymphangitis carcinomatosa. In nearly all the conditions which simulate simple pneumoconiosis, a raised erythrocyte sedimentation rate will be found, and this forms a useful and simple screening test.

Airways' Obstruction

The condition which most commonly causes respiratory symptoms in a miner with simple pneumoconiosis is chronic obstruction of the airways. This is usually due to chronic bronchitis. Its aetiology is still uncertain but a possible association with dust exposure has been shown in miners in early middle age (Rae *et al.*, 1971). Centriacinar emphysema, which often accompanies simple pneumoconiosis, produces neither symptoms nor signs, but emphysema which is sufficiently widespread to be recognized by the clinician or the radiologist (whatever its precise morphology may eventually prove to be) is associated with dyspnoea. There is no evidence that panacinar emphysema is a sequel to dust inhalation; indeed severe emphysema is most frequently found in those lungs which have retained little or no dust (Caplan, 1962).

Pinhead Pneumoconiosis

In recent years attention has been focused on pinhead pneumoconiosis —p. in the I.L.O. classification. Some patients in this group have diffuse interstitial fibrosis accompanied by considerable dyspnoea, cyanosis, clubbed fingers, and basal crepitations (Leathart, 1971a). It is not yet clear whether this represents a true manifestation of dust disease or coincidental fibrosing alveolitis, but inclusion of such patients in a group with pinhead pneumoconiosis may account for the finding of a low transfer factor in this group (Lyons, Clarke, Hall and Cotes, 1967). There is, so far, no statistical support for the suggestion of Gaensler, Hoffman and Elliott (1960), that interstitial fibrosis can be a direct result of exposure to coal dust, nor any certainty that pinhead pneumoconiosis differs from other radiological types of pneumoconiosis.

Management of Simple Pneumoconiosis

The correct management of pneumoconiosis is improved environmental hygiene (see Chapters 8 and 9) and it is assumed, in what follows, that steps will be taken to reduce the respirable dust concentration.

(1) The symptomless miner with pneumoconiosis.

Since simple pneumoconiosis generally causes no symptoms no treatment is needed, and if the miner has no symptoms from other respiratory disease he may continue to work in the same job. He should, however, be recalled for further radiography after an interval which can be as long as five years in the man with Category 1 changes, but should be about two years if the pneumoconiosis is Category 2 or 3. More frequent review is needed in the more advanced cases because of the increased risk of developing massive fibrosis. There is one exception to these generalizations: occasionally a man is seen who shows widespread simple pneumoconiosis after only a short period in the mine (up to ten years). Such a man appears to be a hyper-reactor to coal mine dust and should be advised to leave the industry.

(2) The miner with symptoms (regardless of whether he has pneumo-coniosis or not).

In practice the majority of miners who report to the doctor do so because of symptoms, often because they can no longer manage their present work. If the reason for this is irreversible obstruction of the airways, there is no effective treatment and a transfer to lighter work will be required. This is almost certain to mean a reduction of earnings and in many countries the miner can obtain financial compensation for this. It is the doctor's responsibility to assist the affected man to find lighter work, within the same industry if possible. Physiological tests can reveal the extent of the disability and thus help in deciding the type of job which is within his diminished capabilities. The doctor should also advise the affected man about any financial benefits to which he may be entitled.

Some men must be advised to leave the industry; for example the man who is too disabled to manage even the lightest of jobs within it. The same advice should be given to those men under the age of 40 years who are already unable to do productive work in the mines, and also to the rare individual who develops pneumoconiosis unduly rapidly. These two classes of men will not be able to sustain a full working life within the mines and should be advised to leave while they are still young enough to train for sedentary work.

Progressive Massive Fibrosis

Progressive Massive Fibrosis (P.M.F.) is likely to develop on a back-ground of Category 2 or 3 simple pneumoconiosis in nearly half the men so affected. It is first seen between the ages of 40 and 70, many years after first exposure to coal dust. The early stages of massive fibrosis are usually devoid of symptoms and signs, and the diagnosis is a radiological one. The first appearance of massive fibrosis (A, or ambiguous shadows) on the radiograph should, however, be taken seriously because the shadows may be due to tuberculous or fungal disease or, if unilateral, to bronchial carcinoma. It is therefore essential to undertake a full medical examination and to examine the sputum for malignant cells, fungal hyphae, and by smear and culture, for mycobacteria. If no tubercle bacilli are seen on the smear it is reasonable to allow the miner to continue at work. The chest radiograph should be repeated after one month and then at intervals of 3 or 6 months for the next year. If this is done it is sometimes possible to recognize a bronchial carcinoma at a treatable stage.

More advanced stages of P.M.F. (B and C opacities) are often, but not invariably, accompanied by signs suggesting chronic infection (increased sedimentation rate and loss of weight) and there is also increasing dyspnoea. There are, however, no abnormal signs in the chest despite the extent of the radiological abnormality. It is not until contracture of the diseased lung occurs, late in the disease, that the dyspnoea becomes disabling, and at this time there may be signs of tracheal or mediastinal displacement, inequality of breath-sounds due to bronchial distortion and stenosis (Worth, 1960), or virtual absence of breath-sounds at the bases when compensatory emphysema develops there. The percussion note remains resonant throughout, and only rarely do the breath-sounds become bronchial in type at the site of the fibrosis. The stethoscope gives the doctor very little information in this condition and the progress is recorded in serial radiographs.

One complication of P.M.F., cavitation of a fibrosed mass, gives rise to the only pathognomonic symptom of coal workers' pneumoconiosis —the production of large volumes of inky-black sputum (melanoptysis). This occurs when the necrotic centre of a fibrotic mass breaks into a bronchus, usually as the result of infection. Melanoptysis, therefore, is usually preceded by a day or two of respiratory infection and often by a minor haemoptysis indicating rupture of the bronchial wall. The volume of black sputum (often several hundred millilitres) greatly exceeds the volume of the cavity that appears, presumably because the necrotic material is a powerful secretory agent. This complication is more alarming than serious and the melanoptysis usually stops in a day or two. A fluid level often appears in the "mass" at this time and occasionally the opening into the bronchus becomes valvular so that a fibrotic mass becomes converted, in the course of a few days, into a large lung cyst. Usually the cavity closes after a few weeks leaving a smaller mass of fibrous tissue in the same position as the original P.M.F. (Fig. 1). The classical signs of cavitation are only present when there is free communication with a bronchus.

Massive fibrosis is not invariably progressive but in most cases it advances slowly over the course of five to fifteen years. As this is a disease of the elderly miner death from other causes often cuts short the progress of the condition. When it is allowed to evolve to the end, the gradual attrition of the alveolar surface of the lung and of the pulmonary blood vessels, together with the whittling away of the ventilatory ability by bronchial distortion and stenosis eventually lead to death from cardiac or respiratory failure.

Caplan's Syndrome

The classical syndrome of Caplan (1953) carries much the same prognosis as P.M.F. and follows a similar clinical course; but radio-logical progression is sometimes rapid. It is frequently devoid of

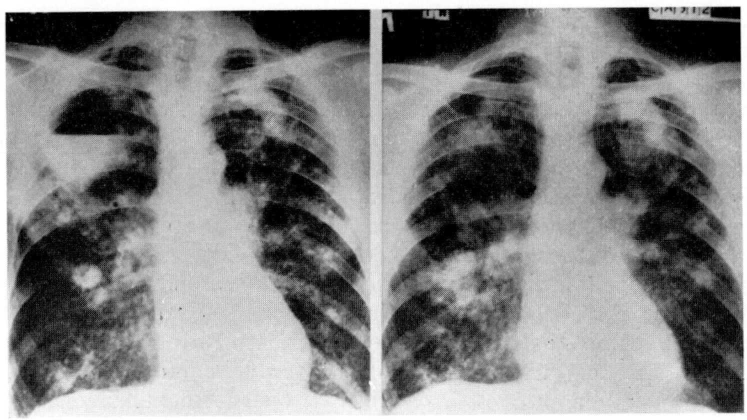

FIG. 1. Cavitation of P.M.F. and subsequent recovery.
Left, February, 1954.   Right, March, 1955.

respiratory symptoms and it is the accompanying arthritis which limits
the employability of the patient. Severe respiratory symptoms in cases
with more diffuse disease (Caplan, Payne and Withey, 1962) suggest
the possibility of cryptogenic fibrosing alveolitis, which has an association with rheumatoid arthritis (Walker and Wright, 1968) but probably
no causal connection with dust exposure. Treatment of a small group
of cases with penicillamine was not beneficial (Wagner, 1971).

Management of P.M.F.
There is no effective treatment for P.M.F. Chemotherapy with anti-
tuberculosis drugs does more harm than good if combined with rest in
bed (Ball, Berry, Clarke, Gilson and Thomas, 1969) and has no effect
if given to out-patients, either in the short term, or after prolonged
observation (McCallum, 1961 and 1971).

Although massive fibrosis may progress without further exposure to
dust it has been shown that progression occurs less frequently if the
miner is transferred to light work underground, or better still, on the
surface (Cochrane, Carpenter, Clarke, Jonathan and Moore, 1956).
Age, however, has the greatest influence on progression (Cochrane,
Moore and Thomas, 1961), which is less of a problem in the elderly
but is sometimes disastrously rapid in miners who develop the condition
under the age of 45. It should, therefore, be our aim to resettle the
miner under 45 in light work on the surface. The older miner with
P.M.F. may continue to work underground if social and economic
circumstances prevent his obtaining light work on the surface, and the
nearer he is to retiring age the less need there is to worry about his
continued exposure to coal dust. Most miners with the later stages of

P.M.F. will accept lighter work because most of them suffer from dyspnoea. Early cases (ambiguous shadows) may feel that a change to lighter work would cause undue financial hardship and may be unwilling to make this change. If they are over the age of 55 years it is reasonable to allow such men to continue in their present work, but between the ages of 40 and 55 each case must be considered on his merits. It is not justifiable to deny a man his ability to earn his living on the grounds that his disease may progress if he continues at work. When radiological progression occurs, then is the time to insist on a change of work.

Resettlement in another job is not the end of the doctor's responsibility. Whether they continue to work in the mines or not, men with P.M.F. should be subject to radiological review every two years at the most, and specimens of sputum should be examined for tubercle bacilli. A rather high incidence of tuberculosis has been reported among the older men with P.M.F., and they may be a source of infection in the community.

Medical treatment of tuberculosis in the presence of pneumoconiosis is usually satisfactory (Fig. 2), the disease being regarded as quiescent in 84 per cent of patients after one year (Medical Research Council/ Miners' Chest Diseases Treatment Centre, 1963 and 1967) but treatment with para-amino salicylate (sodium P.A.S.) and isoniazid must be continued for two years, if relapses are to be avoided. These drugs should be accompanied by daily streptomycin (1 g) for the first three months.

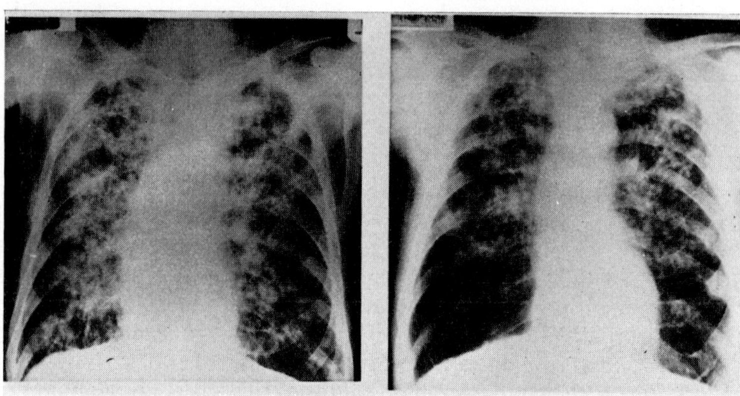

FIG. 2. (Kindly supplied by Dr. R. Y. Keers). Treatment of tuberculosis in a coal miner with P.M.F.

Left, 10 January 1970. Right, 15 March 1971.

These results are not as good as can be expected in tuberculosis without pneumoconiosis. The chest radiograph improves in all patients with simple pneumoconiosis but in only two thirds of those with

P.M.F. (Rolland Ramsay and Pines, 1959). Closure of cavities, however, is rare in P.M.F. and this is particularly true of cases infected by opportunist (anonymous) mycobacteria (Kamat, Rossiter and Gilson, 1961). These organisms are not sensitive to the standard therapeutic agents and surgical removal of the cavitated lesion may be required. On the other hand, if medical treatment achieves a negative sputum, there is no justification for surgical intervention because this may aggravate the pneumoconiosis in as many as 25 per cent of patients (Inoue, Ohta, Ohna, Shimono and Yoshida, 1964).

Once the sputum has become negative to culture for at least six months the patient may return to work in the mines, provided he has sufficient reserve of lung function. In practice, few of these men wish to return to work underground. Treatment, of course, must continue for at least two years.

Severe P.M.F., like other forms of bronchial obstruction, is subject to episodes of secondary infection in which the sputum becomes purulent. These should be treated with a broad-spectrum antibiotic (e.g. oxytetracycline 250 mg 4 times daily) and there is much to be said for continuous therapy, at low dosage, throughout the winter months. Unfortunately, there is no treatment for the fibrosis and although portable oxygen may relieve the dyspnoea of the respiratory cripple, it also shortens his life (Cotes, 1960).

Silicosis

The following account of silicosis is based on experience during the last twenty years and differs markedly from the classical descriptions of silicosis among the knife grinders of Sheffield over 100 years ago. There are probably two reasons for this: dust exposure is now much less intense than it was in the closed workshops of the last century, and tuberculosis is no longer a widespread disease in the community. The occasional patient whose disease pursues a rapid downhill course tends to be regarded as an exceptional hyper-reactor. But in isolated communities where industrial hygiene is inadequate, tuberculosis is common, and radiological facilities are not readily available. Silicosis may still present (as it did in the manufacture of abrasive powders in 1930) as a rapidly advancing massive fibrosis, or "galloping silicosis".

However, this is no longer so in Britain, the United States of America, South Africa or Australia. In these countries silicosis is not common in metal mines, being present, for example, in only 3–4 per cent of working American miners (U.S. Public Health Service Publication, 1963). The clinical presentation and course of the disease are remarkably similar to the mixed dust pneumoconiosis seen in coal miners, possibly because metalliferous mine dust is seldom pure free silica (the silica content varies from 2 per cent to 95 per cent in the U.S.A.). The disease exists in simple and complicated forms, both of which may be devoid of symptoms or signs, but it is generally felt that dyspnoea is rather more marked in Category 3 simple silicosis than in Category 3 pneumoconiosis of coal miners (Posner, 1971). Functional tests support this view for they have demonstrated mild airways' obstruction and loss of transfer factor related to increasing category of simple silicosis (Sartorelli and Scotti, 1962; Nissardi, Sanna-Randaccio, Torazza and Casciu, 1965). In addition to this, however, chronic bronchitis is frequently present, especially in gold miners. McNulty (1968) found evidence of bronchitis almost three times as often in gold miners (i.e. in 27 per cent) as in coal-miners (11 per cent) working in the same area of Western Australia. The bronchitis is related to the combined effects of increasing age, working underground, and the smoking of cigarettes but silicosis itself contributes little to loss of function unless massive fibrosis is present (U.S. Public Health Service Publication, 1963). Similar experience has been reported from South Africa (Sluis-Cremer, Walters and Sichel, 1967).

As with pneumoconiosis of coal workers the diagnosis is a radiological one and there are no abnormal signs in simple silicosis. There are the same difficulties in differential diagnosis, which have been discussed in the preceding section. Progressive massive fibrosis is accompanied by loss of weight and a raised sedimentation rate but severe symptoms and abnormal signs do not appear unless contracture of the lesions leads to bronchial distortion and basal emphysema.

The management of silicosis is similar to the management of coal pneumoconiosis which has already been discussed. The young man who is a hyper-reactor to silica should leave the industry. The older and skilled men should be allowed to continue to work to the limits imposed by their dyspnoea. Treatment of silicosis with polyvinyl-pyridine-N-oxide (Schlipköter, 1970) is still experimental.

There are two special problems of exposure to silica; these are acute silicosis and tuberculosis. Acute silicosis, first described in 1929 (Middleton, 1929) and recently reviewed by Buechner and Ansari (1969), causes alveolar exudation and death within four years of first exposure. The alveolar exudation in this condition is of great interest because of the experimental production of alveolar proteinosis (described in Chapter 2) by silica inhalation in rats (Heppleston 1967; Corrin and King, 1970), but it has not been described in miners.

Fulminating tuberculosis is traditionally associated with silicosis but there is no convincing evidence that tuberculosis behaves in an abnormal way in silicotics (Meiklejohn, 1949); it appears, on the other hand, that tuberculous infection probably potentiates the progression of P.M.F. (certainly in animals). The initial response to medical treatment of tuberculosis in silicotics, whether accompanied by massive fibrosis or not, is satisfactory; sputum conversion was attained within five months of starting treatment with streptomycin (1 g daily) combined with

P.A.S. and isoniazid and all cases were negative at two years (Keers, 1969), but longer term follow-up has not yet been reported.

When successful treatment of tuberculosis has been completed the patient may return to any work that is within his capabilities. Thus miners with simple silicosis may return to mining, but those with P.M.F. may need to take lighter work.

It has been suggested that silicosis pursues a more aggressive course in African natives, but those doctors who have observed the disease in Africa and in Europe (Paul, 1971; Gelfand and Moxton, 1970) state that there is no essential difference between races. Rapid radiological progression in certain races appears to be due to superadded tuberculosis, or to excessively heavy exposure (Czuraj and Szymczykiewicz, 1970).

Diseases asscoiated with Asbestos

The dangers of asbestos are greatest when it is in such a finely divided state that it can readily become airborne. Consequently it is in the factory where asbestos is processed, and in the industries which handle the processed fibre, that it exerts its greatest effect (48 per cent of insulators in New York affected—Selikoff, Churg and Hammond, 1965). Compared with this the mines, especially if open-cast, carry only a small risk of disease (7·2 per cent of miners affected—Becklake, Fournier-Massey, McDonald, Siemiatycki and Rossiter, 1970) but the mills at the minehead carry a substantial risk. It should be remembered that radiological abnormality in an asbestos miner is not necessarily due to asbestosis, but may represent silicosis.

There are six abnormalities associated with asbestos exposure, namely, pleural effusion, hyaline pleural thickening, pleural calcification, pleural and peritoneal mesothelioma, asbestosis and bronchial carcinoma.

Pleural effusion has recently been emphasized in a study of dockyard workers (Harries, 1970) but has not been reported in miners. It is usually a chance finding in radiological surveys and commonly resolves, without treatment, in a number of weeks.

Hyaline pleural thickening is found in about 30 per cent of insulation workers and has been reported in miners. It is thickening, usually bilateral, of the parietal pleura on the postero-lateral wall of the thorax and is diagnosed radiologically. It causes no symptoms or signs and has only a minor effect on lung function (Harries, 1970; Becklake *et al.*, 1970). It appears to be harmless (Leathart and Pumford, 1971).

Pleural calcification is diagnosed radiologically. Calcified plaques develop in the parietal pleura some 20 to 40 years after first exposure to asbestos. They characteristically lie, like a breast-plate, over the antero-lateral regions of the lungs and are also seen on the diaphragm and, more rarely, on the pericardium and mediastinum. Although hyaline pleural plaques can sometimes be recognized in these areas before calcification occurs (Fletcher and Edge, 1970) it is probable that this condition is not the end result of hyaline pleural thickening but is a separate entity (Anton, 1968). It is surprising to find how little this condition interferes with lung function and it produces neither symptoms nor signs. Like hyaline pleural thickening it is visible evidence of past exposure to asbestos but appears to be harmless.

Pleural mesothelioma is a malignant growth of the parietal pleura and appears between 15 and 50 years (mean 42 years) (Whitwell and Rawcliffe, 1971; Elmes, 1966) after first exposure to asbestos, and often many years after exposure has ceased. It spreads by local invasion of the pericardium, diaphragm, chest-wall or liver, and may spread all over the surface of the peritoneum. It may also but less commonly invade other organs by lymphatic or blood-borne metastasis.

This tumour is relatively common in miners of crocidolite in certain areas of South Africa, and in Australia where the mines are now closed. It has only rarely been seen in the chrysotile miners of Canada, and in the amosite mines of the Transvaal (see Chapter 3); it has not yet been reported in the anthophyllite mines of Finland (Wagner, Gilson, Berry and Timbrell, 1971). It is frequently accompanied by a blood-stained effusion, which may conceal the typical lobulated tumour, and in this instance presents as dyspnoea on exertion. Otherwise pain or tightness in the chest is the presenting symptom, and the pain may be very severe if the tumour erodes the ribs or the vertebrae. No treatment is of any value and death from cachexia is usual within two years.

Asbestosis (diffuse fibrosis of the lungs due to asbestos) is a serious condition associated with severe dyspnoea and is eventually fatal. Its onset is insidious with a dry cough and a modest loss of exercise tolerance, usually attributed by the patient to advancing age. As the disease progresses the dyspnoea becomes more marked and the cough becomes productive with mucoid sputum at first. Later, purulent sputum will occur periodically and may become permanent. The dyspnoea at this stage is crippling but respiratory failure, with carbon dioxide retention, is unusual except as a terminal event. Pain is not a common complaint, but short-lived episodes of pleural pain around the costal margins may be recalled on enquiry.

The earliest abnormal sign to develop is crepitation at the lung bases. Initially this is heard in the posterior axillary base, the crepitations being high-pitched ("dry"), heard towards the end of inspiration and intermittent—that is to say they are heard on some but not all inspirations, on some but not all days. They may be heard posteriorly when the patient is supine but not when he is erect. This sign may appear before the patient is aware of any symptoms and before the radiograph has become abnormal (Leathart, 1960). As the disease progresses the crepitations are heard throughout the whole of inspiration, become coarser in character and more widespread in distribution and may eventually fill the whole chest. Towards the end of the disease, the bubbling, musical crepitations of bronchiectasis are sometimes heard. It is only in a small proportion of cases that basal crepitations are absent.

Reduced expansion of the lungs (reflected in the curtailed vital capacity) is not easily recognized and percussion of the chest is normal. Vocal resonance and breath-sounds remain unaltered unless bronchiectasis supervenes.

Cyanosis develops late in the disease while clubbing of the finger-ends is a variable sign, developing early in about one third of patients (Elmes, 1966) but not at all in about one quarter (Williams and Hugh-Jones, 1960).

Early diagnosis of the condition depends firstly on the stethoscope, secondly on the radiograph and thirdly on tests of lung function. Function tests are relegated to third place because the earliest changes in serial observations are a diminution of transfer factor or of vital capacity. These tend to fall with age and also with the development of emphysema or obesity. It is therefore difficult to decide whether an observed loss of function is or is not due to asbestosis until confirmatory crepitations are present or radiological abnormality appears. This difficulty in the assessment of the individual case does not detract from the usefulness of physiological studies in epidemiological work (Leathart, 1968).

Management of Asbestosis

It is not yet established whether the disease can be diagnosed at a stage when progression will halt if further exposure to asbestos is avoided. Nevertheless it is prudent to avoid further exposure once the diagnosis has been made, because the effect of the dust seems to be cumulative and the greater the life-time's exposure the more rapid is the evolution of the disease (Smither, 1965). The miner with asbestosis presents a difficult problem because the disability due to his disease will inevitably make him unfit for heavy manual work. If he is young enough to train for other work, preferably sedentary, he should be advised to leave his present employment. If he is too old to be retrained or to obtain light work in another industry he should be given light work in the mine or the mill, if possible in a situation where there is no airborne asbestos. In either case he should be advised to seek compensation, and it is the doctor's responsibility to help him get settled in suitable work.

The risk of developing bronchial carcinoma is so greatly increased by smoking cigarettes (Selikoff, Hammond and Churg, 1968) that the patient with asbestosis should be persuaded to stop smoking.

There is no satisfactory treatment for asbestosis. Corticosteroids do not influence its progression (Leathart, 1971b; Elder, 1967) and treatment is limited to postural drainage and antibiotics in those individuals who go on to develop bronchiectasis. The outlook is poor and survival for more than 15 years from first diagnosis is unusual. About half of the cases develop bronchial carcinoma (Buchanan, 1965), usually at a time when diffuse fibrosis precludes surgical treatment, but radiotherapy or cytotoxic drugs may be used. Tuberculosis is not a common complication in Britain but there is no reason to suppose that chemotherapy will not be successful.

Conclusion

Each of these three pneumoconioses sets a somewhat similar clinical problem in that there is no effective cure and very little that can be done to delay or alter their progress once they have passed the early stages. There is, however, encouraging evidence that suppression of dust can both delay the onset of disease and reduce its incidence. Control of these diseases demands improved environmental hygiene, and complete eradication should eventually be possible.

References

Anton, H. C. (1968), "Multiple pleural plaques Part II." *British Journal of Radiology*, **41**, 341.

Ball, J. D., Berry, G., Clarke, W. G., Gilson, J. C. and Thomas, J. (1969), "A controlled trial of anti-tuberculous chemotherapy in the early complicated pneumoconiosis of coalworkers." *Thorax*, **24**, 399.

Becklake, Margaret R., Fournier-Massey, Giselle, McDonald, J. C., Siemiatycki, J. and Rossiter, C. E. (1970), "Lung function in relation to chest radiographic changes in Quebec asbestos workers. I. Methods, results and conclusions". *Bulletin Physio-Pathologie Respiratoire*, **6**, 637.

Buchanan, W. D. (1965), "Asbestosis and primary intrathoracic neoplasms." *Annals of the New York Academy of Sciences*, **132**, 507.

Buechner, H. A. and Ansari, A. (1969), "Acute silico-proteinosis. A new pathologic variant of acute silicosis in sandblasters, characterized by histologic features resembling alveolar proteinosis." *Diseases of the Chest*, **55**, 274.

Caplan, A. (1953), "Certain unusual radiological appearances in the chest of coal-miners suffering from rheumatoid arthritis." *Thorax*, **8**, 29.

Caplan, A. (1962), "Correlation of radiological category with lung pathology in coal-workers' pneumoconiosis." *British Journal of Industrial Medicine*, **19**, 171.

Caplan, A., Payne, R. B. and Withey, J. L. (1962), "A broader concept of Caplan's syndrome related to rheumatoid factors." *Thorax*, **17**, 205.

Cochrane, A. L., Carpenter, R. G., Clarke, W. G., Jonathan, G. and Moore, F. (1956), "Factors influencing the radiological progression rate of progressive massive fibrosis." *British Journal of Industrial Medicine*, **13**, 177.

Cochrane, A. L., Moore, F. and Thomas, J. (1961), "The radiographic progression of progressive massive fibrosis." *Tubercle*, **42**, 72.

Corrin, B. and King, E. (1970), "Pathogenesis of experimental pulmonary alveolar proteinosis." *Thorax*, **25**, 230.

Cotes, J. E. (1960), "Respiratory function and portable oxygen therapy in chronic non-specific lung disease in relation to prognosis." *Thorax*, **15**, 244.

Czuraj, H. and Szymczykiewicz, K. (1970), "Pylica krzemowa u pracownikow zatrudinionych przy wydobywaniu i przerobce ziemi krzemionkowej." *Medycyna Pracy*, **21**, 32. (English summary *Excerpta Medica*, Section 15 (1971), **24**, 32.)

DuBois, A. B. and Dautrebande, L. (1958), "Acute effects of breathing inert dust particles and of carbachol aerosol on the mechanical characteristics of the lungs in man. Changes in response after inhaling sympathomimetic aerosols." *The Journal of Clinical Investigation*, **37**, 1746.

Duffield, D. P. and Ashford, J. R. (1960), "A study of the reproducibility of the forced vital capacity of coalworkers at two collieries in Scotland and two collieries in South Wales." *British Journal of Industrial Medicine*, **17**, 122.

Elder, Janet L. (1967), "Asbestosis in Western Australia." *The Medical Journal of Australia*, **2**, 579.

Elmes, P. C. (1966), "The epidemiology and clinical features of asbestosis and related diseases." *Postgraduate Medical Journal*, **42**, 623.

Fletcher, D. E. and Edge, J. R. (1970), "The early radiological changes in pulmonary and pleural asbestosis." *Clinical Radiology*, **21**, 355.

Gaensler, E. A., Hoffman, L. and Elliott, M. F. (1960), "Troubles de la diffusion et fibrose interstitielle dans la silicose." *Le Poumon et le coeur*, **16**, 1137.

Gandevia, B. (1968), "Asthmatic reactions to occupational inhalants." *Proceedings of the First Australian Pneumoconiosis Conference*, 1968, at Sydney University, pp. 429–438. New South Wales Joint Coal Board.

Gandevia, B. and Ritchie, B. (1966), "Relevance of symptoms and signs to ventilatory capacity changes after exposure to grain dust and phosphate rock dust." *British Journal of Industrial Medicine*, **23**, 181.

Gelfand, M. and Moxton, A. S. (1970), "Silicosis in the gold-mining in Rhodesia." *Central African Journal of Medicine*, **16**, 32.

Gilson, J. C. (1971), "Dust and chronic bronchitis." In: *Pneumoconiosis, Proceedings of the International Conference, Johannesburg*, 1969, pp. 315–321. Ed. H. A. Shapiro. Oxford University Press, Cape Town.

Harries, P. G. (1970), "A report on the effects and control of diseases associated with exposure to asbestos in Devonport Dockyard." Royal Navy Clinical Research Working Party. CRWP 1/71.

Heppleston, A. G. (1967), "Atypical reaction to inhaled silica." *Nature*, **213**, 199.

Inoue, G., Ohta, M., Ohna, Y., Shimono, K., Yoshida, M. *et al.* (1964), "End results of surgical therapy for pulmonary silico-tuberculosis with particular reference to more-than-5-year survival." *Bulletin of the Research Institute for Diseases of the Chest*, Kyushu University, **9**, 45.

Kamat, S. R., Rossiter, C. E. and Gilson, J. C. (1961), "A retrospective clinical study of pulmonary disease due to 'Anonymous Mycobacteria' in Wales." *Thorax*, **16**, 297.

Keers, R. Y. (1969), "The treatment of silicotuberculosis." In: *Health Conditions in the Ceramic Industry*, pp. 63–68. Ed. C. N. Davies. Pergamon Press, Oxford.

Leathart, G. L. (1960), "Clinical, bronchographic, radiological and physiological observations in ten cases of asbestosis." *British Journal of Industrial Medicine*, **17**, 213.

Leathart, G. L. (1968), "Pulmonary function tests in asbestos workers." *Transactions of the Society of Occupational Medicine*, **18**, 49.

Leathart, G. L. (1971a), Unpublished observations.

Leathart, G. L. (1971b), "A trial of prednisone therapy in asbestosis: a pilot study." In: *Proceedings of the Second International Conference on Biological Effects of Asbestos*, Dresden, 22–25 April, 1968.

Leathart, G. L. and Pumford, S. (1971), "The prevalence and significance of diffuse pleural thickening following occupational exposure to asbestos." In: *Proceedings of the Second International Conference on Biological Effects of Asbestos*, Dresden, 22–25 April, 1968.

Lyons, J. P., Clarke, W. G., Hall, A. M. and Cotes, J. E. (1967), "Transfer factor (diffusing capacity) for the lung in simple pneumoconiosis of coalworkers." *British Medical Journal*, **4**, 772.

McCallum, R. I. (1961), "Treatment of progressive massive fibrosis in coal miners." In: *Proceedings of the Thirteenth International Congress on Occupational Health,* New York, 1960 pp. 741–744.

McCallum R. I. (1971), To be published.

McDermott, Margery (1962), "Acute respiratory effects of the inhalation of coal-dust particles." *The Journal of Physiology,* **162,** 53P.

McNulty, J. C. (1968) "The prevalence of respiratory symptoms in Western Australian gold miners compared with coal miners." *Proceedings of the First Australian Pneumoconiosis Conference,* 1968, at Sydney University, pp. 411–427. New South Wales Joint Coal Board.

Medical Research Council/Miners' Chest Diseases Treatment Centre (1963), "Chemotherapy of pulmonary tuberculosis with pneumoconiosis. First report." *Tubercle,* **44,** 47.

Medical Research Council/Miners' Chest Diseases Treatment Centre (1967), "Chemotherapy of pulmonary tuberculosis with pneumoconiosis. Second report." *Tubercle,* **48,** 1.

Meiklejohn, A. (1949), "Silicosis in the Potteries. Some observations based on seven hundred and fifty necropsies." *British Journal of Industrial Medicine,* **6,** 230.

Middleton, E. L. (1929), "The present position of silicosis in industry in Britain." *British Medical Journal,* **2,** 485.

Nissardi, G. P., Sanna-Randaccio, F., Torrazza, P. L. and Casciu (1965), "Studio della capacita di diffusione pulmonare a riposo nei silicoti." *Lavoro Umano,* **17,** 367. (English Summary *Excerpta Medica* Section 15 (1966), **19,** 714.)

Paul, R. (1971), Personal communication.

Posner, E. (1971), Personal communication.

Rae, S., Walker, D. D. and Attfield, M. D. (1971), "Chronic bronchitis and Dust Exposure in British Coal-Miners." In Inhaled Particles, III, ed. W. H. Walton. Unwin, London.

Rolland Ramsay, J. H. and Pines, A. (1959), "Results of treatment of pneumoconiosis complicated by tuberculosis." *British Medical Journal,* **2,** 345.

Šarić, M. and Štritof, M. (1969), "Non-specific respiratory effects of dust with a high silica content." In: *Health Conditions in the Ceramic Industry,* pp. 193–200. Ed. C. N. Davies. Pergamon Press, Oxford.

Sartorelli, E. and Scotti, P. (1962), "Rapporti tra funzionalità pulmonare e tipo radiologico della silicosi." *Medicina lavoro,* **52,** 569.

Schlipköter, H-W. (1970), "Possibilities of causal prophylaxis and therapy of pneumoconiosis." *Archives of Environmental Health,* **21,** 181.

Selikoff, I. J., Churg, J. and Hammond, E. C. (1965), "The occurrence of asbestosis among insulation workers in The United States." *Annals of The New York Academy of Sciences,* **132,** 139.

Selikoff, I. J., Hammond, E. C. and Churg, J. (1968), "Asbestos exposure, smoking and neoplasia." *Journal of the American Medical Association,* **204,** 106.

Sluis-Cremer, G. K., Walters, L. G. and Sichel, H. S. (1967), "Chronic bronchitis in miners and non-miners: an epidemiological survey of a community in the gold-mining area in the Transvaal." *British Journal of Industrial Medicine,* **24,** 1.

Smither, W. J. (1965), "Secular changes in asbestosis in an asbestos factory." *Annals of The New York Academy of Sciences,* **132,** 166.

Stratton, T. (1838), "Case of anthracosis or black infiltration of the whole lungs." *The Edinburgh Medical and Surgical Journal,* **49,** 490.

U.S. Public Health Service (1963), "Silicosis in the metal mining industry. A revaluation 1958–1961." *U.S. Public Health Service Publication No. 1076.* Washington.

Wagner, J. C. (1971), "Complicated coalworkers' pneumoconiosis." In: *Pneumoconiosis, Proceedings of the International Conference, Johannesburg,* 1969, pp. 306–308. Ed. H. A. Shapiro, Oxford University Press, Cape Town.

Wagner, J. C., Gilson, J. C., Berry, G. and Timbrell, V. (1971), "Epidemiology of asbestos cancers." *British Medical Bulletin*, **27**, 71.
Walker, W. C. and Wright, V. (1968), "Pulmonary lesions and rheumatoid arthritis." *Medicine*, **47**, 501.
Whitwell, F. and Rawcliffe, Rachael M. (1971), "Diffuse malignant pleural mesothelioma and asbestos exposure." *Thorax*, **26**, 6.
Williams, R. and Hugh-Jones, P. (1960), "The significance of lung function changes in asbestosis." *Thorax*, **15**, 109.
Worth, G. (1960), "The bronchi in silicosis." In: *Proceedings of the Pneumoconiosis Conference held at the University of Witwatersrand, Johannesburg*, February, 1959, pp. 187–192. Ed. A. J. Orenstein, J. and A Churchill, London, 1960.

Chapter 7

Hazards of Mining Uranium, Some Rarer Ores and the Use of Vibrating Tools

Uranium Mining

Essentially, uranium mining is no different from other forms of hard rock mining. Ore may be extracted by typical deep mining (Fig. 1), a small operation to extract high-grade ore (Fig. 2), or the open pit method (Fig. 3). In deep mining in the Canadian Precambrian shield, for example, once the ore body has been identified a shaft is sunk in the vicinity of the ore veins, and crosscuts are driven horizontally to the veins at various levels, usually every 100 to 150 metres. Similar tunnels, known as drifts, are driven along the ore veins from the crosscut. To win the ore, the next step is to drive tunnels, known as raises, up the deposit from level to level. These raises are subsequently used to develop the stopes where the ore is mined in the veins. The stope, which has been described as the workshop of a mine, is the excavation from which the ore is being extracted. Two methods of stope mining are commonly used. In the "cut-and-fill" method the space remaining following the removal of the ore after blasting is filled with waste rock or, sometimes, with tailings from the mill which contain the radium originally present in the ore. The "shrinkage" method involves the removal of just sufficient broken ore via the chutes below to allow the miners to work from the top of the pile to drill and blast for the next layer to be broken off; eventually a large hole is left.

Drilling the holes for blasting in crosscut or drift mining is usually done with a light-weight, fast "Jack-leg" drill (Fig. 4). This is hand-guided, but supported by the single Jack-leg. In some larger operations automatic machines capable of drilling several holes simultaneously may be used. In raises and stopes the stope drill is used for drilling upwards; the Jack-leg may also be used for horizontal drilling in stopes.

The ore from the stopes is moved in cars, pulled by an electric or diesel locomotive, to the ore pass which leads to the jaw crusher at the bottom of the mine; from there it is hoisted to the mill at the surface. As natural ventilation is never adequate for uranium mining, fans are used to deliver air through rigid or flexible tubing to all areas of the mine. Ventilation air is conserved by bratticing (isolating) inactive areas of the mine. In a large mine fans are capable of delivering several hundred cubic metres of air per second.

A small high-grade operation is usually worked by two or three

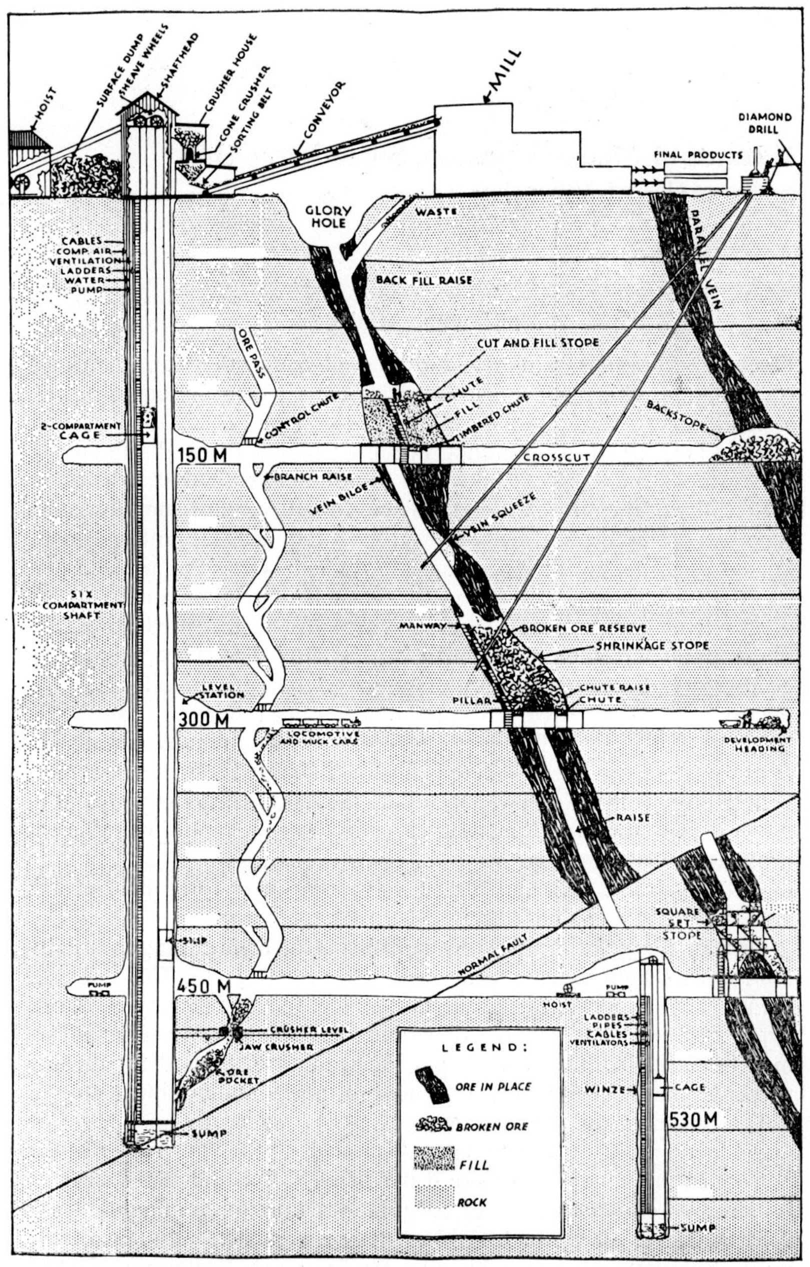

FIG. 1. Sketch of idealized section through the workings of a typical small hard rock mine. The drifts are not shown; these are in the opposite plane, being driven along the ore veins from the crosscuts. (Reproduced from *Mining Explained*, with permission, Northern Miner Press Limited, Toronto, Canada.)

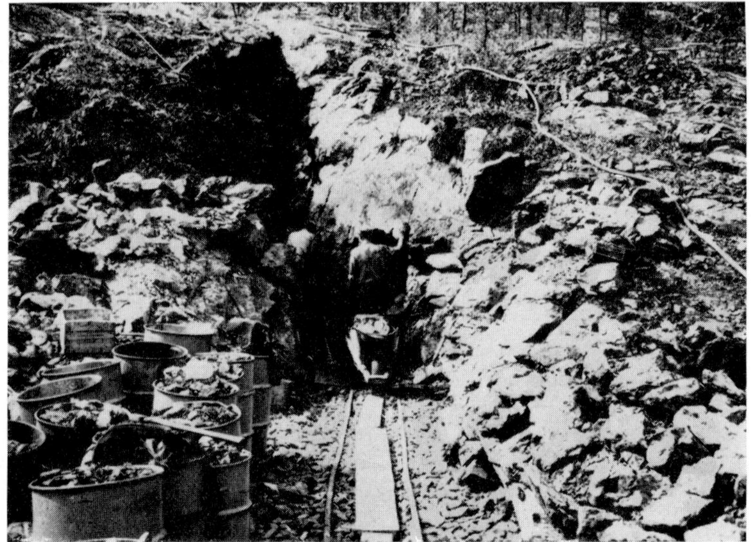

FIG. 2. High-grade uranium mining in northern Saskatchewan. This is a surface operation, but, if necessary, a short drift would be driven into the hillside to follow the ore body.

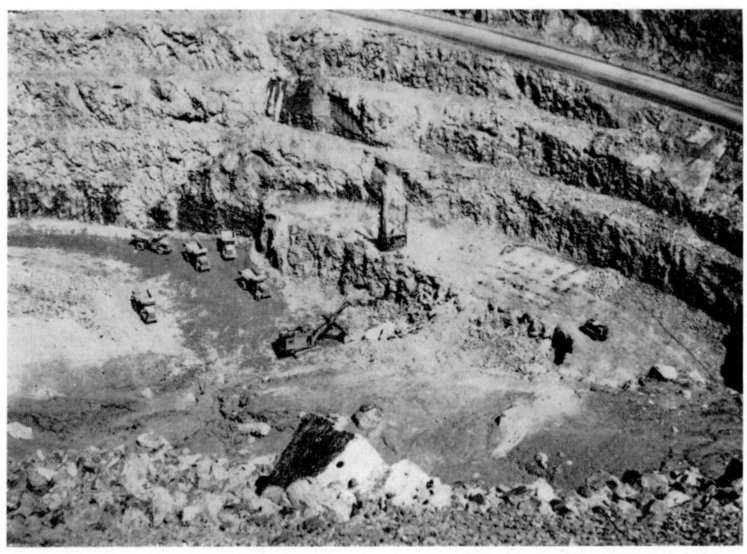

FIG. 3. Open pit uranium mining in northern Saskatchewan.

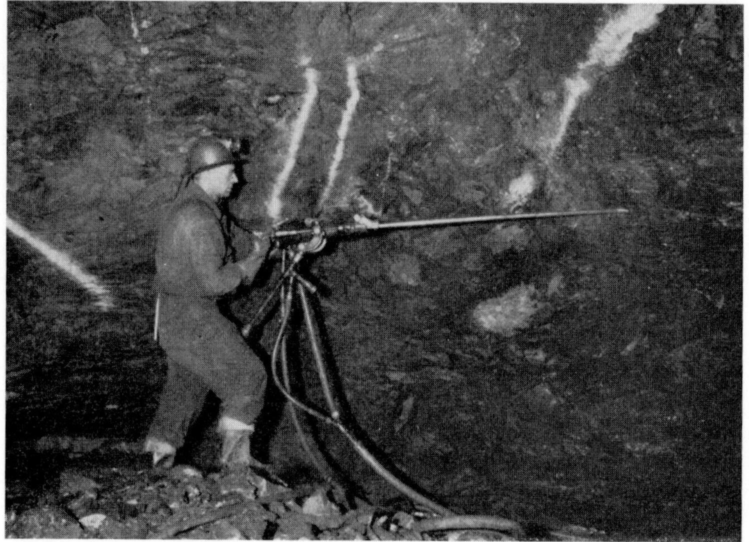

Fig. 4. Uranium miner using a Jack-leg drill.

miners working independently. The ore, which is on the surface or a limited distance below it, is rich (5 per cent or more), but present in quantities insufficient to be mined economically by a large company. The ore can generally be mined from the surface, but sometimes a short drift is developed into a hillside. The miners sell their high-grade ore to a local uranium mill where it is mixed with lower grade ore.

The Radiation Hazard

Although deliberate mining for radioactive ores, first for radium, and more recently for uranium, has been going on for only 70 years, miners must have been exposed for centuries to air in the mines with higher than normal background levels of radioactivity. Lorenz (1944) cited old chronicles which make it apparent that the metal miners of Schneeberg and Joachimsthal (Jáchymov), situated in the Ore Mountains dividing Saxony and Bohemia, were aware as early as the 16th century that many of the miners died of a respiratory disorder "Bergkrankheit", or mountain sickness. The symptoms were cough, chest pain and shortness of breath. It is probable that it represented more than one disease, and included lung cancer, silicosis and silico-tuberculosis. Lung cancer was first diagnosed as an occupational disease of the Schneeberg miners by Harting and Hess (1879). They found that 75 per cent of the deaths of the miners were due to lung cancer, generally occurring after 20 years' work in the mines. Unaware of radioactivity, which was not discovered until nearly 20 years later, they attributed the lung cancer hazard to the arsenic which was present in the ore. They mistakenly made a histological diagnosis of lymphosarcoma. The tumours were later recognized to be epithelial in origin, squamous cell carcinomas (Arnstein, 1913; Rostoski, Saupe and Schmorl, 1926). A similar situation was not apparent at Joachimsthal until Lowy (1929) and Sikl (1930) reported their investigations. Sikl found that 8 out of 15 miners and pensioners coming to autopsy had squamous cell or small cell carcinoma of the lung.

Ludwig and Lorenser (1924) were the first to suggest that airborne radon in the Schneeberg mines might be responsible for the high lung cancer death rates. This view was supported by Sikl (1930). However, in a critical review of the hazard at Schneeberg and Joachimsthal, Lorenz (1944) expressed the opinion that radon was not the sole cause of lung cancer in the miners; he listed pneumoconiosis, chronic respiratory disease, arsenic and hereditary susceptibility as other contributing factors.

Uranium ores generally contain less than 0·5 per cent of uranium; occasionally pockets of ore with 5 per cent, or even more, are found. The most abundant isotope is uranium 238, which decays through a series of solid elements to radium 226, which has a half life of 1,620 years and decays to the gas radon 222 with a half life of 3·82 days. The decay chain of radon 222 to stable lead 206, ignoring the parallel branches which account for only a fraction of 1 per cent of the decay, is shown in Table 1. It will be noted that in addition to radon 222, three of the radon daughters, polonium 218, polonium 214 and polonium 210 are alpha emitters.

Table 1

Decay characteristics of members of the uranium series important in uranium mining

Isotope	*Historical name*	*Half life*	*Radiation*
Radium 226	Radium	1,620 years	$\alpha\ \gamma$
Radon 222	Radon	3·82 days	α
Polonium 218	Radium A	3·05 minutes	α
Lead 214	Radium B	26·8 minutes	$\beta\ \gamma$
Bismuth 214	Radium C	19·7 minutes	$\beta\ \gamma$
Polonium 214	Radium C′	164×10^{-6} seconds	α
Lead 210	Radium D	22·0 years	$\beta\ \gamma$
Bismuth 210	Radium E	5·0 days	β
Polonium 210	Radium F	138·4 days	α
Lead 206	Radium G	Stable	Stable

The radon gas diffuses from the surface of the uranium bearing rock into the mine air, but perhaps more important in some situations, such as the Newfoundland fluorspar mines, is the release of this gas from solution in ground water flowing into a mine (de Villiers and Windish, 1964).

8

Uranium 235 comprises less than 0·7 per cent of the mass of natural uranium. It decays through radon 219, with a half life of 3·92 seconds, which will therefore not diffuse from the ore in sufficient quantities for its daughters to make a significant contribution to airborne radioactivity in the mines.

In still air radon 222 will be in equilibrium* with its short-lived daughters in 3 hours, but in working areas of mines equilibrium is not reached except with polonium 218, the first daughter produced. The polonium 218 atom formed by the decay of radon 222 and the other radon daughters exist as free ions in air for less than a minute. Chamberlain and Dyson (1956) have shown that they quickly become attached to moisture or dust particles which may be inhaled and retained in the lungs.

It can be calculated that the major radiation dose to the lungs, where the radon daughters are deposited, is derived from the alpha particles emitted by polonium 218 and polonium 214, and to a lesser extent by the alpha particles from radon 222. Alpha particles have a very short range. This is the reason why external alpha radiation of the skin is of no consequence; the particles do not penetrate through the superficial layers of the epidermis to the basal layer where a biological effect could be exerted. The range, in tissue, of the alpha particle produced by radon and its daughters has been reported by Lea (1955) (Table 2). The heavy

Table 2

Range of radon and radon daughter alpha particles in tissue
(after Lea, 1955)

Nuclide	Energy (MeV)	Range in tissue (Microns)
Radon 222	5·49	41·1
Polonium 218	6·00	47·0
Polonium 214	7·68	70·8
Polonium 210	5·30	38·9

[MeV—million electron volt.]

alpha particle (the nucleus of the helium atom, consisting of 2 protons and 2 neutrons) causes dense ionization along its path; this is particularly intense when the energy is reduced to less than 2 MeV* towards the end of its track—the Bragg effect. This has special significance because the energies of alpha particles are such that they will have been reduced to 2 MeV by passage through mucus and cilia by the time they reach the basal cells of the bronchial epithelium. Thus the nucleus of the basal cell is likely to be subjected to damage by ionization, and current evidence leads to the assumption that such damage can result

* See Appendix.

in malignancy. Although the main target of alpha particles is considered to be the bronchial epithelium, other lung tissues could be similarly affected by emissions from radon and, more important, its daughters deposited elsewhere in the lung.

For the practical control of radiation levels in mines the United States Public Health Service (USPHS) has adopted the concept of the Working Level (WL), which is defined as any combination of radon daughters in 1 litre of air which will result in the ultimate emission of $1 \cdot 3 \times 10^5$ MeV of potential alpha energy. This is equivalent to the alpha energy released by the total decay of the short-lived radon daughters at radioactive equilibrium with 100 picocuries* (pCi) of radon 222 per litre of air. In its epidemiological studies the USPHS has used the Working Level Month (WLM) to express total exposure of miners. One WLM is equivalent to the exposure to 1 WL for 1 month of 170 working hours.

Many of the isotopes of the uranium series decay with the emission of gamma-rays. In the U.S.A. where the average $U_3 O_8$ content of processed ore is $0 \cdot 23$ per cent (Federal Radiation Council, 1967a), it has been estimated that the external gamma radiation intensities to which miners are exposed seldom reach $2 \cdot 5$ mR† per hour, and that the average intensities are only a fraction of this (Federal Radiation Council, 1967b). The maximum permissible dose recommended by the International Commission on Radiological Protection (1966a) for occupational exposure is an average of 5 rems* per year for the whole body. Such a dose might be received by a miner exposed to $2 \cdot 5$ mR per hour for a working year, an unlikely event even in high-grade mining (Fig. 2) or stope mining in consistently rich ore. The ordinary radiation film badge worn by a miner will enable his gamma exposure to be measured. In Saskatchewan uranium mines, film badge surveys indicated exposure rarely exceeding 20 mR per week, and routine monitoring was therefore discontinued.

A considerable body of knowledge is now available to support a cause and effect relationship between exposure to radon and radon daughters, and an increased risk of developing lung cancer. Based on admittedly incomplete data, it has been calculated that the miners at Schneeberg and Joachimsthal had a lung cancer mortality twenty times expected, associated with an estimated exposure of 30–150 WL (Federal Radiation Council, 1967c).

Starting in 1950 the USPHS initiated an epidemiological and environmental study at the uranium mines in the western mountain states (Colorado, Utah, Arizona and New Mexico). In the early years of this study measurements of airborne radioactivity were infrequent in the mines; in some, where no surveys had been undertaken, exposures were

* See Appendix.
† See Appendix.

estimated by reference to surveyed mines with similar ore bodies and ventilation. The most recent report of the lung cancer mortality of the uranium miners, up to 1967, was published by Lundin, Lloyd, Smith, Archer and Holaday (1969). Of the 3,414 white uranium miners, 62 had died of malignant respiratory neoplasm. If they had had the mortality experience of white males of similar age in these western states, only 10 deaths would have been expected from this cause. Most of the deaths occurred 10 years after mining uranium; there was no excess mortality in the first 5 years. They were able to demonstrate a clear relationship between exposure to airborne radiation, expressed in WLM, and lung cancer deaths. With exposures from 840 to 1,799 cumulative working level months (CWLM) there was a marked progressive lung cancer risk. Below 840 CWLM there were 25 deaths against 7·2 expected. But most important was the observation that there was an excess of deaths, 10 observed against 2·4 expected, most unlikely to be due to chance, among miners with 120 to 359 CWLM. This could be interpreted as a fourfold risk for miners exposed to 1 working level for 10 to 30 years. The synergistic effect of cigarette smoke was clearly demonstrated. Smoking uranium miners experienced an excess of lung cancer 10 times greater than non-smoking miners. There was some suggestion that the non-smoking miner was subject to an increased risk—2 lung cancer deaths were reported compared with 0·5 expected.

Saccomanno, Archer, Auerbach, Kuschner, Saunders and Klein (in press) have studied the pathological material from 150 uranium miners with lung cancer. At high radiation exposures (greater than 1,500 CWLM), over 50 per cent of carcinomas in uranium miners were small anaplastic, World Health Organization 2B cell type, compared with 8 per cent in the controls. The ratio of small cell undifferentiated types to epidermoid cell types increased rapidly with exposure up to 2,000 CWLM, after which the ratio remained relatively constant. They thought that previous hard rock mining, with some exposure to airborne radiation, was a factor in the rather short period between first mining uranium and the development of the small cell undifferentiated carcinomas in men under 55 years of age. Only 1 of these 150 uranium miners was not a cigarette smoker, whereas 32 per cent of all miners did not smoke cigarettes (Saccomanno, 1970). The conclusion that cigarette smoking and inhaled radon daughters act as synergistic carcinogens can hardly be avoided. Other studies among the Newfoundland fluorspar miners (Report of Royal Commission, 1969a), and the Joachimsthal uranium miners (Horacek, 1969), confirm the higher incidence of small cell undifferentiated carcinomas in airborne radiation induced tumours.

There is therefore convincing evidence to support a cause and effect relationship between airborne radiation and the incidence of lung cancer. The role of ionizing radiation is further supported by the unusually high proportion of small undifferentiated cell type carcinomas in exposed workers.

Other Biological Effects of Airborne Radiation

There are grounds to suspect that there may be pulmonary effects other than lung cancer associated with the retention of airborne radio-activity. Uranium miners have been shown to have a decrement in various parameters of pulmonary function which corresponds with the estimated cumulative exposure to airborne radiation, and is greater than that which would be expected on the basis of age and smoking history. Archer, Brinton and Wagoner (1964) made the puzzling observation that exposure to high radon levels resulted in a transient improvement in pulmonary function. Trapp, Renzetti, Kobayashi, Mitchell and Bigler (1970) stated that their pulmonary function studies of the miners were indicative of a widespread pathological process, probably fibrotic in nature, and suggested that alpha radiation enhanced the fibrotic effect of silica.

When radon is inhaled it is quickly dispersed throughout the body, with a predeliction for fatty tissue. It has been a matter of conjecture what effect, if any, radon and its daughters have on various organs and body systems. Study of the blood picture in uranium miners, for example, has shown minor variations, but still within normal values (Vich and Kriklava, 1970). Single cases of other disorders have been reported, but there is no evidence to substantiate their relationship to airborne radiation exposure. Epidemiological studies of the USPHS have not, so far, indicated that uranium miners have an increased disease mortality experience other than for lung cancer and possibly neoplasms of the gastrointestinal tract.

A Safe Exposure to Airborne Radiation

There is insufficient data available to arrive at an accurate figure for a "safe" exposure. Moreover, in view of the current assumption for protection purposes that there is no threshold for radiation effects (International Commission on Radiological Protection, 1966b), one is left with the problem of selecting a level of exposure which will not subject a miner to an unreasonable hazard. The difficulty is compounded if consideration is given to the synergistic effects of other exposures—cigarette smoking, and other potentially hazardous substances in mine air. Holaday, Rushing, Coleman, Woolrich, Kusnetz and Bale (1957a) suggested a working level of $1\cdot3 \times 10^5$ MeV of potential alpha energy per litre of air for radon daughter products, polonium 218, lead 214 and bismuth 214 (i.e. 1 WL), this being based on theoretical calculations, animal studies and human exposure. This has been the standard applicable to the control of exposure to radon 222 and its short-lived daughters in the U.S.A., Canada, Australia, Spain and the U.S.S.R.

(Tompkins, 1968). However, in the U.S.A. an advisory committee, after reviewing all available data, came to the conclusion that there was a statistically significant increase in the lung cancer risk for miners with approximately 100 to 400 CWLM exposure (Federal Radiation Council, 1968). [In consequence, the U.S. Department of Labor made a regulation reducing the permitted WL by a factor of 3, allowing a maximum of 4 WLM exposure in 1 year and 2 WLM in any 3 month period. This would permit a miner to work for 25 years without being subjected to a significantly increased lung cancer risk. Evans (1969) is of the opinion that a "practical threshold" exists in distinction to the biological threshold. He feels that a cumulative life-time exposure of 300–400 WLM would carry only a negligible risk of developing lung cancer from radiation.

In Newfoundland, the current regulations for underground mines are a little more strict. No miner is permitted to receive an exposure of more than 1·8 WLM in any consecutive 3 month period, and no more than 3·6 WLM in any consecutive 12 month period.

It has been demonstrated that it is possible in the Newfoundland fluorspar mines to comply with these strict standards. The average concentration during a 6 month period in 1968 was 0·325 WL, giving an annual exposure of 3·90 WLM; prior to the introduction of mechanical ventilation in the mines, the average level was 32·5 WL with a range of 193 to 1 WL (Report of Royal Commission, 1969b).

Control of the Radiation Hazard

While the potential hazard in a uranium mine is now obvious, the possibility of a similar situation in other types of mines may be overlooked. It is therefore recommended that periodic radon or radon daughter determinations be made in all mines. The frequency will depend on the geological features in the vicinity of the mine, and previously measured levels of airborne radioactivity.

The methods of measuring radon and radon daughters in mine atmospheres have been described by Holaday *et al.* (1957b). Because the radiation dose to the lung is derived mainly from the short-lived radon daughters, it is logical to measure these. Figure 5 shows the equipment used for sampling air for radon daughters in many Canadian mines. A known volume of air is drawn through a molecular filter by a battery operated pump for a period of 5 or 20 minutes. The time of collection is noted, and after an interval of about 1 hour (range 40 to 90 minutes) the filters are placed in a portable alpha scintillation counter, and the number of disintegrations per minute read from the meter. A correction has to be made in calculating the radiation level in the sampled air if the reading is not made exactly 1 hour after collection.

The field method for radon measurement involves the use of an evacuated portable chamber coated on the inside with zinc phosphide.

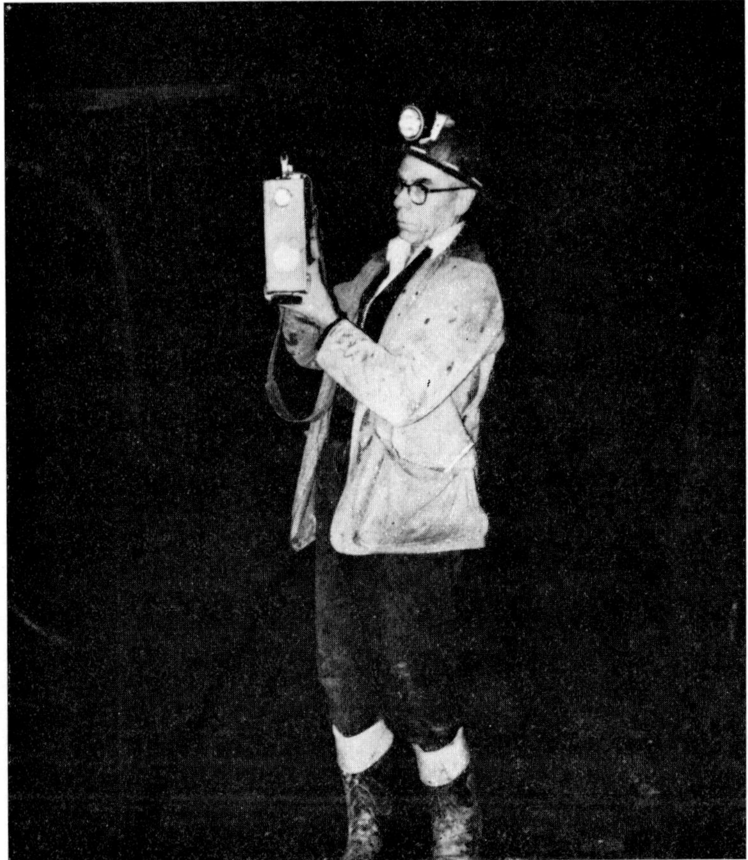

FIG. 5. Sampling mine air for radon daughters using battery operated
pump and molecular filter.

Samples of mine air are collected in these chambers which are then taken
to the surface where, after equilibrium is reached, the scintillations are
counted using a standard photomultiplier tube and scaler combination.
This method has also been used to measure airborne radioactivity in
coal mines where an electric motor driven pump would be unsafe
(Duggan, Howell and Soilleux, 1968).

Determination of airborne radiation levels by means of what are
essentially grab samples is useful for routine surveys and evaluating the
efficiency of control measures, but they may not reflect the exposure of
individual miners. A film badge, comparable to those carried by X-ray
and gamma-ray exposed workers, would be the ideal, and considerable
progress has been made in the development of a small, rugged and

inexpensive badge which will integrate alpha particle exposure over long periods of time (Geiger, 1967; Rock, Lovett and Nelson, 1969; Lovett, 1969). The routine determination of polonium 210 and lead 210 in urine and blood samples of miners to estimate cumulative exposure appears promising (Holaday *et al.*, 1957c; Blanchard, Archer and Saccomanno, 1969).

Engineering Control

Once a potentially hazardous level of airborne radiation has been found in a mine, the responsibility for reducing the levels in working areas of the mine to an acceptable figure rests with mine engineers. Some, or all of the following methods may be applicable:

1. If a significant source is identified as radon dissolved in ground water seeping into the mine, steps should be taken to prevent it flowing through the mine. If possible, it should be collected near its source and pumped to the surface; it must not be used for mining machines or wetting down in the mine.

2. Seal or brattice all unused mine areas which are a source of radon.

3. Plan mine ventilation in advance of the development of the ore bodies. Fresh air must be brought to working areas by means of fans and portable ducts. This is particularly important after blasting ore in view of the observations of Vuchot, Berger, Duhamel, Pradel, Billard and Granier (1963) that levels of airborne radiation were up to 50 times greater immediately after blasting and 5 times greater after an interval of 15 minutes. The economics of uranium mine ventilation in American uranium mines is discussed by the Federal Radiation Council (1967d). At three mines it was calculated that total costs over a 6-year period to reduce the average WL to 1·5 was $1,012,000 compared with an estimated cost of $178,000 if they had followed normal ventilation practices for hard rock mines.

4. A slight increase in barometric pressure in uranium mines will reduce the diffusion of radon from rock and water (Schroeder, Evans and Kraner, 1966; Pohl-Ruling and Pohl, 1969). It has been suggested that an increased pressure in working areas combined with a reduced pressure in an adjoining unused part of the mine would induce a flow of radon away from the work spaces. The effectiveness of this method of control remains to be proved in an operating mine.

5. Avoid having miners work regularly in areas where airborne radiation levels are consistently high, and which are difficult to ventilate adequately. There should be a rotation of miners through high level areas in order to achieve time weighted average exposures within legal limits.

6. Respirators are available which will reduce considerably the level of inhaled radon daughters. In fact, the Federal Radiation Council (1967e) states that the ordinary surgeon's mask would give a 2 to 5 fold

reduction. The practical value of a respirator as a means of protection will be doubted by many industrial physicians when it is known that hard rock miners spend many hours each day performing physically arduous labour without immediate supervision. A dust respirator will not give protection against radon exposure.

Medical Supervision

All miners should be under regular medical surveillance. In situations where miners of uranium, or any other ores, are exposed to airborne radiation levels resulting in more than 2 WLM exposure per year the following special medical supervision programme should be instituted:

1. Men should not be accepted for employment who have evidence of chronic respiratory disease at pre-employment medical examination.

2. If possible, at the time of employment, an estimate should be made and recorded of the previous exposure to ionizing radiation in mining or other work.

3. Each miner should have an annual chest X-ray for the first 5 years of mining, thereafter twice yearly.

4. In an attempt to improve the present poor prognosis for lung cancer by earlier diagnosis, the miners' sputum should be examined cytologically every 6 months for the first 5 years of mining, thereafter every 3 months. Saccomanno, Saunders, Ellis, Archer, Wood and Beckler (1963) have described the procedure for collecting sputum, and the preparation of the slide smears. Needless to say, the slides will have to be examined by an experienced cytologist. As more experience is gained with the interpretation of the cytological appearances it may be possible to predict with a reasonable degree of certainty those miners which are going to develop lung cancer. Saccomanno, Saunders, Archer, Auerbach, Kuschner and Beckler (1965) followed 24 uranium miners by sputum cytology for up to 8 years before they developed lung cancer. They came to the conclusion that Class II, Stage III metaplasia was the last step before malignancy, and that miners with this cytology should avoid further potential carcinogenic exposure. In uranium miners this would imply giving up smoking and stopping uranium mining.

5. In view of the greater risk among heavy cigarette smokers, the physician should give serious consideration to recommending that such individuals should not be employed. In any event, the physician should conduct an educational programme, individually and in groups, to encourage the miners to give up smoking.

6. As part of new miners' orientation, they should be told of the hazards of uranium mining and the means of preventing them. This should include the health surveillance programme, the importance of the mine ventilation system and the hazards of smoking.

7. Good medical and radiation exposure records must be kept, in such a manner that the information is readily retrievable for research

purposes. Physicians in the mining industry can contribute to knowledge of its hazards and their control.

8. In the event that a uranium miner dies from any cause, the physician should attempt to arrange for an autopsy. There may be medico-legal reasons for this, but contribution to knowledge of the airborne radiation dose/response relationship is of primary importance. Saccomanno *et al.* (in press) have shown that lead 210 content of bone can be used to estimate cumulative working level months of exposure to radon and radon daughters. It may be possible to have this radio-chemical analysis performed in the laboratory of a large uranium mine; otherwise a university or government laboratory should be contacted. The objective would be to publish findings on a series of cases, perhaps in collaboration with physicians associated with uranium mining in other areas.

Other Health Hazards

Other health hazards of uranium mining include silicosis, occupational deafness, and Raynaud's phenomenon. The free silica content of the Precambrian shield ore bearing rock in northern Saskatchewan ranges from 10 to 20 per cent. In the United States, uranium is found in sandstone, and the free silica content of the rock may be over 50 per cent. However, in a uranium mine the ventilation required to control the radiation hazard, combined with wet drilling and watering of muck and ore piles, will also control the silicosis hazard.

Noise of great intensity is produced by many machines used in hard rock mining; potash mining machines are not as noisy, but do present an occupational deafness hazard. Table 3 includes material from a

Table 3

Noise Levels of Some Underground Mining Equipment in Saskatchewan and Manitoba

Level in decibels (re 0·0002 microbar)

Machine	Overall C scale	Frequency Range (c/s)						
		20–75	75–150	150–300	300–600	600–1,200	1,200–2,400	2,400–4,800	4,800–9,600
Leyner Drill	117	99	107	111	109	110	110	105	105
Jack-leg Drill	119	115	114	112	106	106	106	103	103
2 Jack-leg Drills	126	113	117	117	116	119	119	117	114
Stoper Drill	125	115	115	119	118	115	113	113	115
Diamond Drill	111	77	82	104	100	104	107	101	96
Diamond Drill (with muffler)	110	75	70	75	92	102	104	104	103
Mucking Machine	113	98	109	100	96	101	104	105	106
Scram	110	98	103	101	102	104	98	91	89
Rock Bolting	114	110	98	106	104	108	109	106	103
Continuous Mining Machine (Potash)	107	94	104	101	96	99	98	90	79

report by Elias (1968) on the measured noise levels of machines in Saskatchewan and Manitoba hard rock mines. Prior to the introduction of hearing conservation programmes in Saskatchewan it was patently obvious that many miners in their late twenties had difficulty in following a conversation.

Uranium Milling

The hazards in the crushing area of the mill are similar to those in the mine itself—the dust may be a pneumoconiosis hazard, and the workers can be exposed to airborne radioactivity. Control is achieved by enclosure and ventilation.

Various methods are used to extract the uranium from the ore, but whichever is used the end product of the uranium mill is "yellowcake", a uranate salt (Harris, Breslin, Glauberman and Weinstein, 1959). This may be in the form of a powder or pellets. The weighing and packing of the yellowcake into drums can lead to exposure to hazardous dust levels of uranium. Although experience with human toxicity is limited, animal studies have clearly demonstrated that uranium is highly toxic. The 1969 Threshold Limit Value of the American Conference of Governmental Industrial Hygienists is $0{\cdot}2\ \mathrm{mg/m^3}$ (the same as lead). The target organ is the kidney, the tubules being damaged as a result of the uranyl ion combining with the protein of the tubular cells.

The hazard can be prevented by enclosure and exhaust ventilation of the drum filling and weighing process (Fig. 6). Unless it has been

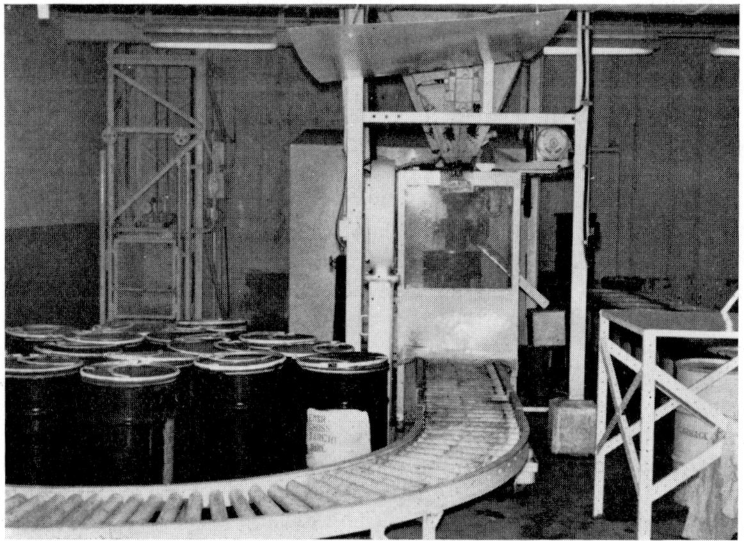

FIG. 6. Enclosure and exhaust ventilation prevent the escape of dust when packing and weighing yellowcake.

demonstrated by repeated industrial hygiene surveys that exposure is consistently well below the Threshold Limit Value, the workers in this area should be under medical surveillance. The routine procedure is to determine the amount of uranium in urine. There is no "safe" excretion level. Butterworth (1955) suggested that a level in excess of 100 μg/litre of urine indicated an undesirable risk; he advised that workers with over 100 μg/litre should have a urine test for protein. Harris *et al.* (1959) found that uranium millers exposed to the 1959 Maximum Permissible Concentration of uranium in air (0·25 mg/m^3 for insoluble uranium) excreted an average of 15 μg/litre, with a maximum of 50 and a minimum of 5 μg/litre. In Saskatchewan a level of 30 μg/litre has been used as a warning, and 60 μg/litre as an indication for immediate removal from exposure; over a period of several years using these standards, there has been no evidence of renal damage among the drum fillers. An additional precaution has been to keep a worker on this job for a period of 3 months only, when first employed in the mill, after which he is transferred to another job, and never works again as a drum filler. This prevents the possibility of any significant deposition in bone, although, provided exposure is kept within the Threshold Limit Value, the hazard from a lifetime exposure is negligible.

To avoid contamination of the urine specimen with dust from work clothes, the specimen should be collected at the time the worker comes "on shift" wearing his ordinary clothes. In a stabilized work environment a monthly sample is adequate. Methods of analysis for uranium in air and urine are listed in the Hygienic Guide Series (1969).

If other potentially hazardous substances are present in the uranium ore, precautions will be necessary to protect mill workers. Carnotite, a common uranium ore in the U.S.A., also contains vanadium, which has caused respiratory illness in workers welding or cutting vanadium coated pipes or metals (Miller, Holaday and Doyle, 1956).

Potash

Potash mining has been undertaken for many decades in Germany and the U.S.A. In the 1960's a new potash mining industry developed in Saskatchewan. The potash beds which are being mined are 2·5–3 metres thick, and situated nearly 1,200 metres below the surface. The air temperature in the mines is generally below 31°C, but may be up to 34°C in the vicinity of the continuous mining machines. The very low humidity, combined with adequate air movement, accounts for the absence of a heat stress problem.

The usual method of mining had been drilling and blasting, but by the time the Saskatchewan mines opened, electric powered, self-propelled continuous mining machines had been developed (Fig. 7). These machines cut the ore from the bed by means of numerous bits fixed to cylinders which rotate in either a horizontal or vertical plane, according

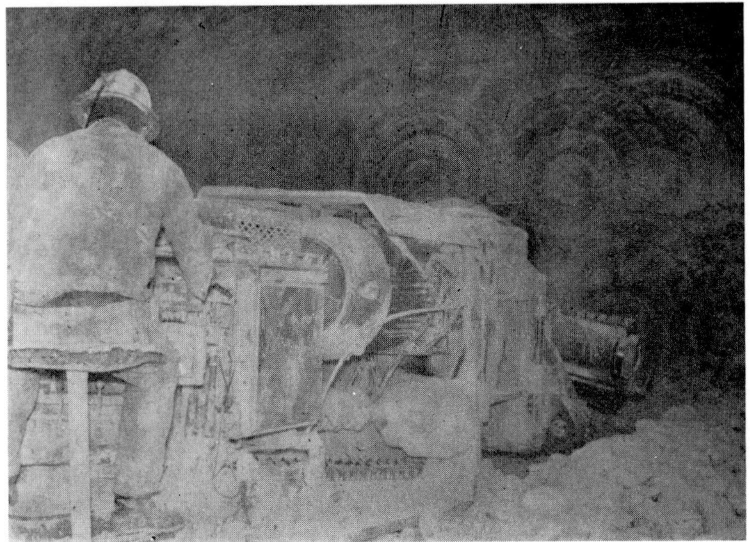

FIG. 7. Continuous potash mining machine. The indistinctness of the
photograph is due to suspended potash dust.

to the design of the machine. Blunt cutting bits not only reduce efficiency,
but create more dust. The broken ore is automatically pushed onto a
conveyor on the machine, to be discharged behind it. From there it is
moved to the roof-bolted mine conveyor belt system by either mobile
conveyor belts or large electric powered dump vehicles.

Machine mining produces very high levels of airborne dust. Without
a dust control system, the level at the breathing zone of a machine
operator has been measured at over 2,000 mg/m^3; the operator of the
ore loading equipment, situated behind the continuous mining machine,
was exposed to 1,900 mg/m^3. The dust levels in the mine away from
the ore face were below 10 mg/m^3. The two main constituents of the
ore (Saskatchewan) are sodium chloride and potassium chloride,
generally present in the ratio of about 2:1. Also present in the ore are
clays and some iron oxide. Traces of other metals are present but no
chromium or arsenic has been detected.

Within a year of starting mining in Saskatchewan it was evident that
perforation of the nasal septum was a hazard, particularly for the
operators of the continuous mining machines, and to a lesser extent
those working in the vicinity of these machines (Williams). At one mine
10 out of 159 underground workers were found to have perforations
of the nasal septum. It was unusual to find perforations occurring in
miners who had been employed for more than one year. In the following

2 years only 2 more cases occurred in the 159 miners previously examined, whereas 6 more occurred in 180 new miners.

Generally, the first symptoms appeared within 1 to 3 months of mining potash. These were: nasal discharge, bleeding, soreness and the development of troublesome crusts in the nose. If untreated, perforation followed in a few days. Once this occurred it rarely extended, was confined to the cartilagenous septum, and the edges healed with healthy mucous membrane (Fig. 8). The size of the perforation ranged from a pin hole to the greater part of the septum; the anterior and lower borders were never destroyed. The only inconvenience was an embarrassing nasal whistle when breathing and talking if the perforation was of a critical small size.

Among the many known occupational exposures capable of causing perforation of the nasal septum are certain hygroscopic dusts, including sodium chloride. Perhaps potassium chloride should be added to this list because nasal septum perforation developed in one man who worked only with the refined potassium chloride (99 per cent pure) in the potash mill. The ability of potassium chloride, in the form of enteric coated tablets, to cause ulcers of the small intestine in a small proportion of those on this medication is well documented (Raf, 1967). Potassium chloride is highly toxic when its extracellular concentration rises even slightly above the normal level. It is therefore possible that it is this specific effect, rather than the hygroscopic action, which is responsible for perforation of the nasal septum in potash miners and mill workers.

Prevention

Dust control is achieved by means of a heavy curtain extending from the roof to the floor, which creates a temporary duct at one side of the passage immediately behind the continuous mining machine. A fan in the duct draws air from behind the machine, across the ore face where the dust is produced, and into the duct where it is filtered before being released well behind the operator and loader (Figs. 9 and 10). The curtain is moved forward as mining progresses. Care has to be taken in the design of the system, otherwise too rapid an air flow picks up potash ore dust from the floor and increases the dust levels. Dust exposures of the machine operators have been reduced to 40 mg/m^3, substantially reducing the nasal septum perforation hazard.

Dust respirators are impractical due to the irritation of the skin by a combination of sweat and ore dust. Air supplied hoods have been tried, but are unpopular with the operators as they restrict their freedom of movement (Fig. 11).

Education of the miners concerning the hazard is of some help in reducing the incidence of perforation of the nasal septum. They should be advised to seek medical advice if they have nasal discharge, bleeding

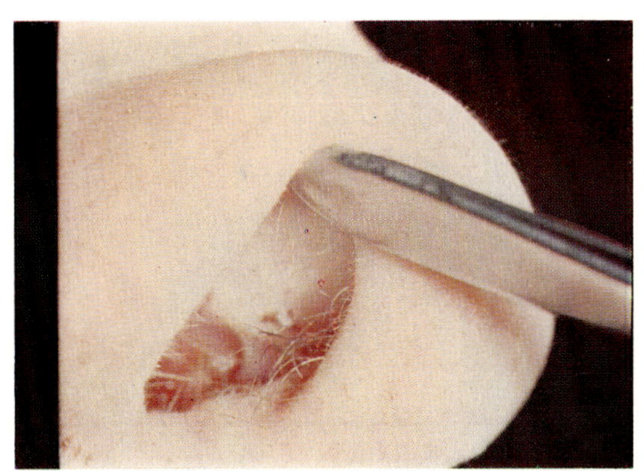

Fig. 8

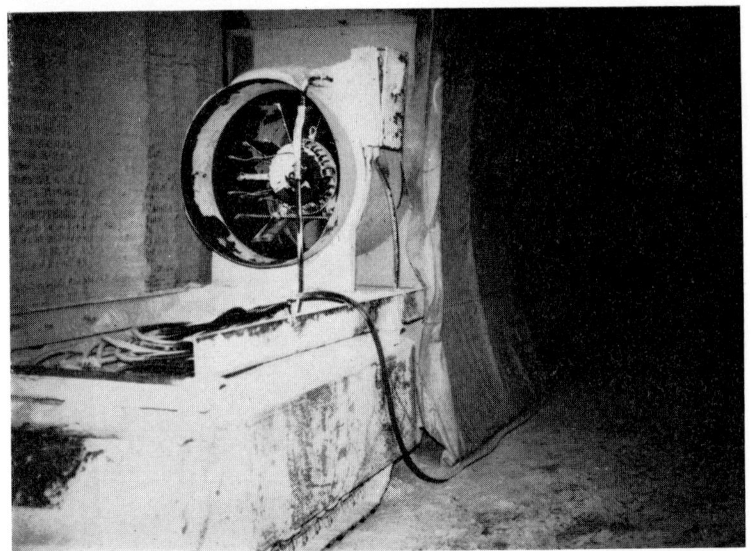

FIG. 9. Curtain and fan used for dust control in Saskatchewan potash mine.

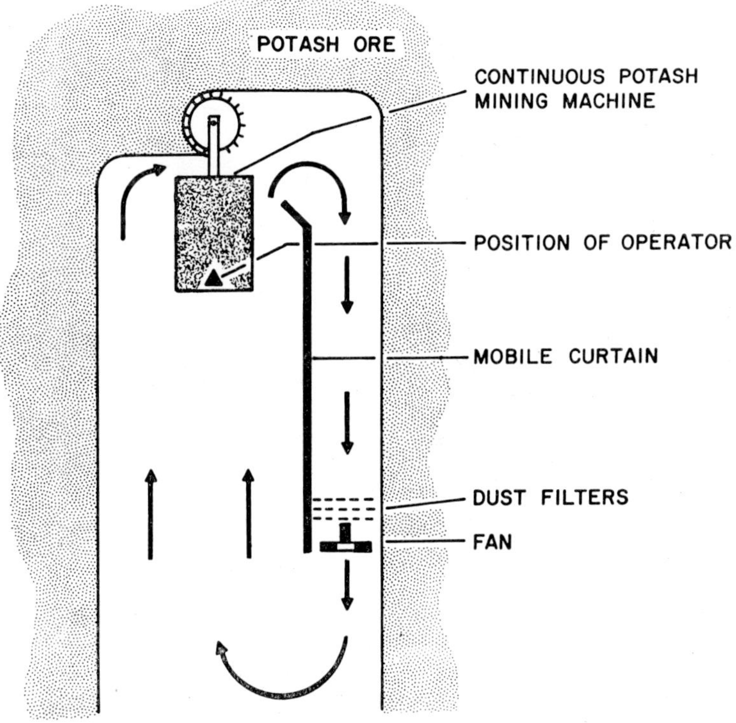

FIG. 10. Diagrammatic plan of dust control system at potash face. Arrows show direction of air flow.

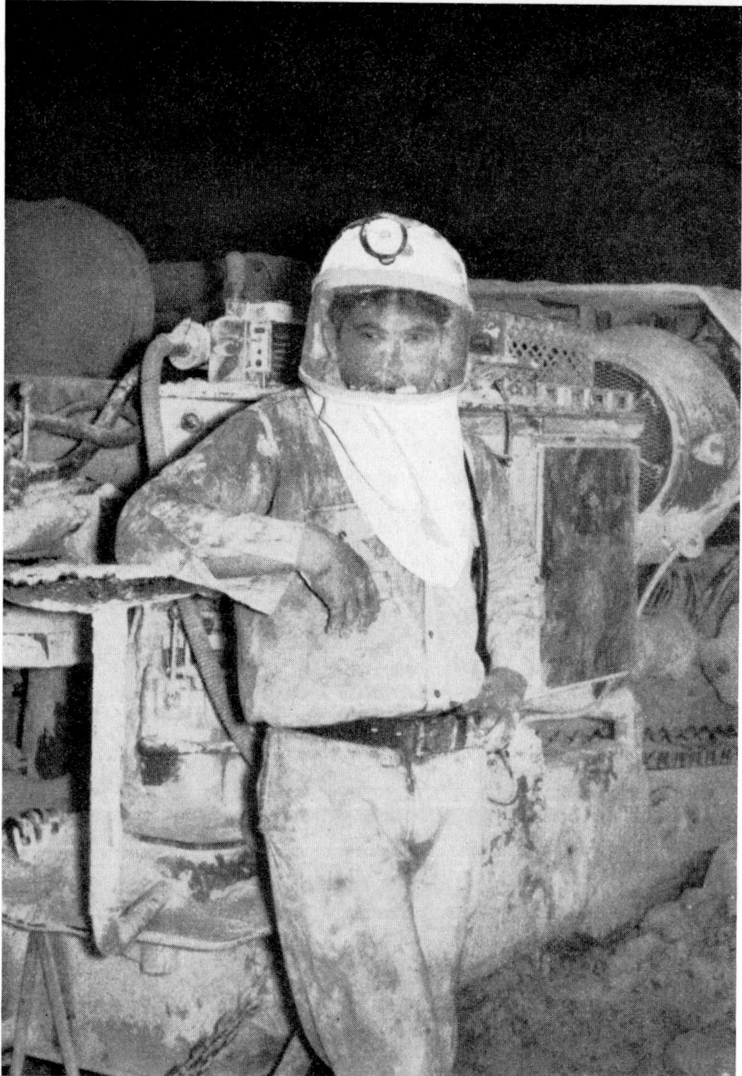

FIG. 11. Operator of continuous potash mining machine wearing air
supplied hood. Dust is removed from the mine air used, by means of
a cyclone and mechanical filtration.

or soreness. Periodic irrigation of the nose with plain water during the
shift has been tried, but it is difficult to evaluate its effectiveness as dust
exposures have been reduced at the same time.

Other than altering the size and shape of the perforations of those
who have an embarrassing nasal whistle, no treatment is necessary.

Manganese

Most reports of manganese poisoning among miners refer to situations where drilling has been undertaken dry due to a shortage of water, resulting in dust exposures obviously well above the accepted safe level.

Several authors have described the features of manganese poisoning among manganese miners in various parts of the world (Jimenez, Uiberall and Escudero, 1947; Avila and Ballina, 1953; Rodier, 1955; Schuler, Oyanguren, Maturana, Valenzuela, Cruz, Plaza, Schmidt and Haddad, 1957; Neogi, 1958; Murphy, 1968).

Manganese can affect the nervous or respiratory systems; the most crippling manifestations are related to the extrapyramidal system. The initial features of nervous system involvement are: weakness, somnolence, apathy, sweating, sexual stimulation soon followed by impotence, paraesthesiae, sialorrhoea, hallucinations, flight of ideas, psychic excitement, euphoria and compulsive acts. The intermediate effects are clumsiness, disturbance of speech, a fixed and jovial facies and exaggeration of the reflexes of the lower limbs. The established phase is characterized by tremors, hypertonia in extension causing the miner to walk on the metatarsophalangeal joints, high stepping gait, and propulsion and retropulsion. The unfortunate victims of the disease are by this stage completely incapacitated.

The average reported period of exposure prior to the symptoms has ranged from 2–8 years. Rodier (1955) detected symptoms in some Moroccan miners with less than 2 months exposure; 60 per cent were affected within 2 years. Manganese dust levels in these mines were not measured. In Chilean mines, where Schuler *et al.* (1957) reported exposures as high as 46 mg/m^3 while drilling, the earliest onset was 9 months after first exposure, the average being 8 years. Experience with manganese mill workers who developed manganism with exposures of 10–173 mg/m^3 (Flinn, Neal, Reinhart, Dallawalle, Fulton and Dooly, 1940) justifies the 1969 American Conference of Governmental Industrial Hygienists Threshold Limit Value of 5 mg/m^3; this is a ceiling value which must not be exceeded at any time.

Manganese pneumonitis seems to occur infrequently. Schuler *et al.* (1957) reported no cases in their miners. Rodier (1955) found very few miners with pneumonitis. Those he did see had marked dyspnoea and shallow respiration; facilities for radiography were not available. The author has seen a case of pneumonitis in a worker in a base metal concentrator who shovelled the dry powdery concentrate, containing about 3 per cent manganese, for a shift when mechanical equipment broke down. A few hours after exposure he developed severe dyspnoea; a chest radiograph revealed patchy opacities scattered throughout both lung fields.

9

Prevention

Wet drilling and spraying ore piles with water will control the dust and prevent manganism (Murphy, 1968). Where water is not available, dust respirators are a possible alternative, though Rodier (1955) had little faith that the miners would use them.

All manganese miners should be under medical surveillance. The frequency of examinations, at which the early symptoms and signs of manganism are looked for, will vary according to the environmental conditions in the mines. Rodier (1955) found it necessary at intervals of 2 months at mines with a severe dust hazard. There is at present insufficient evidence to justify the routine use of any laboratory studies to predict the development of manganism.

Treatment

Although Rodier, Mallet and Rodi (1954) have reported the successful use of ethylenediaminetetraacetic acid (EDTA) in animals poisoned with manganese, suggesting that this drug might be used in early occupational manganese poisoning with a view to preventing severe and total permanent neurological disability, experience in human cases has been conflicting. Mena, Marin, Fuenzalida and Cotzias (1967), using the radioisotope ^{54}Mn, studied the excretion of manganese in healthy manganese miners and in pensioned miners with chronic manganism. They interpreted their findings as indicating that the healthy miners had actively exchanging large stores of manganese, whereas those with chronic manganism had largely eliminated their body stores of manganese after leaving the mines. They concluded that there was no compelling reason for treating these patients with EDTA. A far more promising therapeutic approach has appeared with the success of Mena, Court, Fuenzalida, Papavasiliou and Cotzias (1970) in the treatment of chronic manganese poisoning with oral L-dopa in doses up to 8 g per day. In a series of 6 patients, 5 showed striking improvement, with reduction or disappearance of rigidity and hypo-kinesia, significant improvement in postural reflexes and restitution of balance. The sixth case became worse with L-dopa but was helped by D,L-5 hydroxy-tryptophane, 3 g daily.

Prior to the use of L-dopa the prognosis in cases where neurological manifestations were present was not good, though Jimenez *et al.* (1947), found that the psychiatric symptoms often disappeared.

Vibration

Prior to the 1950's drilling in hard rock mine drifts was done with machines which were relatively heavy, cumbersome and slow; once set up they did not have to be held by hand. When the lightweight (20–25 kg) Jack-leg drill (Fig. 4) which had a faster drilling rate, became available, it was quickly adopted by mines throughout the world. Within a few years of its use Williams and Riegert (1960), Anda (1960) and St. Clair Renard (1963) described cases of Raynaud's phenomenon in hard rock miners in Saskatchewan, Norway and Sweden respectively. In many respects the environmental conditions and the clinical features were similar. The average time using the drill before the onset of symptoms was about 5 years. Over 70 per cent of the Scandinavians who had used the drill for more than 5 years had the disorder. In a further study of the Saskatchewan miners, Ashe and Williams (1964) came to the conclusion that the majority of Jack-leg drillers would develop Raynaud's phenomenon. A major difference in the groups was the presence of pathological changes in the bones and the joints of the hands in half the Norwegian miners, whereas decalcification and cyst formation in the carpi was seen in none of the Swedes and only one of the Saskatchewan miners. Previous studies of individuals exposed to vibration in factories have shown that Raynaud's phenomenon and carpal bone changes can occur independently of each other.

The ambient temperatures prevailing when the hands are exposed to vibration appears to determine whether Raynaud's phenomenon of occupational origin will occur. Lloyd Davies, Glaser and Collins (1957) failed to detect a single case in the Singapore dockyard workers using a tool which produced many cases in Britain. No cases were found among miners who had worked with the Jack-leg drill only at a large uranium mine in northern Saskatchewan where waste heat from diesel engines was used to maintain underground temperatures at 16°C (Ashe and Williams, 1964). There are apparently a few exceptions; George and Cumpston (1964) reported symptomatic Raynaud's phenomenon of occupational origin in an Australian uranium mine where the underground temperature was 21°C.

The drilling position may have a bearing on the development of the disease. It is rarely reported in miners sinking shafts using the Jack-hammer which exposes the operator's hands to similar vibration, often in low environmental temperatures. In this work the arms are in the lowered position. The Jack-leg driller spends part of his shift holding the drill above shoulder height.

The mechanism by which a finger or hand exposed to vibration can become oversensitive to cold has never been satisfactorily explained. Some of the affected Saskatchewan miners were subjected to detailed study in an effort to elucidate the mechanism involved (Ashe, Cook and Old, 1962; Ashe and Williams, 1964). No significant neurological effects were observed, even with electromyographic studies. Digital and pedal arteries were biopsied. Three of the miners, those more severely affected, had subintimal fibrosis of their digital arteries. This was not seen in their pedal arteries, nor in the digital arteries of 3 less severely affected, in a non-affected miner or the cadaver controls. It was suggested that there were two phases of occupational Raynaud's phenomenon; the first was a functional overreaction, which was concurrent with the second, fibrotic change in the arteries.

Typically, the left hand is involved more frequently than the right, and the condition develops in the third and fourth digits, later extending to other fingers, but rarely involving the thumb. In some cases the whole hand may be affected. Usually the attacks of blanching are triggered by exposing the hand to cold (Fig. 12). If the hand is simultaneously exposed to vibration using the Jack-leg drill, or gripping something such as a car steering wheel or the handle of a lunch pail, attacks are induced more readily. Attacks in the mine can present a safety hazard, due to inability to grip adequately and a reduction of sensitivity of the hand.

Gangrene of the fingers is generally considered not to occur in Raynaud's phenomenon of occupational origin. This has been confirmed with the 42 Saskatchewan miners who have suffered from Raynaud's phenomenon.

Almost as troublesome to many Jack-leg drillers as Raynaud's phenomenon, is the nocturnal pain and burning sensation in the arms, extending up to the shoulders. This frequently wakes a miner at night. Some relief is obtained by hanging the arms down outside the bed. No neurological or bone disorder has been found to account for these symptoms.

Within a year of ceasing Jack-leg drilling the pain in the arms at night disappears. There has been little or no change in the Raynaud's phenomenon during the 3 or 4 years the Saskatchewan miners have been followed, even after the hands have lost their calluses, which would be in conflict with the theory of Stewart and Goda (1970) that calluses play a major role in occupational Raynaud's phenomenon. St. Clair Renard (1963) followed cases for several years after they had ceased to use Jack-leg drills; only 17 per cent were free of Raynaud's symptoms, 61 per cent had diminished symptoms and 22 per cent were unchanged.

Prevention

In view of the fact that the majority of miners using this drill in cold mines ultimately develop Raynaud's phenomenon, it would probably be wise to consider the use of some other type of drill for work in drifts, crosscuts and stopes which does not have to be held in the hand. It is unlikely that mines would revert to the use of the old Leyner drill, but other fast drills have since been developed which are capable of drilling several holes simultaneously.

If the Jack-leg drill is used, the miners should be educated concerning the hazard. They should be advised to hold the drill only when collaring a hole. Warm gloves should be worn inside the rubber or plastic outer

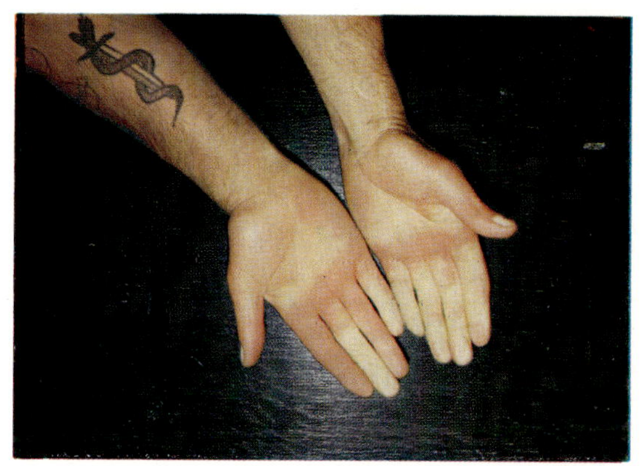

Fig. 12

gloves. A spare set of dry gloves should be taken on shift. If possible, underground temperatures should be maintained at 16°C. Economic considerations may preclude this in very cold climates unless waste heat is available. The miners should be under medical surveillance. Symptoms should be carefully evaluated. Immersion of the hands in cold water sometimes fails to cause blanching. Some men who had no blanching with the test have returned a short while later with blanching after starting to walk home in a temperature of minus 35°C in full winter clothing holding a lunch pail. Whole body cooling is not usually practical as a routine examination procedure.

Those found with Raynaud's phenomenon should not necessarily be recommended to give up Jack-leg drilling. They are usually reluctant to change to other less well paid jobs in the mine. Some have been able to continue provided their drilling is restricted to the lower, and warmer levels of the mine. Below 1,000 metres the temperature is usually above 16°C in Canadian sub-arctic mines. But if the disorder progresses the physician will probably have to recommend transfer to another job; otherwise the miner will become disabled to an extent which makes it impossible to perform manual work in a cold environment.

The role of specific frequencies and amplitudes of vibration in the aetiology of Raynaud's phenomenon has been discussed in the literature. This suggests that alteration of the vibration characteristics might reduce or eliminate the hazard. The author would agree with von Gierke (1965) who came to the conclusion that there was insufficient evidence to draw anything resembling quantitative conclusions with respect to vibration levels, frequencies and exposure times concerning or contributing to Raynaud's phenomenon.

Treatment

No effective treatment is known. Two miners treated for a year with papaverine hydrochloride and nicotinamide failed to improve (Ashe and Williams, 1964). One of the miners who had a digital biopsy found that he had no blanching in the biopsied finger when other fingers were affected, but this relief persisted for only one year. None of the other miners had a similar experience. Sympathectomy is not recommended for the treatment of Raynaud's phenomenon of occupational origin (de Takats, 1959). While many drugs have been used for the treatment of the non-occupational condition, none has won a lasting place in clinical medicine. It remains to be seen whether two more recent methods of treatment—oral or intra-arterial reserpine, and oral griseofulvin—which have helped some cases of severe Raynaud's disease and Raynaud's phenomenon, will have any value in Raynaud's phenomenon of occupational origin.

Appendix

equilibrium: the state that prevails, in a radioactive series, when the ratios between the amounts of successive members of the series remain constant.

ion: an atom or group of atoms which is electrically charged because of the gain or loss of electrons.

MeV: million electron volts, a unit of energy. One electron volt is the energy gained by an electron when accelerated through a potential difference of one volt.

mR: milliroentgen. One thousandth of a roentgen. One roentgen, a unit of radiation exposure, equals 2.58×10^{-4} coulomb per kilogram of air.

picocurie: one millionth of a curie. One curie, a unit of radioactivity, equals 3.7×10^{10} nuclear transformations per second.

quality factor: a factor which relates biological effects of different types of radiation The quality factor for X-rays and gamma-rays is 1.0, for alpha particles 10.

rad: a unit of energy absorbed by a material, such as a tissue. 1 rad is 100 ergs per gram.

rem: a unit of dose equivalent. The dose in rems equals the absorbed dose in rads multiplied by the quality factor, the distribution factor and sometimes other factors.

(The reader requiring further information should consult a radiological health text.)

References

Anda, B. (1960), "Incidence of vasospastic disturbances of hands in miners." *Nordisk Hygienisk Tidskrift*, **41**, 123.

Archer, V. E., Brinton, H. P. and Wagoner, J. K. (1964), "Pulmonary function in uranium miners." *Health Physics*, **10**, 1183.

Arnstein, A. (1913), "Über den sogenannten 'Schneeberger Lungenkrebs'. Verhandlungen der Deutschen." *Pathologischen Gesellschaft*, **16**, 332.

Arnstein, A. (1913), "Über den sogenannten 'Schneeberger Lungenkrebs'." *Wiener Klinische Wochenschrift*, **26**, 748.

Ashe, W. F., Cook, W. T. and Old, W. J. (1962), "Raynaud's phenomenon of occupational origin." *Archives of Environmental Health*, **5**, 333.

Ashe, W. F. and Williams, N. (1964), "Occupational Raynaud's II." *Archives of Environmental Health*, **9**, 425.

Avila, M. G. and Ballina, R. P. (1953), "Manganese poisoning in the mines of Cuba." *Industrial Medicine and Surgery*, **22**, 220.

Blanchard, R. L., Archer, V. E. and Saccomanno, G. (1969), "Blood and skeletal levels of ^{210}Pb–^{210}Po as a measure of exposure to inhaled radon daughter products." *Health Physics*, **16**, 585.

Butterworth, A. (1955), "The significance and value of uranium in urine analysis." *The Transactions of the Association of Industrial Medical Officers*, **5**, 36.

Chamberlain, A. C. and Dyson, E. C. (1956), "The dose to trachea and bronchi from decay products." *British Journal of Radiology*, **29**, 317.

de Takats, G. (1959), *Vascular Surgery*, p. 428. W. B. Saunders Company, Philadelphia and London.

de Villiers, A. J. and Windish, J. P. (1964), "Lung cancer in a fluorspar mining community, I. Radiation, dust and mortality experience." *British Journal of Industrial Medicine*, **21**, 94.

Duggan, N. J., Howell, D. M. and Soilleux, P. T. (1968), "Concentrations of radon-222 in coal mines in England and Scotland." *Nature*, **219**, 1149.

Elias, J. D. (1968), "Noise levels of underground mining equipment." *Technical Report, No. 18*. Province of Manitoba Department of Health.

Evans, R. (1969), In Report of Royal Commission, Respecting Radiation, Compensation and Safety at the Fluorspar Mines, St. Lawrence, Newfoundland, p. 114.

Federal Radiation Council (1967a), Report No. 8 revised, Guidance for the Control of Radiation Hazards in Uranium Mining, p. 3.

Federal Radiation Council (1967b), Report No. 8 revised, Guidance for the Control of Radiation Hazards in Uranium Mining, p. 9.

Federal Radiation Council (1967c), Report No. 8 revised, Guidance for the Control of Radiation Hazards in Uranium Mining, p. 24.

Federal Radiation Council (1967d), Report No. 8 revised, Guidance for the Control of Radiation Hazards in Uranium Mining, pp. 35 and 36.

Federal Radiation Council (1967e), Report No. 8, revised, Guidance for the Control of Radiation Hazards in Uranium Mining, p. 38.

Federal Radiation Council (1968), Radiation Exposure of Uranium Miners, p. 21. A Report of an Advisory Committee from the Division of Medical Sciences: National Academy of Sciences—National Research Council—National Academy of Engineering, Washington, D.C.

Flinn, R. H., Neal, P. A., Reinhart, W. H., Dallavalle, J. M., Fulton, W. B. and Dooly, A. E. (1940), "Chronic manganese poisoning in an ore-crushing mill." *Public Health Bulletin No. 247*, 77.

Geiger, E. L. (1967), "Radon film badge." *Health Physics*, **13**, 407.

George, W. E. and Cumpston, A. G. (1964), Personal Communication referred to in Ashe, W. F. and Williams, N. (1964), "Occupational Raynaud's II." *Archives of Environmental Health*, **9**, 425.

Harris, W. B., Breslin, A. J. Glauberman, H. and Weinstein, M. S. (1959), "Environmental hazards associating with milling of uranium ore." *A.M.A. Archives of Industrial Health*, **20**, 365.

Harting, F. H. and Hesse, W. (1879), "Der Lungenkrebs, Die Bergkrankheit in den Schneeberger Gruben." *Vierteljahrsschrift für gerichtliche Medicin und öffentliches Sanitäswesen*, **30**, 296; **31**, 102 and 313.

Holaday, D. A., Rushing, D. E., Coleman, R. D., Woolrich, P. F., Kusnetz, H. L. and Bale, W. F. (1957a), *Control of Radon and Daughters in Uranium Mines and Calculations on Biologic Effects*, p. 20. Public Health Service Publication, U.S. Department of Health, Education and Welfare, No. 494.

Holaday, D. A., Rushing, D. E., Coleman, R. D., Woolrich, P. F., Kusnetz, H. L. and Bale, W. F. (1957b), *Control of Radon and Daughters in Uranium Mines and Calculations on Biologic Effects*, pp. 21–44. Public Health Service Publication, U.S. Department of Health, Education and Welfare, No. 494.

Holaday, D. A., Rushing, D. E., Coleman, R. D., Woolrich, P. F., Kusnetz, H. L. and Bale, W. F. (1957c), *Control of Radon and Daughters in Uranium Mines and Calculations on Biologic Effects*, p. 43. Public Health Service Publication, U.S. Department of Health, Education and Welfare, No. 494.

Horacek, J. (1969), "The lung cancer of Joachimstal after the Second World War. A report of 55 cases." *Zeitschrift für Krebsforschung*, **72**, 52.

Hygienic Guide Series (1969), "Uranium (natural) and its compounds." *American Industrial Hygiene Association Journal*, **30**, 313.

International Commission on Radiological Protection (1966a), Radiation Protection, Recommendations of the International Commission on Radiological Protection (Adopted September 17, 1965), p. 10, Publication 9, First Edition. Pergamon Press, Oxford.

International Commission on Radiological Protection (1966b), Radiation Protection, Recommendations of the International Commission on Radiological Protection (Adopted September 17, 1965), p. 6, Publication 9, First Edition. Pergamon Press, Oxford.

Jimenez, J. A., Uiberall, E. and Escudero, E. (1946), "La intoxicación por manganeso en Chile. (Estudio sobre 64 casos.)" *La Prensa Médica Argentina*, **33**, 1684.

Lea, D. E. (1955), *Actions of Radiations on Living Cells*, p. 25, Second Edition. The Syndics of the Cambridge University Press, London.

Lloyd Davies, T. A,. Glaser, E. M., and Collins, C. P. (1957), "Absence of Raynaud's phenomenon in workers using vibratory tools in a warm climate." *Lancet*, **1**, 1014.

Lorenz, E. (1944), "Radioactivity and lung cancer: a critical review of lung cancer in the miners of Schneeberg and Joachimsthal." *Journal of the National Cancer Institute*, **5**, 1.

Lovett, D. B. (1969), "Track etch detectors for alpha exposure estimation." *Health Physics*, **16**, 623.

Lowy, J. (1929), "Über die Joachimstaler Bergkrankheit." *Medizinische Klinik*, **25**, 141.

Ludwig, P. and Lorenser, E. (1924), "Untersuchungen der Grubenluft in den Schneeberger Gruben auf den Gehalt an Radiumemanation." *Strahlentherapie*, **17**, 428.

Lundin, F. E., Jr., Lloyd, J. W., Smith, E. M., Archer, V. E. and Holaday, D. A. (1969), "Mortality of uranium miners in relation to radiation exposure, hard rock mining and cigarette smoking—1950 through September 1967." *Health Physics*, **16**, 571.

Mena, I., Court, J., Fuenzalida, S., Papavasiliou, P. S. and Cotzias, G. C. (1970), "Modification of chronic manganese poisoning." *New England Journal of Medicine*, **282**, 5.

Mena, I., Marin, O., Fuenzalida, S. and Cotzias, G. C. (1967), "Chronic manganese poisoning." *Neurology*, **17**, 128.

Miller, S. E., Holaday, D. A. and Doyle, H. N. (1956), "Health protection of uranium miners and millers." *A.M.A. Archives of Industrial Health*, **14**, 48.

Murphy, G. (1968), "Intoxication cronica por manganeso. Parkonsonismo manganico." *La Prensa Medica Argentina*, **55**, 564.

Neogi, T. P. (1958), "Chronic manganese poisoning and its prevention." *Alumni Association Bulletin* (Calcutta), **7**, 39.

Pohl-Ruling, J. and Pohl, E. (1969), "The radon-222 concentration in the atmospheres of mines as a function of the barometric pressure." *Health Physics*, **16**, 579.

Raf, L. E. (1967), "Enteric-coated potassium chloride tablets and ulcer of the small intestine." *Acta Chirurgica Scandinavica Supplementum*, **374**, 79.

Report of Royal Commission (1969a), Respecting Radiation, Compensation and Safety at the Fluorspar Mines, St. Lawrence, Newfoundland, 104.

Report of Royal Commission (1969b), Respecting Radiation, Compensation and Safety at the Fluorspar Mines, St. Lawrence, Newfoundland, p. 63.

Rock, R. L., Lovett, D. B. and Nelson, S. C. (1969), "Radon-daughter exposure measurement with track etch films." *Health Physics*, **16**, 617.

Rodier, J., Mallet, R. and Rodi, L. (1954), "Étude de l'action détoxicante de l'éthylénediaminetétraacétate de calcium dans l'intoxication expérimentale par le manganèse." *Archives Des Maladies Professionnelles De Médecine Du Travail Et De Sécurité Sociale*, **15**, 210.

Rodier, J. (1955), "Manganese poisoning in Moroccan miners." *British Journal of Industrial Medicine*, **12**, 21.

Rostoski, Saupe and Schmorl (1926), "Die Bergkrankheit der Erzbergleute in Schneeberg in Sachsen ('Schneeberger Lungenkrebs')." *Zeitschrift Für Krebsforschung*, **23**, 360.

Saccomanno, G., Saunders, R. P., Ellis, H., Archer, V. E., Wood, B. G. and Beckler, P. A. (1963), "Concentration of carcinoma or atypical cells in sputum." *Acta Cytologica*, **7**, 305.

Saccomanno, G., Saunders, R. P., Archer, V. E., Auerbach, O., Kuschner, M. and Beckler, P. A. (1965), "Cancer of the lung: the cytology of sputum prior to the development of carcinoma." *Acta Cytologica*, **9**, 413.

Saccomanno, G. (1970), Personal Communication.

Saccomanno, G., Archer, V. E., Auerbach, O., Kuschner, M., Saunders, R. P. and Klein, M. G. "Histologic Types of lung cancer among uranium miners." *Cancer* (in Press).

Schroeder, G. L., Evans, R. D. and Kraner, H. W. (1966), "Effect of applied pressure on the radon characteristics of an underground mine environment." *Transactions of the Society of Mining Engineers of AIME*, **235**, (1), 91.

Schuler, P., Oyanguren, H., Maturana, V., Valenzuela, A., Cruz, E., Plaza, V., Schmidt, E. and Haddad, R. (1957), "Manganese poisoning. Environmental and medical study at a Chilean mine." *Industrial Medicine and Surgery*, **26**, 167.

Sikl, H. (1930), "Über den Lungenkrebs der Bergleute in Joachimstal (Tschechslowakei)." *Zeitschrift Für Krebsforschung*, **32**, 609.

St. Clair-Renard, K. G. (1963), "Vibration injuries in the fingers of miners in Northern Sweden." Proceedings, International Mining Congress, Saltzburg.

Stewart, A. M. and Goda, D. F. (1970), "Vibration syndrome." *British Journal of Industrial Medicine*, **27**, 19.

Tompkins, P. C. (1968), "Radiation protection and uranium mining." *Journal of Occupational Medicine*, **10**, 702.

Trapp, E., Renzetti, A. D., Jr., Kobayashi, T., Mitchell, M. M. and Bigler, A. (1970), "Cardiopulmonary function in uranium miners." *American Review of Respiratory Disease*, **101**, 27.

Vich, Z. and Kriklava, J. (1970), "Erythrocytes of uranium miners: the red blood picture." *British Journal of Industrial Medicine*, **27**, 83.

von Gierke, H. E. (1965), "On noise and vibration exposure criteria." *Archives of Environmental Health*, **11**, 327.

Vuchot, L., Berger, C., Duhamel, Pradel, Billard, J. and Granier (1963), "Preventive measures against radiation hazards in underground mining." Proceedings, International Mining Congress, Saltzburg.

Williams, N. and Riegert, A. L. (1960), "Raynaud's phenomenon of occupational origin in uranium miners," p. 819. Proceedings, 13th International Congress on Occupational Health, New York.

Williams, N. (to be published).

Chapter 8

The Control of Dust in Mining

Introduction

The aim of this chapter is to outline the general principles of dust control and to give an indication of techniques which may be used, rather than to describe details peculiar to one method of mining.

Dust formation is an inherent feature of most mining processes. The control of fine particles once they have become airborne in a mine is usually more difficult than in surface industry because both men and machinery must operate in the same ventilation currents, frequently under cramped conditions and in an essentially temporary environment. Dust control apparatus must be rugged, preferably simple to use and to maintain, and must also be safe to use in a potentially explosive atmosphere.

The main objective of dust control in mines is recognized as that of obtaining acceptable levels of concentration of airborne respirable dust, and to this end the great majority of countries with mining industries have defined "approved conditions" of dust concentration in which men may work, and which provide targets for dust control. The very fine particles which are usually regarded as respirable are typically in the size range 0·5–10 microns, with median falling speed in air of the order of 1 millimetre/second, so thay they remain suspended in the mine ventilation for long periods; for this reason they can penetrate the defences of the human respiratory system and are difficult to "suppress".

It is perhaps useful to explain briefly the various methods of underground mining in use. Coal mining involves winning a fairly weak material from a continuous seam varying in thickness from less than one to a hundred or so metres, and usually, but not always, fairly horizontal. In Europe coal seams are thin and "long wall" mining is most commonly used: a narrow coal face, usually 50 to 300 metres in length is advanced between two parallel tunnels and when the coal has been removed the roof is allowed to collapse. In the United States and other countries where coal seams are thicker, and less deep, various forms of "pillar mining" are used. Here a pattern of tunnels or headings is driven to extract the coal from the seam, leaving large "pillars" of coal to support the overlying strata. Other soft minerals, such as potash, may be mined in this way. Although coal is still sometimes "won" from the seam by shot-firing and hand-loading, mechanization is now the rule and various types of machine break down the coal using sharp cutter picks. Metalliferous mining involves in general the extraction of a hard "ore body" by driving "stopes" or tunnels following the mineral and a very wide variety of mining methods is in use, depending on the thickness and inclination of the ore body. The breaking down of rock is normally carried out by shot-firing and mechanical loading of the broken material.

The attainment of acceptable dust concentrations must usually involve the application of one or more of the following lines of attack:

(*a*) The removal and dilution of dust by ventilation.

(*b*) The control of the formation and dispersion of dust by attention to the method of mining and the way in which machines are operated.

(*c*) The application of water, either to limit the dispersion of dust into the air, or to suppress airborne particles.

(*d*) The use of exhaust ventilation to contain dust sources, followed either by ducting the dusty air to unoccupied parts of the mine, or by filtration before returning it to the main ventilation current.

Ventilation

Mine ventilation, apart from assisting in dust control, is used to help provide reasonable working conditions in terms of heat and humidity, and in coal mines to give dilution to safe levels of methane and in some cases of carbon monoxide. Since every part of a mine must be provided with "through" ventilation, men may obviously be protected by remaining on the "upwind" side of a dust source. In gold mining, for example, it is normal practice to fire the explosive charges in the ore body throughout the mine in succession from "return" to "intake" of the ventilation at a certain time of day, and operators do not return until sufficient time has elapsed for all airborne dust to have been carried away from the mine (Beadle, 1968). Ventilating air may be used to dilute dust concentration, but the effect of air velocity is also important and under certain conditions, increasing air volume may result in excessive dispersion of dust. At air speeds less than 1·0 metre/second (200 ft/min) the concentration of dust from a particular source is progressively diluted as the volume of air flow is increased, but as air speed rises higher, there is an increased tendency for dust to be picked up, until at speeds above 2·0 metres/second (400 ft/min) this effect may begin to outweigh that of dilution.

A number of measurements have been made of the relationship between respirable dust concentration and air velocity, and some of these are shown plotted as one graph in Figure 1 (Breuer, 1969; Hall, 1955; Hodkinson, 1960). All the measurements show the same general pattern, but the nature of the dust source itself has an effect on the "critical" air speed at which increased "pick-up" of dust begins to outweigh dilution.

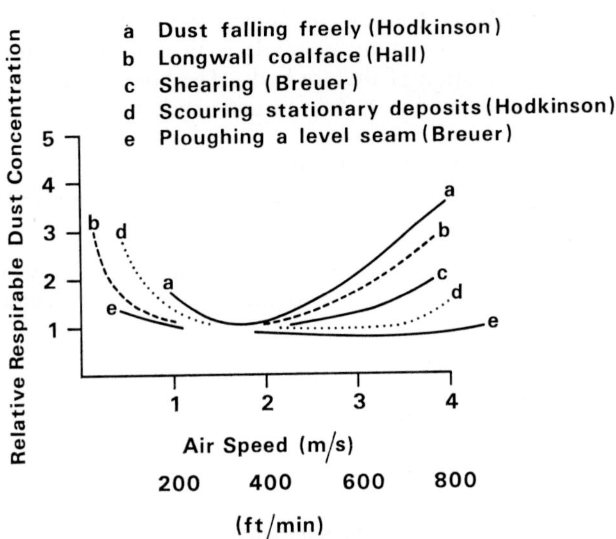

FIG. 1. Relationships between dust concentrations and air speed
for different types of dust source.

This critical air speed is lowest when dust is falling freely across the airstream, as for example, on a steeply sloping coal face, and is highest when dust is being "scoured" from stationary deposits. There is in addition, a tendency for particles, somewhat too coarse to be respirable, but which give reduced visibility and uncomfortable working conditions, to be picked up in high air speeds more readily than finer respirable particles.

The Control of Dust Formation and Dispersion

When a brittle material is broken, a wide "spectrum" of different sized particles is produced, and below a particle size of about 0·2 millimetre, there is a constant size distribution of breakage product which includes the potentially respirable dust and is peculiar to the type of rock being broken and virtually independent of the method of breakage (Hamilton and Knight, 1958). The proportion of the fine dust in the total breakage product is reduced by increasing the proportion of coarse material by, for example, increasing the top size of debris. Thus in rotary drilling a deeper penetration per revolution, obtained by increasing the thrust on the drill, results in the production of coarser debris and less fine dust. Similarly, a cutter pick produces minimum dust when taking deep bites, when a sharp, rather than a blunt pick is used, and when there is adequate lateral spacing between following picks for each to work efficiently. The possibilities of reducing dust formation when breaking down rock by the use of explosives are more limited, although by using charges in the most efficient patterns (and also economizing in the use of explosives) and by ensuring that there is effective "stemming", some reductions in dust may be obtained. In recent years there have been moves to examine "wedging" actions to break rock in metalliferous mining, and there also appears to be a possibility of using forms of cutter pick machines for this work (Beadle, 1968). In this last case reduction in dust make would be obtained by restricting mining more closely to the ore body itself.

In practice a relatively small fraction of the very fine particles produced in most mining processes is dispersed into the air, because of the tendency of the finest dust particles to agglomerate with larger particles very soon after their formation. The strength of the rock broken, to some extent, affects the dispersion of dust; stronger rocks tend to break more explosively, thus giving less chance for agglomeration. An important factor in dust dispersion from cutter pick machines is the speed of the picks: although a fast moving pick produces no difference in breakage pattern and thus makes no more dust than when it moves slowly, its rapid motion causes a greater proportion of the dust to be dispersed into the air, roughly in proportion to its speed: Figure 2 shows the results of experiments with a single pick, and the relationship between depth of cut, pick speed and airborne dust (Hamilton, Levin and McKinlay, 1962). The effect on dust concentration of reducing the pick speed of a mining machine such as an Anderton Shearer can be most marked because, provided the rate of movement along the coal face (haulage rate) is maintained, a reduction of, for example, 25 per cent in pick speed results also in a one third increase in the depth of cut taken by each pick. Studies of dust production by mining machines in routine use (Evans and Hamilton, 1964) have shown enormously wide variations in dust due to the factors mentioned above.

A recent development in coal mining which has been found to result in significant reductions in dust has been that of multi-speed gearboxes for coal face machines so that a cutter drum may be used at slow speed under suitable conditions, when, for example, it is being employed to "load" debris, and at a higher speed for hard cutting.

The proportion of dust dispersed from cutter picks is controlled by external air movement, particularly in longwall coal mining, in which the machine operates in a ventilation current which may have a high volume flow, and hence velocity, because of the need to limit methane concentration. Close fitting cowls (used also to facilitate the loading of coal from the drum), give some protection from the ventilation and reduce dust dispersion. Another important requirement is to avoid cutting at such a slow haulage speed that the drum is but lightly loaded and the debris more exposed to the ventilation.

In addition to the dust produced in the actual mining process, the

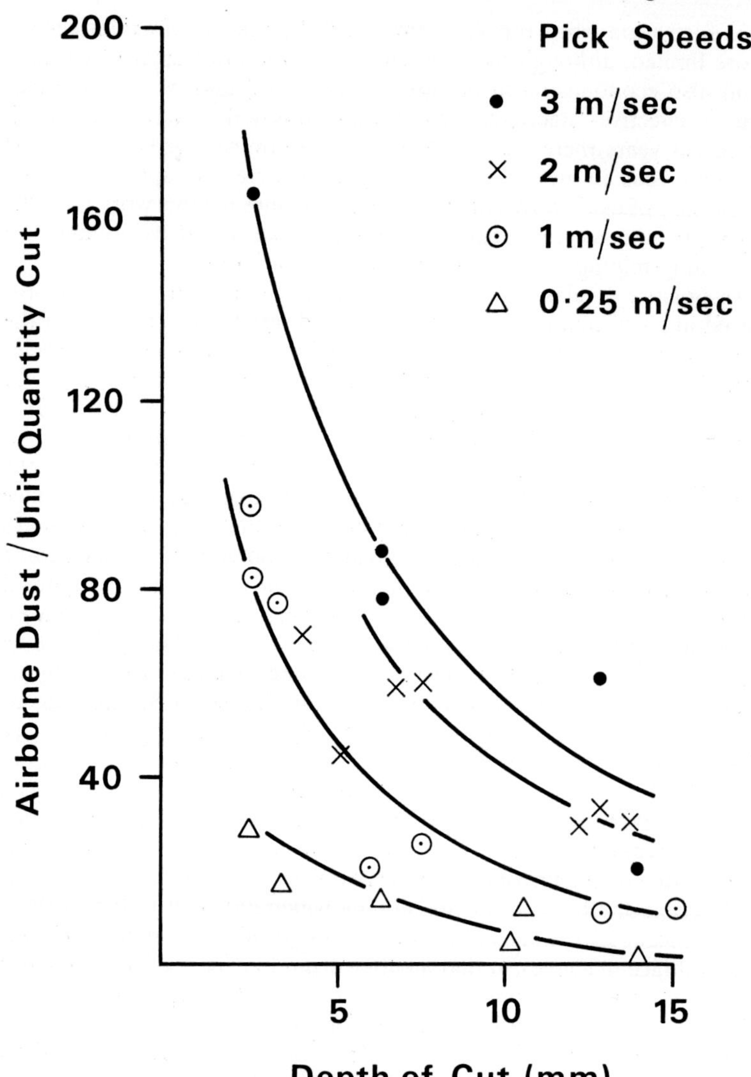

FIG. 2. The relationship between pick depth of cut, pick speed and dust.

loading of broken material, and its transport, can give rise to excessive dust, both because of fresh breakage and from the dispersion of dust already present. Often a simple engineering solution can be effective, for example, by the use of chutes to avoid free fall of material into hoppers and at conveyor loading and transfer points. Dust sometimes is dispersed from the conveyor belt itself. If this is out of alignment there may be spillage, and unsealed belt joints can result in a continuous shower of fine dust as they bump over the support rollers. The pattern of the relationships between dust and ventilation, first in dilution and, as it increases in velocity, in the dispersion of more dust has already been mentioned. When rock or coal is carried on open conveyors in a direction against the ventilation current, it is the relative air velocity that matters: and unfortunately in coal mining, where conveying in intake roadways is often the rule, high dust concentrations may be carried on to the coal faces for this reason. Conveying in the same direction as the ventilation ("homotropal" working) has many advantages for dust control.

The Use of Water in Dust Control

The Wetting of Broken Material

Water, for maximum effect, should be employed to minimize the dispersion of dust. For example, in dealing with broken rock, "wetting down" before movement has long been recognized as good practice, and similarly for rock in transit, its thorough wetting, even by quite crude spraying methods, at the start of travel, can be effective in preventing dust dispersion, since the movement of the material tends to result in more or less uniform spreading of moisture, so that dust is held in contact with the coarser material (Hamilton and Knight, 1964). The effective application of water to prevent dust dispersion when breaking down rock from the solid is more difficult. In shot firing, the use of plastic bags, or "ampoules" filled either with water, or with an aqueous "gel" for "stemming" the explosive charges in the drill holes can result in significantly lower dust concentrations than when conventional stemming materials (clay or sand) are used (Schramm, 1961), although whether this is due to the ampoules providing more effective stemming or to the actual presence of water is not entirely clear. "Wet" rotary or percussive drilling, in which water is fed down the drill shaft and out through holes in the drill bit is very effective, and is used at the same time to flush debris from the drill hole. Drills fitted with external sprays directed to suppress airborne dust as it emerges from the drill hole are also used, but this method of dust suppression is usually less effective than true "wet drilling".

"Water infusion" has been used for a number of years in coal mining, and consists of injecting water under pressure into the coal seam before mining takes place. As used originally in South Wales and described by Jenkins (1943) the technique consisted of the daily drilling of 1·5 to 2 metre holes into the coal face and pumping water into each hole for a few hours at 50–70 atmospheres pressure (A in Fig. 3). Later work showed that under some circumstances much longer holes (20 metres or more in length) could be used, with water pumped in under very high pressure (100–300 atmospheres). The main advantage of this method (B in Fig. 3), which is usually known as long hole infusion, was that the treatment would be effective for some days and might be carried out at the weekend, to cover the week's work. There are local variations of long hole infusion such as, in place of self-sealing infusion guns, which may be difficult to remove from the drill holes, the use of a flexible hose sealed permanently into the drill hole with cement. More recently there has been developed (Breuer, 1969) a method of water infusion which is particularly applicable to a modern system of longwall mining, in which prior to the mining of coal two parallel tunnels are driven, one on each side of a panel of coal, which is then worked "on retreat" (C in Fig. 3). Holes

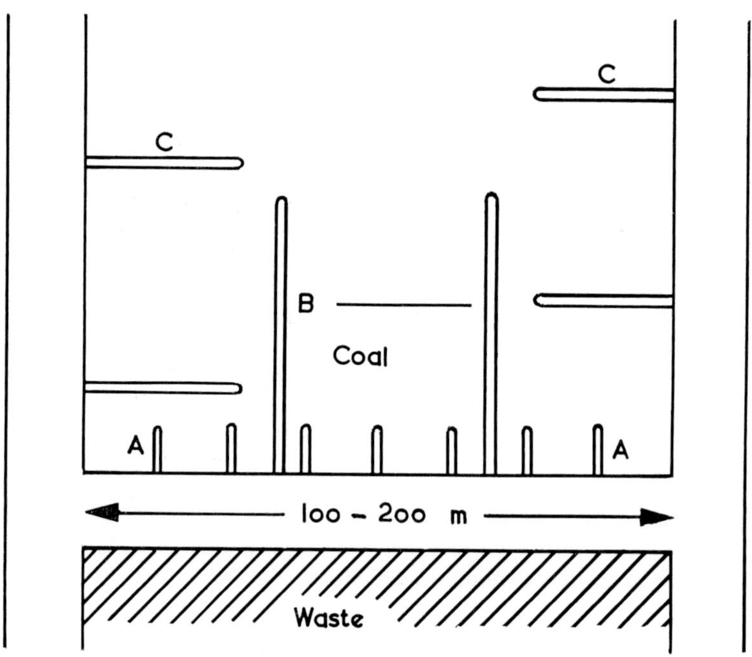

FIG. 3. Three types of water infusion.

20 metres or so in length are drilled into the coal from the two headings, and water at moderate pressure (60–80 atmospheres) is pumped in at a low flow rate for some weeks. This last technique has proved successful in France, Germany and Great Britain, has the advantage of not interfering with other mining operations and appears to be effective in reducing dust. Some success has also been achieved in France and Holland in infusing a coal seam through vertical holes drilled from

tunnels in a higher seam. Although this last technique is difficult to apply, it is reported to give effective results.

Water infusion is an obligatory technique of dust suppression in coal mines in France, Germany and the U.S.S.R., but is used to a lesser extent in Great Britain. Its success appears to be related to the nature of coal seams, and a well defined crack structure may be a pre-requisite for its effective use. It is employed, in general, only in longwall mining and with the exception of the method described for use in retreat working, is becoming increasingly difficult to apply under present-day mechanized mining conditions.

Water Applied to Cutting Elements

The problem of applying water effectively to the cutter picks of mining machines has presented many practical problems: it has long been known that for maximum effectiveness the water should be applied to the rotating elements themselves and for several years sprays mounted on shearer drums have been in fairly common use in Great Britain and Germany (Hamilton *et al.*, 1962).

Water applied in this way is in general more effective in suppressing dust than if it is applied by "external" sprays, but in the past rotating water seals have been unreliable and the jets themselves are more susceptible to blockage both from dirt in the water supply, and by fine debris than are fixed sprays. Recently these problems have been overcome, and now "pick face flushing" is being applied on various types of cutter pick machine—Figure 4 shows water flowing down a cutter pick from a jet mounted on the pick box. Figure 5 shows a shearer loader with jets mounted in front of each pick, which is also fitted with a "phasing" distribution system to restrict flow to the cutting side of the drum only. For this application jets must be protected by some form of shroud and there must also be incorporated in the water supply an effective filtration system to stop blockage of the jets. Pick face flushing has been found to result typically in a 70 per cent reduction in the dispersion of respirable dust, compared with "dry" cutting, as against the 25–40 per cent reduction in dust when external water sprays are used. The optimum amount of water applied appears to be between about 2 per cent by weight of coal mined (20 litres/tonne, 4·5 gallon/ton).

Water Sprays

Water sprays are not uncommonly used in mining, in order to "knock down" particles from the air, or to form "spray curtains" and "barriers". No doubt such sprays have some effectiveness due to the impaction of water droplets with coarse particles, but with respirable particles effectiveness is very small (Walton and Woolcock, 1960). It has been shown, for example, that in order to capture 90 per cent of three micron

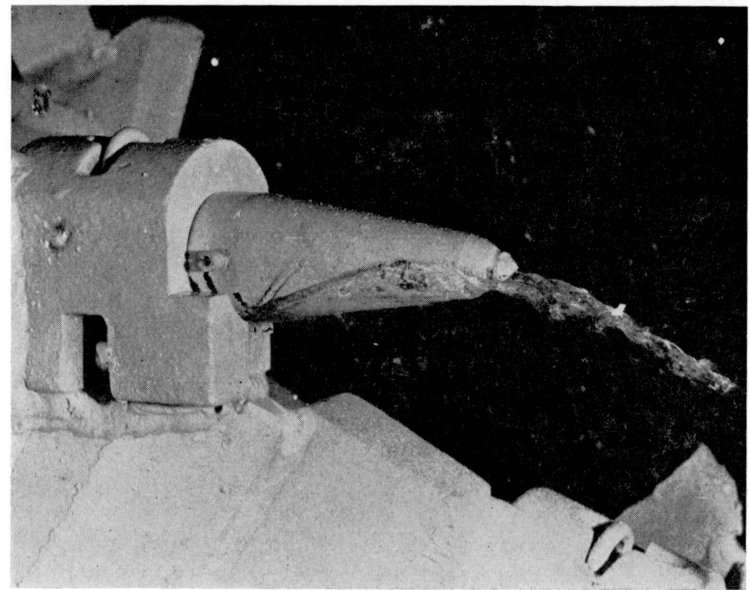

FIG. 4. Pick face flushing.

diameter particles in a dust cloud moving at 30 metres per minute through a mine roadway, it would be necessary to spray some 1200 litres per minute of water. There are other problems connected with the use of atomizing sprays: for greatest efficiency, water droplets should be small and move as fast as possible—necessitating the use of high pressure atomization. However, the smaller the droplet the more rapidly it slows down to its free falling speed in air and an atomizing spray also gives rise to considerable air movement, which can in turn result in an increased dispersion of dust. An effective application, however, of airborne capture is in an enclosure, such as a hopper, or at the bottom of a drop shaft where very fine mist sprays or even wet steam may be used to provide a saturated atmosphere and most effective dust control.

When sprays are used to suppress the dust from mining machines this function should be regarded as supplying water to the dust producing zone in order to inhibit the dispersion of dust, rather than capturing airborne particles. For this purpose jets of various types, or coarse droplets are more effective than finely atomized water sprays.

Wetting Agents, Foam and "Dust Proofing" Agents

The use of detergents or "wetting agents" for increasing the effectiveness of water for dust suppression has been investigated in some detail. There is some evidence that in infusion a detergent solution or even

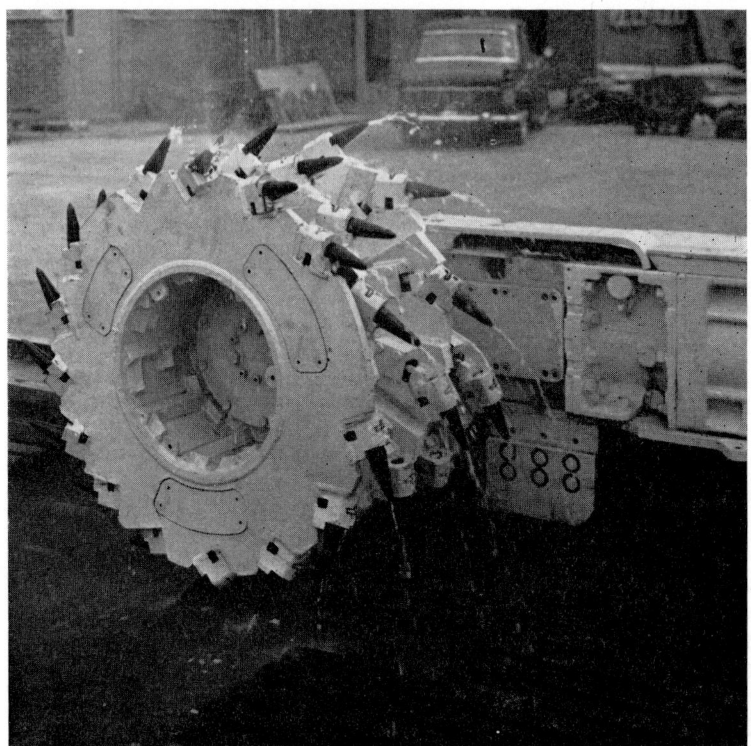

FIG. 5. A shearer loader equipped for pick face flushing.

calcium chloride (Bauer, 1970) allows easier penetration of the coal seam than does water alone, and these agents can also sometimes be of help in wetting static heaps of coal (but not other types of rock). However, in the majority of applications of water for dust suppression, the addition of a wetting agent is of no practical advantage. Most rocks are wetted equally well by water alone, and although some types of coal, particularly steam and coking coals, are admittedly more readily wetted by a detergent solution than by water, with possibly some short term advantage, the inevitable mechanical movement of coal on a conveyor belt or in a loading operation serves to spread untreated water over the surfaces of the coal with the result that after a very short time no significant difference in effect can be observed. At various times aqueous foams have also been tried for dust suppression, in the hope that as in firefighting, a "blanket" would be formed to inhibit dispersion of dust into the atmosphere. Presumably where there is little mechanical disturbance the application of foam in this way might be successful. Laboratory and underground experiments have, however, shown that very large amounts of foam are required to maintain effective dust control under practical mining conditions because of the continuous rupture of the foam by moving cutter picks and broken material. The best type of foam for dust control work proved to be a low expansion wetting agent type which was mobile enough to close gaps made by the moving rock or coal (Hamilton and McKinlay, 1961) unlike the typical "stiff" high expansion foam used for fire fighting.

Sometimes "dust proofing" or long term dust suppression is needed for the consolidation of mine roadways and the treatment of surface stockpiles. Here water alone evaporates too quickly, but effective dust control may be obtained by the application of hygroscopic salt solutions such as calcium chloride—sometimes used in conjunction with non-ionic wetting agents or of aqueous solutions of "soluble oils" (Hamilton and Knight, 1964) or of mineral oil by itself.

Exhaust Ventilation

When mining consists of driving "blind" tunnels or headings, the use of exhaust ventilation provides the most effective form of dust control. Dusty air is removed continuously from the face of the heading so that work is carried out in the clean air stream drawn in round the mining machine. There are various ways in which this can be done: in "room and pillar" coal mining in the United States (Morse, 1970) a popular system involves dividing the heading itself by a vertical screen, or "line brattice", and arranging for the air to course round the working places with the aid of "stoppings" set up in previously excavated roadways (Fig. 6). An alternative system is to extract the dusty air through a ventilation duct, as shown in Figure 7 (*a*). For effective dust control the entry to the exhaust system must be kept as close to the working place as possible: with some machines it may be convenient to incorporate the forward end of the exhaust ducting into the machine itself, and an air speed forward in the machine operators position of at least 0·4–0·5 metres/second, 80–100 feet/minute (Robinson, 1961; Kingery, Doyle, Harris, Jacobson, Peluso, Shutack and Schlick, 1969) must be maintained. Even if these requirements are fulfilled, there is some "backing up" of dust cloud caused by air movements produced by the mining process, and by the inherent air flow pattern into the exhaust entry. In coal mining enough air must be exhausted to maintain methane concentration in the main body of the air at well below the explosive level (5 per cent) and since an exhaust system is essentially ineffective in "scouring" the face of the heading, it may also be necessary to use supplementary forcing air jets to clear stagnant zones which may contain high methane concentrations and which typically occur in the corners and roof. If this is done, it will be necessary to increase the volume of exhaust air in order to counter-balance the extra air movement produced by these jets.

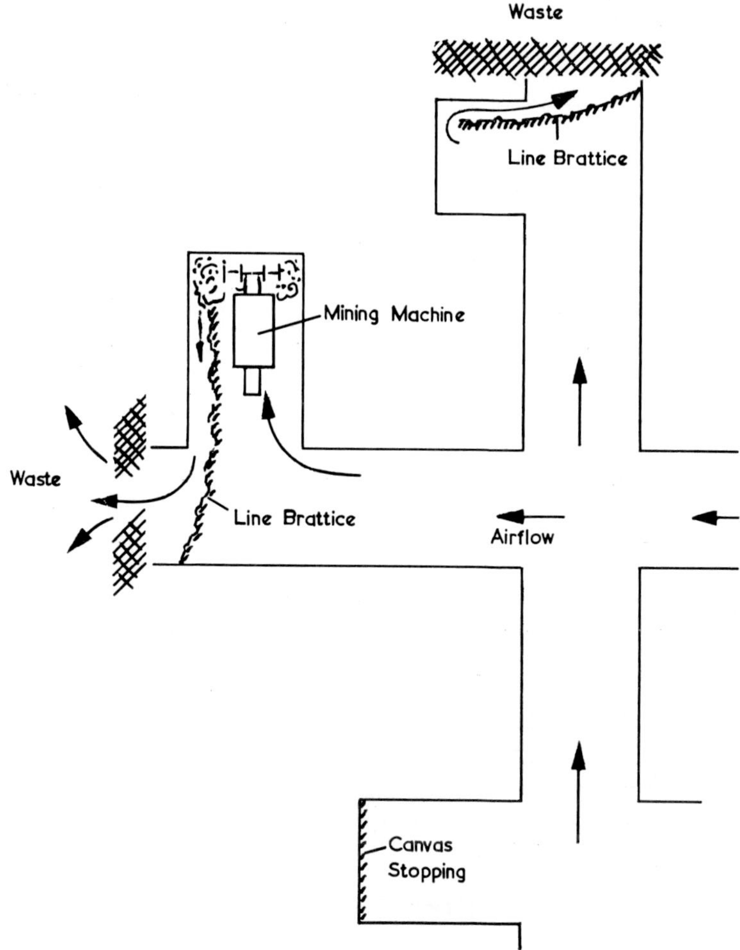

FIG. 6. Dust control by line brattice in room and pillar mining.

It will be appreciated that the greater the proportion of cross-section of the tunnel taken up by the mining machine, the higher will be the forward air velocity round the machine and the more effective the control of dust. This is particularly so if there is a bulkhead behind the cutting tools, as in some tunnel driving machines, where the cutting takes place in front of an advancing shield.

As an alternative to a "total exhaust" system an overlap arrangement (Hamilton, 1965; Breuer, 1969) may be used, as shown in Figure 7 (*b*). The basic method of ventilation is in this case by forcing air, which is

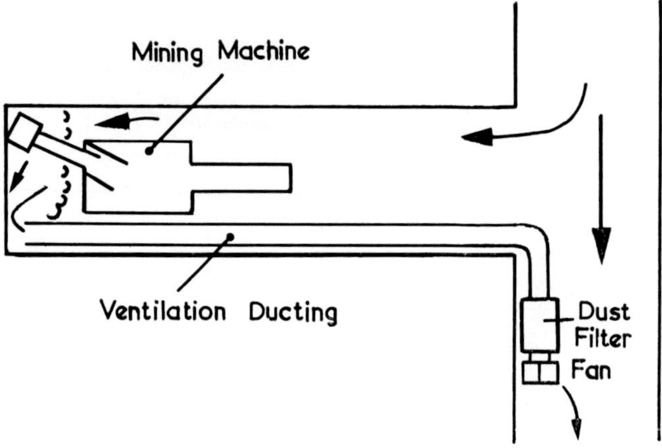

FIG. 7 (*a*). Dust control using ducted exhaust ventilation.

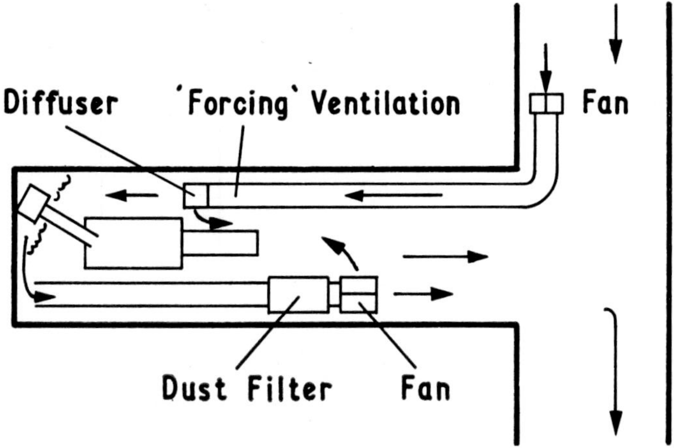

FIG. 7 (*b*). Overlap ventilation system for dust control.

carried in a duct terminated by a special "diffuser" with a variable area
shutter and annular baffles, to produce as far as possible uniform
"diffusion" of air out sideways. With the shutter open the heading may
be adequately ventilated by forcing air alone. A short exhaust system
is carried forward by the mining machine, and incorporates a dust filter.
When this is operated the shutter on the forcing diffuser is adjusted to
allow effective dust control by the exhaust system.

The "overlap" system is particularly useful in controlling dust at the
end of long tunnels—since the forcing air may be carried forward using

simple flexible ducting. It is also of value when the heading drivage is carried out in front of a bulkhead.

Exhaust ventilation and air cleaning can be used to control dust from localized sources such as rock crushers, loading plants and skip winding installations and has for many years been used in gold mining (Rees, 1947) and coal mining (Engels, 1961). It is necessary to enclose the dust source as far as possible, and the air extracted must be sufficient in volume to ensure a velocity entering the enclosure through any openings to be at least 0·5 metres/second–1·0 metres/second, 100–200 feet/minute.

An interesting application of exhaust ventilation on a different scale is the removal of drilling debris, including dust, either through hollow drill rods, or by use of a seal at the mouth of the drill hole. Percussive type rock drills are very suitable for this approach, since only fine debris is produced, and a compressed air driven ejector forms an effective suction device—dust collection is usually by a bag filter, which may be preceded by one or more cyclones, the whole being mounted in a portable container. This method of dust control is invaluable for such operations as drilling for roof-bolting, for here, as in other cases where the drill hole is rising, the use of water is unacceptable.

Experiments have been carried out in the control of dust from mining machines used in through ventilation currents, as in longwall coal mining. The difficulty here is that since the air velocities into an exhaust duct entry fall off rapidly with distance (thus at one duct diameter from the entry the air velocity is one tenth of that in the duct) there must in consequence be efficient shrouding of the dust-producing zone from the main ventilation, a requirement which usually interferes to some extent with the operation of the machine. Some success has however been achieved with this technique in controlling dust produced by roadway ripping machines.

Dust Filtration

A high proportion of the dust control by exhaust ventilation in mines is successfully carried out without any need for filtration, since the dusty air can often be released either into a large volume of "waste" as in room and pillar coal mining, or diluted into a high volume air stream. However, in some cases it may be desirable to ventilate working places in series, so that some form of dust filtration is necessary.

In coal mining the majority of filters used are of the wet scrubber type. These have the advantages of operating continuously without much maintenance, being safe in methane laden atmospheres and being somewhat smaller, although in the form normally used in mines, less efficient than conventional dry "bag" filters. A typical wet dust collector designed for mining is shown in Figure 8. Units such as this usually have a dust-water mixing stage, which may be, for example, a sprayed

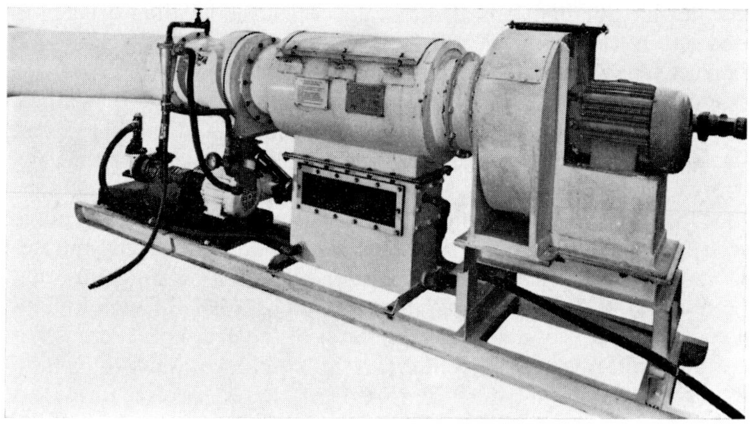

Fig. 8. A typical wet dust collector.

wire screen, or a form of venturi, and this is followed by a water removal system, typically of cyclone form.

A problem with any wet dust filter is that of dealing with the water, and most units are now fitted with some form of recirculation system. A very simple form of wet dust "filter" with no water removal system, but which can give an adequate performance in a coal mine, under certain conditions, consists merely of an axial flow fan fitted with an upwind water spray.

In hard rock mining the mass concentration of dust is normally lower than in coal mining, but more efficient removal of the very finest particles is required. Electrostatic precipitators may be used or alternatively high efficiency filters which incorporate either a shaking mechanism for cleaning the filter bags when no air is flowing or "reverse air jets" to dislodge the dust layers either continuously, or when sections of the unit are isolated in turn for cleaning. The fibre of which the filter bags are made may be natural, such as wool or cotton, or synthetic as for example terylene (dacron) or glass fibre, and the fabric is normally used in the form of sausage shaped bags or flat envelopes. Filters of this type can accept fairly low rates of airflow, ranging from 1·5 to 5 cubic metres/minute/square metre of filter area, and as a result are much larger than "wet" dust filters.

Another form of filter, which has obvious application to mining, uses either a plastic foam or synthetic fibre felt filtration medium. These materials are inexpensive and can tolerate air velocities through them of up to 1·5 metre/second, 300 feet/minute, so that they can be used in compact units and can either be cleaned, usually by washing after use, or thrown away. The efficiency of dust collection is lower than for cloth filters and more equivalent to that of wet scrubbers, but these materials have the advantage of tolerating moisture, unlike a closely woven cloth which blocks up under damp conditions. It is probable that in the next few years dust filters of this kind will find wide application for dust control in many types of mining.

Personal Protection

The prime object of dust control is to protect the individual, and although normally acceptable conditions can be obtained by the use of the various techniques described above, in some cases it may be desirable to provide miners with personal protection, particularly where they are exposed to high dust concentrations for short periods.

Dust respirators are described elsewhere in this book and there is no doubt that they can play a most important role in providing a measure of personal protection, better than can often be achieved by conventional dust control methods. Unfortunately they are uncomfortable to wear for long periods, and the protection of the man is dependent on his own action. It is doubtful also if the use of "life support suits" as described by Burgess (1970) and employed in nuclear energy installations, are practicable for mining conditions. However, the provision of clean air enclosures for men occupied as mining machine operators, who are not infrequently exposed to the highest dust concentrations, might well be feasible. Some work has already been carried out along these lines to protect men operating remote control consoles. The enclosure itself can be relatively simple; a small fan and dust filter carried on the mining machine itself supplies the clean air. There is little doubt that as all mining techniques become more highly mechanized and employ fewer men, such techniques must become increasingly important.

References

Bauer, H. D. (1970), "Tranken mit Calciumchloridzusatz, Eine moglichkeit zur Verbesserung der Trankwirkung." *Bergfreiheit*, **35**, 26.

Beadle, D. G. (1968), "Dust sampling and dust control in metalliferous mines." *Proceedings of First Australian Pneumoconiosis Conference*, p. 225. New South Wales Joint Coal Board, Sydney.

Breuer, H. (1969), "Problems der staubbekampfung bei der Betriebszusammenfassung." *Gluckauf*, **23**, 1158.

Burgess, W. A. (1970), "Life support systems." *Proceedings of Symposium on Respirable Coal Mine Dust*. p. 229. Information Circular 8458. U.S. Bureau of Mines, Washington.

Engels, L. H. (1961), "Installing and testing fixed filtration installations for underground use in coal mines." *Staub*, **21**. 315.

Evans, C. G. and Hamilton, R. J. (1964), "Production of dust by Anderton Shearers." *Colliery Guardian*, **209**, 445.

Hall, D. A. (1955), "Factors affecting airborne dust concentrations with special reference to the effects of ventilation." *Transactions Institute Mining Engineers*, **115**, 245.

Hamilton, R. J. (1965), "Control of dust in coal mines." *Mining Electrical and Mechanical Engineer*, **45**, 472.

Hamilton, R. J. and Knight, G. (1958), "Some studies of dust size distribution and the relationship between dust formation and coal strength." *Proceedings of Conference on non-Metallic Brittle Materials*. Butterworth Scientific Publications, London.

Hamilton, R. J. and Knight, G. (1964), "Laboratory studies of the suppression of dust from broken coal and shale." *International Journal of Rock Mechanics and Mining Sciences*, **1**, 105.

Hamilton, R. J., Levin, M. L. and McKinlay, K. W. (1962), "Research into the formation and suppression of dust by fast moving cutter picks." *Mining Engineer*, **21**, 590.

Hamilton, R. J. and McKinlay, K. W. (1961), "Dust suppression investigations." *Colliery Engineering*, **38**, 448.

Hodkinson, J. R. (1960), "Relation between ventilation airspeed and respirable airborne dust concentration in coal mines." *Colliery Engineering*, **37**, 236.

Jenkins, P. T. (1943), "Suppression of dust by system of water infusion." *Colliery Guardian*, **66**, 213.

Kingery, D. S., Doyle, H. N., Harris, E. J., Jacobson, M., Peluso, R. G., Shutack, J. B. and Schlick, D. P. (1969), "Studies on the control of respirable coal mine dust by ventilation." Mineral Industry Health Program, Technical Progress Report 19. U.S. Bureau of Mines, Washington.

Morse, K. M. (1970), "Dust control practices in the bituminous coal mining industry." *American Industrial Hygiene Association Journal*, **31**, 160.

Rees, J. P. (1947), "Development of silicosis suppression methods on the Witwatersrand: ventilation and dust suppression." *Proceedings at 1947 Conference in London on Silicosis Prevention and Dust Suppression in Mines*, p. 112. Institute of Mining Engineers, London.

Robinson, R. (1961), "Ventilating and dust extraction with the Joy continuous miner at Easington Colliery." *Mining Engineer*, **9**, 718.

Schramm, G. (1961), "Reduction of the dust content of mine airs during blasting when using water as stemming material." *Bergbau Technik*, **11**, 260.

Walton, W. H. and Woolcock, A. (1960), "The suppression of airborne dust by water spray." *Aerodynamic Capture of Particles*, p. 129, ed. E. D. Richardson. Pergamon Press, London.

Chapter 9

The Measurement of Airborne Dust

Introduction

The health hazard of airborne dust in mining is now generally recognised, and most countries with substantial mining industries have established dust 'standards' either by law or by agreement. Such standards are usually derived from consideration of past experience and observed relationships between dust concentrations and disease incidence, having regard to the lowest dust levels which can be obtained by good practice. There is no finite level of dust concentration which will ensure zero retention, but the aim of dust standards must be that a workman will not be seriously affected in a normal working life-span.

Measurements of dust concentration are required to ensure compliance with these dust standards, for the assessment of the exposure of individuals, and to aid the development of methods of dust control. A dust sampling technique should be used in which the parameter of dust concentration measured is related to the health hazard and the samples obtained should be truly representative of the airborne dust cloud.

Numerous methods of dust measurement have been used at various times in different countries since 1905, the year when dust control was imposed by law in the South African gold mines. At first dusty air was simply aspirated through a filter and the dust which was collected was weighed, no account being taken of particle size or composition. It is doubtful if the early collecting devices effectively retained the finer particles. Later, in 1913, McCrae showed that it was very fine dust particles that caused silicosis, and in 1915 Collis identified crystalline silica (quartz, flint) as being the most injurious of all dusts. Mavrogordato (1929) considered that particles with a diameter less than 5 microns (μm) were associated with disease. This early recognition that measurements should be directed towards a particular fraction of the dust led to the development of new sampling procedures. Methods have continued to evolve and to provide a better index of the hazard, in parallel with improved understanding of the disease process.

Free crystalline silica in the form of quartz constitutes more than 10 per cent of the earth's crust and is present in most mine dust clouds; it stands alone among common mineral dusts encountered in mining in having high toxicity to alveolar phagocytes and producing a strong pathogenic reaction. Hence it is not surprising that acceptance that other mineral dusts may cause lung disease came tardily. Indeed it was not until 1943 that coalworkers' pneumoconiosis was made a compensable industrial disease in Great Britain. Coal and the silicate dusts when retained in the lungs cause comparatively little fibrosis (asbestos is a notable exception), although when they are present in sufficient quantity they can produce significant lesions—these are discussed in other chapters. Finally, recent work reported by Robock and Klosterkötter (1971) and Schlipköter, Hilscher, Pott and Beck (1971) has indicated that quartz itself may vary in toxicity, and that the presence of other minerals may inhibit its activity. The uncertainty concerning the relative contributions of different minerals, especially of quartz, to the hazard of mixed dusts has been one major reason for the differences between methods of dust assessment used in different countries.

The Physical Principles of Dust Measurement

A dust sampling instrument almost always consists of some form of pump or aspirator which draws a known quantity of air through a dust collecting device. The overriding consideration which governs the design of sampling instruments is the chosen method of analysis of the collected dust. One of the three basic parameters of dust concentration may be studied: the number of particles, the surface area of the dust, or the mass of dust, in a measured volume of air.

Dust Count Assessment

It is not surprising that until recently a very high proportion of all measurements of dust in mines was made in terms of the number concentration, since the importance of the very fine particles in the aetiology of silicosis was recognised, and there were obvious practical advantages in having instruments which sampled only small volumes of air. Moreover, the microscope was a readily available scientific tool.

The original 'dust-count' instrument development by Kotze in 1916 (Union of South Africa, 1937), the Konimeter, is still used in modified form, in, for example, South Africa, Canada, Germany and Poland. This instrument collects dust from a small volume of air, almost instantaneously, and the dust particles with a diameter less than 5 microns are counted by low power microscopy. Later dust-count instruments are the Impinger (Greenburg and Smith, 1922), the Owens Jet (Owens, 1922), the Thermal Precipitator (Green and Watson, 1935), the Long-Running Thermal Precipitator (Hamilton, 1956). With the exception of the Impinger, in which the particles are dispersed in a liquid, the dust collected by all these instruments is deposited on glass slides or cover slips. A recent development has been the collection of dust on 'membrane' filters; the filter material is rendered transparent to facilitate dust evaluation by microscopical counting. For evaluation, the filter is wetted on both sides with an oil of matching refractive index (e.g. glycerine triacetate), sandwiched between a microscope slide and cover slip, and counted by microscope using a 4 mm objective. The optical quality of the specimen is inferior to that of thermal precipitator samples. The method is particularly useful for measuring fibrous asbestos dust, for which phase-contrast microscopy is desirable (Addingley, 1966). Membrane filters are also suitable for gravimetric sampling.

Dust counting by microscope is tedious and subject to considerable personal bias; counts of the same sample by different observers may vary widely unless careful precautions are taken (Holdsworth, Price and Tomlinson, 1954). This problem is in part associated with the question whether particle clumps should be counted as single particles or a number; also artificial clumping may occur if too many particles are deposited together. When counting takes place in a liquid (as in samples from the Impinger) the natural clumps are broken up and the count is quite different from that obtained from a thermal precipitator slide.

The majority of dust-count instruments are short period samplers; the Long Running Thermal Precipitator, however, is designed to sample over a working shift.

Gravimetric Assessment

A growing weight of evidence has suggested that the hazard of the dust collected in the lungs is best reflected by its mass. Mavrogordato (1939–40) concluded that the number and size of particles comprising the mass of fibrosis producing dust were of no particular significance, and although there have been suggestions that the toxic action of quartz is a surface phenomenon and that therefore the most appropriate measurement for this mineral is the surface area of the 'respirable' particles (Orenstein, 1960), subsequent animal experiments with quartz dust of various particle sizes (Goldstein and Webster, 1966) showed that the mass of quartz dust correlates at least as well as its surface area with fibrosis production. For coal dust Bedford and Warner (1943) considered that the mass of particles finer than 5 microns gave the best measure of hazard; a result more recently confirmed by post mortem studies of mineworkers' lungs (Rossiter, Rivers, Bergman, Casswell and Nagelschmidt, 1967) and by epidemiological research studies (Jacobsen, Rae, Walton and Rogan, 1970) in which correlations were demonstrated between the mass of lung dust and the radiological category of pneumoconiosis, and between the concentration of respirable dust and the progression of disease among the exposed population. The use of a mass parameter was also advocated by the pneumoconiosis conference arranged by the World Health Organisation in Katowice (1968).

The Selective Sampling of Respirable Dust

Most dust clouds in mines, and particularly those in coal mines, contain a proportion of particles coarser than those deposited in the lungs, and it is therefore usually necessary to segregate in some way the respirable fraction from the gross airborne sample. Indeed this is essential when the mass of respirable dust is to be measured.

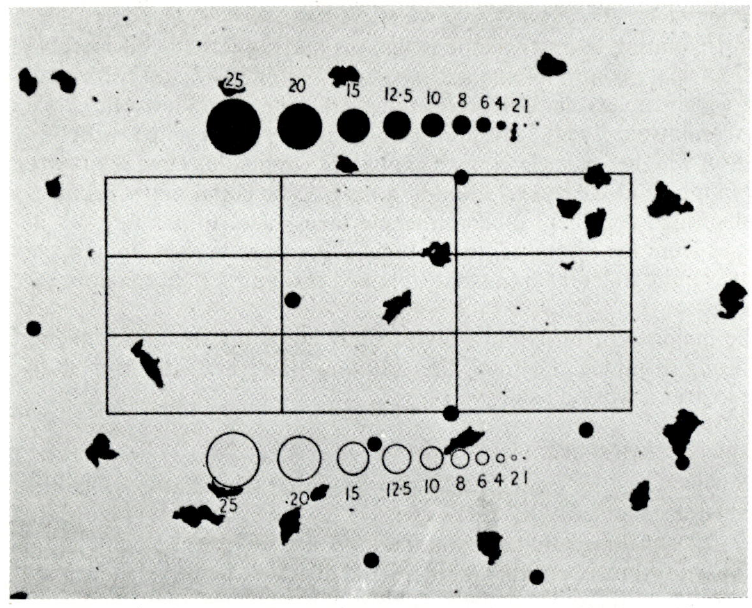

FIG. 1.   A photomicrograph, with graticules, of a 'conifuge' sample showing coal dust particles and spheres of density 1·4 g/cm³, all having the same falling speed (Hamilton, 1954).

Whether or not an airborne particle penetrates into the lungs depends on its falling speed in air, and this in turn depends on its size, shape, density and degree of aggregation. The relationship between particle size and falling speed has been studied in some detail (Timbrell, 1954; Hamilton, 1954), and coal particles and spheres of equal falling speed are shown in Fig. 1: the irregular coal dust may have diameters as great as three times that of a sphere of equal falling speed and intrinsic density. Fibres, such as those of asbestos, have falling speeds almost independent of their length, but related only to their diameter (Timbrell, 1965)—a feature which explains the presence of asbestos fibres up to 100 μm in length in lungs.

It is clearly desirable to incorporate in the sampling instrument an 'artificial nose' in which the selection of the respirable fraction can take place, simulating the action of the human nose and upper respiratory passages. A simple method of obtaining such a selection is by drawing the dust laden air through a horizontal rectangular section channel in which dust settles out under streamline flow conditions (Walton, 1954; Hamilton and Walton, 1961). The British Medical Research Council panels in 1952 (Hamilton and Walton, 1961) specified a selection curve for respirable dust based on the performance of a horizontal elutriator of this type. This recommended selection curve does not allow the penetration of any particles with falling speeds greater than that of a 7·1 μm sphere of unit density (that is, greater than 1·5 mm/s) and 50 per cent penetration of particles of falling speed equal to that of 5 μm spheres of unit density (0·75 mm/s).

The Medical Research Council panels' recommendations were endorsed by the 1959 Johannesburg International Conference on Pneumoconiosis (Orenstein, 1960). A somewhat different selection curve, based on the use of a cyclone pre-selector, was proposed by the United States Atomic Energy Commission (Lippman and Harris, 1962)— this provided 100 per cent acceptance of 1μm unit density spheres, 50 per cent at 3·5 μm, and complete rejection for all particles of falling speed greater than 10 μm unit density spheres. Cyclones had also been used previously in Germany, but with an even finer selection curve (Breuer, 1961). The Medical Research Council/Johannesburg selection curve for spheres of unit density is shown in Fig. 2, together with the U.S. A.E.C. curve, in comparison with the alveolar deposition curve of Brown, Cook, Ney and Hatch (1950). Fig. 3 illustrates how the separation of coal dust, in terms of particle diameter, differs from the curve for unit density spheres, due to the shape factor effects depicted in Fig. 1.

New dust standards, based on the mass concentration of respirable dust according to the MRC/Johannesburg selection curve were established for coal mines in Britain in April 1970 (Jacobsen *et al.*, 1970; Jacobsen, Rae, Walton and Rogan, 1971) and in the U.S.A. from June 1970 (Schlick, 1971). The technique is also attracting increasing interest elsewhere, for example, in West Germany (Breuer, 1971) and Czechoslovakia (Kubālek and Šimeček, 1968).

Compositional Analysis

Knowledge of the pathological effects of different minerals has encouraged the development of analytical techniques for the measurement of dust composition. Detailed mineralogical analysis is usually preceded by incineration to remove carbonaceous material. (In several countries the dust standard for coal mines is adjusted for the ash content.) In metal mines the ash is usually washed with acid to remove soluble minerals derived from the water used for dust suppression.

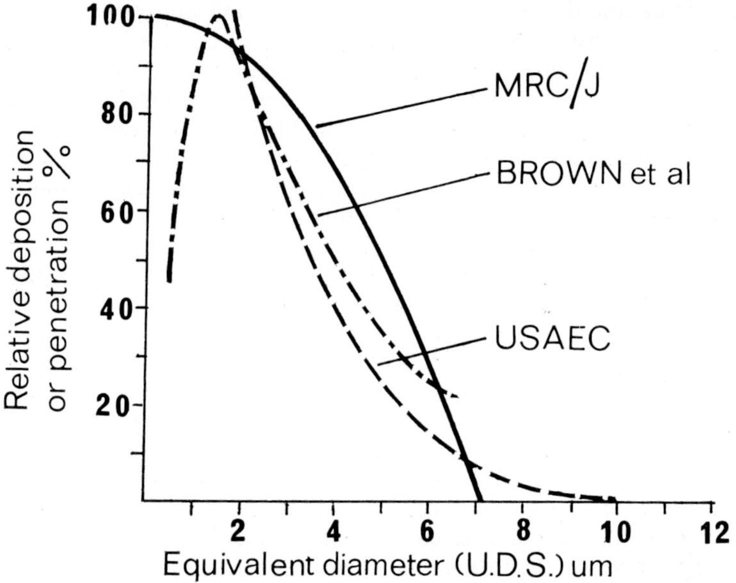

FIG. 2. Medical Research Council/Johannesburg and U.S.A.E.C. selection curves for respirable dust in comparison with the alveolar deposition curve of Brown *et al.* (1950).

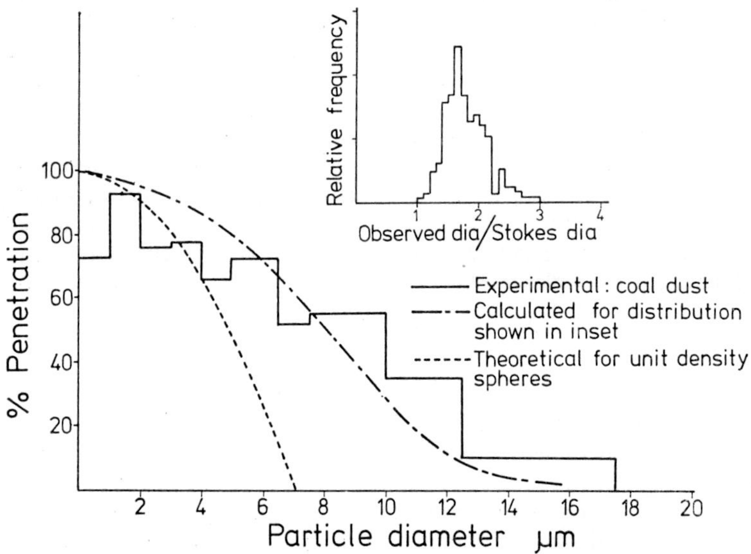

FIG. 3. Selection curve for respirable coal dust compared with unit density spheres (After Hamilton and Walton, 1961).

The proportion of free silica in respirable dust is, of course, of particular importance and has been incorporated into a number of mine dust standards (Walton, 1970).

Chemical Methods

Classical chemical methods were first adapted for dust analysis, the measurement of free silica being determined in rather large samples of ashed dust (100-500 mg) digested with phosphoric acid (Talvitie, 1951). Recently the sensitivity of the technique has been improved by such means as colorimetric determination (Talvitie, 1964), allowing the use of as little as 2 mg of ashed dust, and by emission spectroscopy or atomic absorption analysis by elemental assay. For example, Kennan and Lynch (1970) describe the use of the last named method, using magnesium assay, for the measurement of chrysotile asbestos in dust samples weighing less than 0·1 milligram.

Physical Methods

Physical methods of analysis are now widely employed, and provide in general greater sensitivity than chemical methods, although sometimes particle size effects are important, requiring the grinding of dust to below 5 μm: selective sampling of respirable dust however, usually eliminates this need. X-ray diffraction is usually regarded as the standard method for the analysis of a wide range of crystalline minerals (Klug and Alexander, 1954), allowing mineral identification by the position of the diffraction peaks produced by X-ray scattering, and quantitive determination by the measurement of peak intensity. Gordon, Griffin and Nagelschmidt (1952) described the use of X-ray diffraction for quartz determination in coal mine dust, and Crable and Knott (1966) its application in the analysis of asbestos dust. Although originally X-ray diffraction required dust samples weighing several milligrams, recent refinements of technique allow the use of samples weighing less than 1 milligram (Talvitie and Brewer, 1962).

Infra-red spectrophotometry (Hunt, Wisherd and Bonham, 1950) in which the absorption of infra-red radiation at specific wavelengths is measured is used for the determination of quartz (Gade and Luft, 1963) and of kaoline and mica (Dodgson, Hadden, Jones and Walton, 1971). Samples of dust below 1 milligram in weight are incorporated in discs of potassium bromide—the technique is simple and apparatus relatively inexpensive. However, problems can arise due to interference between the absorption bands of different minerals. Differential thermal analysis consists of the study of the cooling curves of thermally active minerals in comparison with those of an inert substance such as alumina. The technique has the disadvantage of requiring large

II

samples of dust, although Weiss, Boettner, Stenning and Arbor (1970) describe a method using sample weights as low as 50 milligrams. Neutron activation techniques, involving the measurement of X-ray activity of dust, in comparison with that of similarly treated standards, induced by irradiation with neutrons in a reactor, are very accurate and sensitive. Morgan and Holmes (1969) describe the use of this method in the characterisation of asbestos dust.

Microscopical Methods

Identification of quartz and various other mineral particles may be made by their colour when examined by dark field (Dodge, 1948), phase contrast (Schmidt, 1955) and interference microscopy (Dodgson, 1963) after immersion in liquids of high optical dispersion (Crossman, 1949). These techniques are, however, subjective and liable to the errors inherent in ordinary microscope counting and sizing of dust. Electron microscopy can be used for the identification of very small particles and fibres, employing either electron diffraction or X-ray microprobe analysis; in the latter case by analysis of the characteristic x-radiation excited by an electron beam (Kay, 1965). The identification of asbestos fibres by this method has also been carried out (Pooley, Oldham, Chang-Hyun and Wagner, 1969).

Dust Sampling Instruments

The Konimeter

Present-day forms of this instrument are similar in the principle of their operation to the original Kotze model. The standard German Konimeter is illustrated schematically in Fig. 4. Release of the spring-loaded piston of a small pump draws a $5\ cm^3$ sample of air into the instrument through a small-diameter (0·5 mm) orifice. The incoming high-velocity jet of dust laden air impinges on a glass plate coated with adhesive, giving a 'spot' of dust particles which can be examined and counted microscopically, usually by light field illumination at × 200 magnification. Some models have a built-in microscope. 30 samples can be taken on one circular plate, which can be rotated to bring different positions under the jet orifice, or the dust spots under the microscope. South African practice is to incinerate and wash the slides in acid before microscope evaluation under dark field illumination (Transvaal Chamber of Mines, 1947).

The konimeter has a low collection efficiency for particles below 1 μm in diameter. Aggregate particles tend to be disrupted in the jet and large particles may bounce off the slide or be shattered, thus giving a spurious high count of small particles—this may be alleviated by using an adhesive film of vaseline of appropriate thickness (Hamilton,

Wainwright and Walton, 1951). It is a convenient instrument for rapid assessment of dust in mine air but it is unsuited for accurate estimation of mean concentrations.

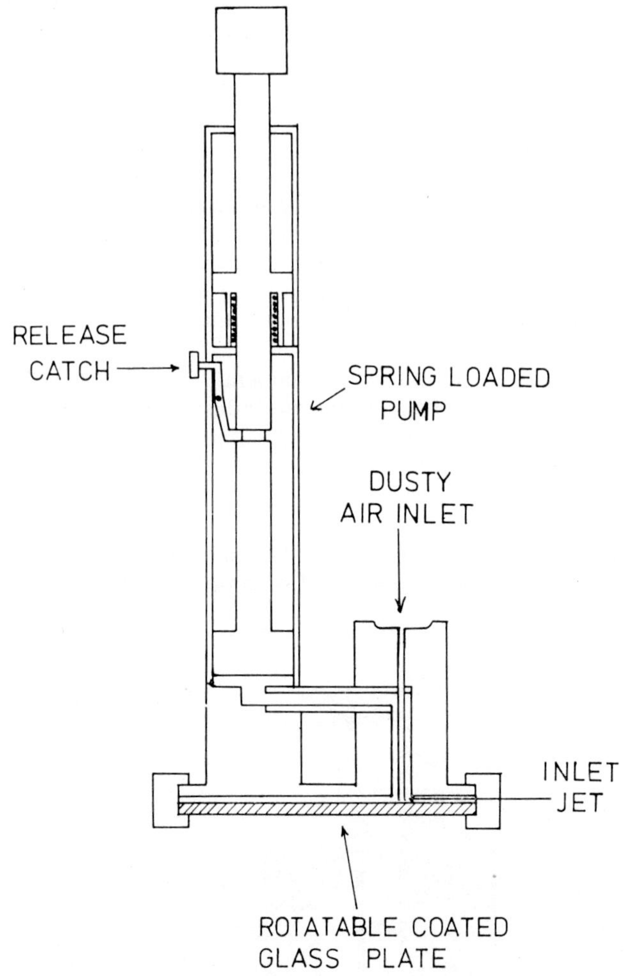

Fig. 4. Diagram of Konimeter.

The Impinger

The instrument hitherto generally used for dust measurements in the United States is the midget impinger (Littlefield, Feicht and Schrenk, 1937).

The air sample enters through a central glass tube which terminates in a 1 mm diameter jet situated 5 mm from the base of an outer glass vessel containing water, isopropyl alcohol or other suitable liquid. Particles are collected by impaction on the constantly wetted floor of the outer vessel, and accumulate in suspension in the liquid. The source of suction is commonly a hand pump with crank handle, or a mechanically driven pump. Particles are counted in liquid, on the floor of a 1 mm deep haemocytometer cell after allowing at least 30 minutes settlement time. Samples should be counted within 36 hours after collection.

The collection efficiency of the impinger is poor for particles smaller than 1 μm diameter and the settlement of such particles in the counting cell may be incomplete. There may be some shatter of large particles. Aggregate particles are dispersed in the liquid and a proportion of the fine particles counted may have been airborne as constituents of large non-respirable particles. The sampling time is flexible and may be up to several hours and the samples can be diluted before evaluation to give a suitable concentration of particles in the counting cell.

The threshold limit values for mineral dusts published by the American Conference of Governmental Industrial Hygienists (1970) are presently expressed in millions of particles per ft^3, measured by impinger, though a change to gravimetric units is probable.

The Thermal Precipitator

The sampling head of the Standard Thermal Precipitator (Green and Watson, 1935) is shown in Fig. 5a. The sampled air is drawn vertically

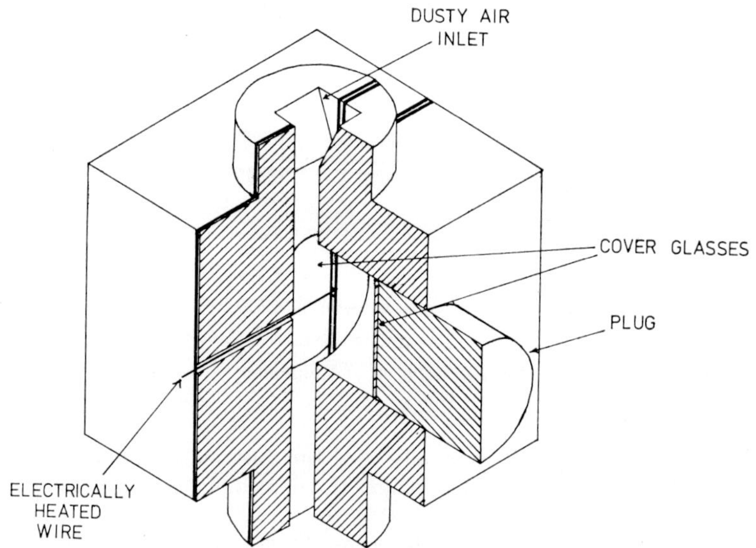

Fig. 5a. Diagram of Standard Thermal Precipitator Head.

downwards through a narrow channel, between two microscope cover glasses. Stretched horizontally and centrally across this channel is an electrically heated wire, and as the dust-laden air passes between it and the cover glasses, differential molecular bombardment in the thermal gradient causes the particles to be deposited on the glasses. The deposits are evaluated microscopically, usually with a 2 mm oil immersion objective.

The sampling rate of the thermal precipitator is 7 cm³/min. The instrument is provided with a water aspirator and powered electrically by a miners cap-lamp battery with controls in the battery top. It is safe for use in gassy mines. A sampling time of about half an hour is typical, depending on the dust concentration.

The outstanding feature of the thermal precipitator is that it samples particles less than about 10 μm in size with 100 per cent efficiency (thermal deposition becomes more effective the smaller the particle size) and without breakage or disruption of aggregates. With minor modifications it is suitable for electron-microscope studies of sub-micron particles (Walton, 1947). At the large-size end of the spectrum beyond the respirable size range errors arise from the combined effects (which compensate one another to some extent) of gravitational fall-in of particles and failure of the thermal forces to cause deposition. Like most other dust counting instruments, thermal precipitator dust deposits are subject to particle overlap if too dense, with consequent underestimation of the concentration (Roach, 1959). This was not fully appreciated in much early work with the instrument. The thermal precipitator was for many years the standard dust measuring instrument used in British coal mines, but was superseded by the M.R.E. gravimetric dust sampler (*vide infra*) in 1970.

The South African Modified Thermal Precipitator (Kitto and Beadle, 1952) operates on the same principle as the standard instrument, but the heated wire is supported on an insulating block so that only a single dust deposit, on one side of the wire, is obtained. Deposition takes place on a 75 mm × 25 mm glass slide which can be moved to different positions to accommodate up to 12 samples at one loading. The horizontal air entrance channel is designed to exclude, by settlement, particles larger than 10 μm diameter. A mechancial aspirator is provided. The modified thermal precipitator has been widely used for investigatory work in South African gold mines, and is used for routine dust sampling in the coal mines. In this latter application the samples are assessed by their light obscuration, measured photo-electrically (Beadle, 1954; Kitson and Winer, 1960).

Another variant is the Long Running Thermal Precipitator (Hamilton, 1956) shown in Fig. 5b. Like the South African instrument, it gives a single deposit and has an entrance channel designed to exclude large particles—in this case in accordance with the MRC/Johannesburg selection curve. The slide is horizontal and the dust passes over an area where first there is gravitational deposition of particles before they reach the heated wire. There the residual small particles are collected by thermal deposition. The sample is thus spread out over a length of about 12 mm within which there is a large measure of particle size segregation. These features simplify the counting and diminish particle overlap. The electrically driven linear reciprocating pump draws air in

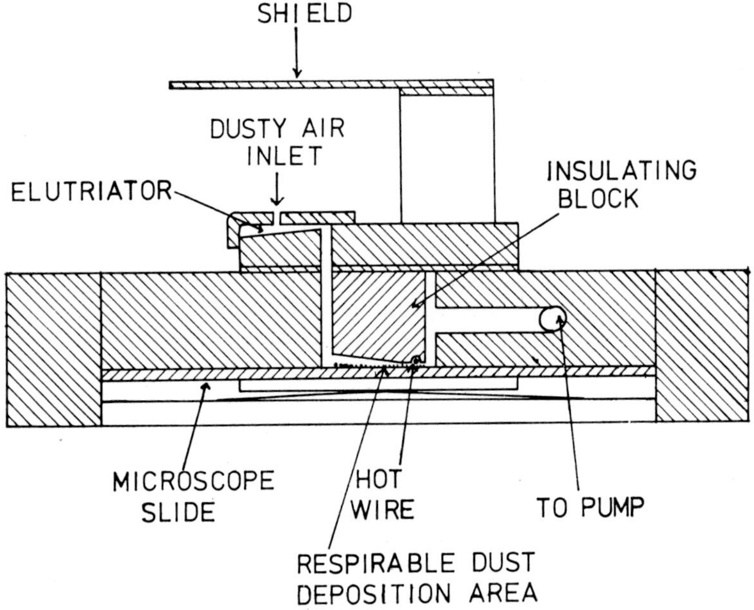

FIG. 5b. Diagram of Long Running Thermal Precipitator.

only in alternate half-minutes, which further increases the possible duration of the sample. Under normal conditions the instrument will operate satisfactorily over an eight-hour shift; the mean sampling rate is 2 cm³/min.

Membrane Filters Samplers

The introduction of micro-porous membrane filters (of cellulose ester, polyvinyl chloride and similar materials) with a variety of pore sizes down to less than 1 μm simplified dust sampling by particle counting techniques. The particles can be counted in situ on the filter after rendering the material transparent with a suitable medium. A number of instruments are now available which consist mainly of a filter holder, a pump or aspirator, and an airflow meter. An advantage of this type of instrument is that the airflow rate, and the filter size, can be chosen to suit a wide variety of requirements of concentration and sampling time.

The Tyndalloscope

This instrument consists of a chamber into which dusty air passes, a light source and a photometer. The intensity of light scattered by the airborne particles is compared with that of light from a reference source. A measurement of concentration related to the surface area of the dust is obtained, but corrections for the composition of the particles are necessary (rock and coal particles of the same size give a different response) and aerosols such as diesel fumes also affect its accuracy. The Tyndalloscope is in common use in Germany, Japan and Sweden.

A light scattering measurement technique has obvious attractions for continuous monitoring of airborne dust concentrations in mining and various instruments are now being developed for this purpose.

The Hexhlet Selective Gravimetric Sampler

The Hexhlet sampler (Wright, 1954), shown in Fig. 6, was the first to incorporate a horizontal elutriator size selector designed to the Medical Research Council specification (Walton, 1954; Hamilton and Walton, 1961). The original version operated at a flow rate of 100 l/min, but this was subsequently reduced to 50 l/min to avoid the risk of some settled particles being removed from the elutriator plates by the high velocity air (Hamilton and Walton, 1961). Suction is by a compressed air ejector and the flow is controlled by a critical orifice. It is suitable for use in mines where compressed air is available and a relatively large sample is required. A very similar instrument has been developed in Germany (Landwehr, 1962).

The MRE Gravimetric Dust Sampler (Type 113A)

This portable gravimetric sampler, seen in Fig. 7, was developed at the National Coal Board's Mining Research Establishment (Dunmore, Hamilton and Smith, 1964) and has been adopted as the standard dust sampling instrument for coal mines in Britain (Chamberlain, Makower and Walton, 1971) and the United States (Schlick, 1971). It is provided with an MRC/Johannesburg elutriator, and samples at 2·5 l/min for an 8 hour shift. It is powered by a rechargeable electric battery; the weight is 4·3 kg. The respirable dust penetrating the elutriator is collected on a glass-fibre or membrane filter for weighing and analysis. The instrument is intrinsically safe for use in atmospheres containing methane.

Gravimetric Samplers with Cyclone Size Selectors

Cyclone dust separators are well-known in industry (McCormick, Lucas and Wells, 1963) and miniature designs have been used by a

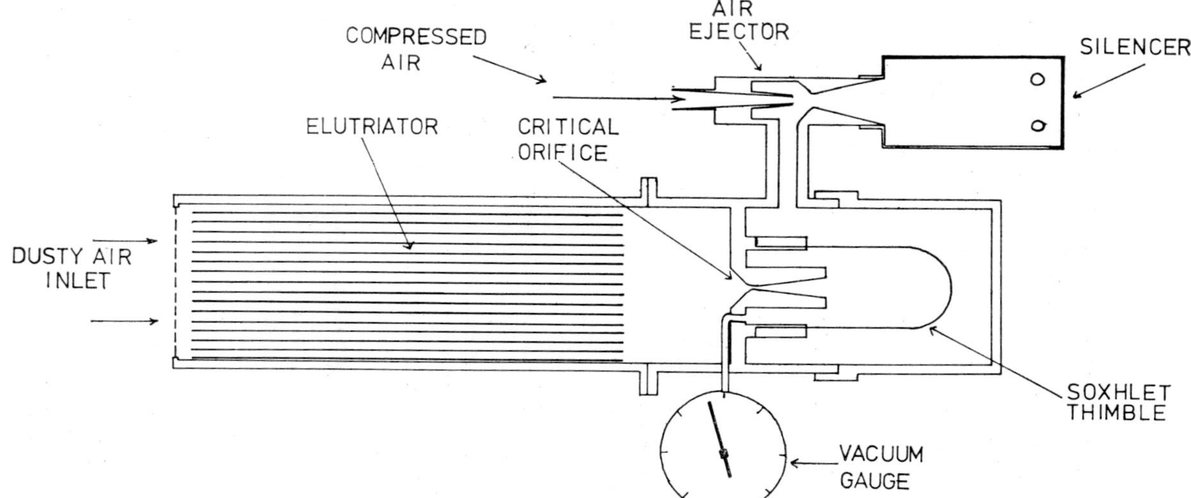

Fig. 6. Diagram of Hexhlet Sampler.

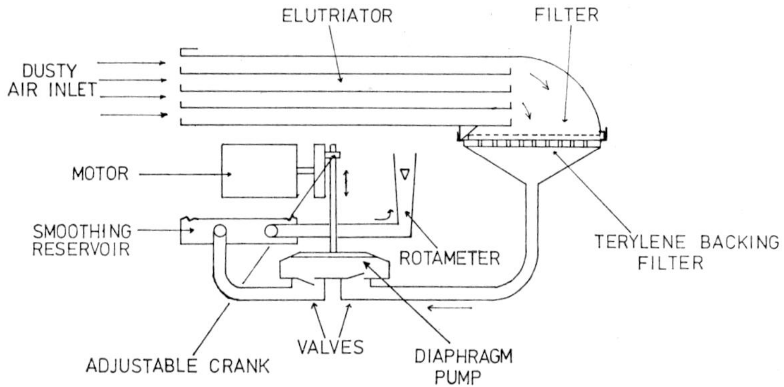

Fig. 7. Diagram of M.R.E. Gravimetric Sampler.

number of workers as size selectors for dust sampling instruments. In the cyclone, illustrated in Fig. 8a, air enters a cylindrical chamber tangentially and follows an inwards spiral path with increasing velocity as it approaches the axis before escaping through a smaller diameter axial outlet tube. Large particles are removed from the air stream by centrifugal force and collect in a receptacle at the bottom of the lower conical section of the cyclone chamber. Respirable dust penetrating the cyclone is collected on a filter. The cyclone is smaller than the equivalent elutriator and its orientation is not critical. It is, however, an empirical device and, unlike the elutriator, its performance cannot be precisely calculated. The selection curve is characteristically of the form shown in Fig. 8b, and differs from the elutriator curve in having a long 'tail' instead of a sharp cut-off. A cyclone has been designed to simulate as far as possible the performance of the MRC/Johannesburg elutriator (Higgins and Dewell, 1967) and has also been incoporated in the 'Simpeds' sampling instrument designed for mine use (Harris and Maguire, 1968; Maguire, Barker and Badel, 1971). In this instrument, the motor and pump are contained in the upper compartment of a miner's cap-lamp battery and the sampling head comprising cyclone and membrane filter is attached to the lamp worn on the miner's helmet. Personal samplers for colliery use, incorporating cyclones simulating the Atomic Energy Commission selection curve (Lippmann and Harris, 1962) are being widely used in United States coal mines. Cyclone instruments operating at higher flow rates, powered by compressed air ejectors, have been developed in Germany (Breuer, 1961; 1971).

The Errors and Statistical Aspects of Dust Sampling

The measurement of dust concentrations in mining is subject to a number of errors. Briefly these are connected with (1) the design and operation of the instrument and the evaluation of the sample, (2) the spatial variability of the dust clouds in the mine, and (3) the variation of dust concentration with time.

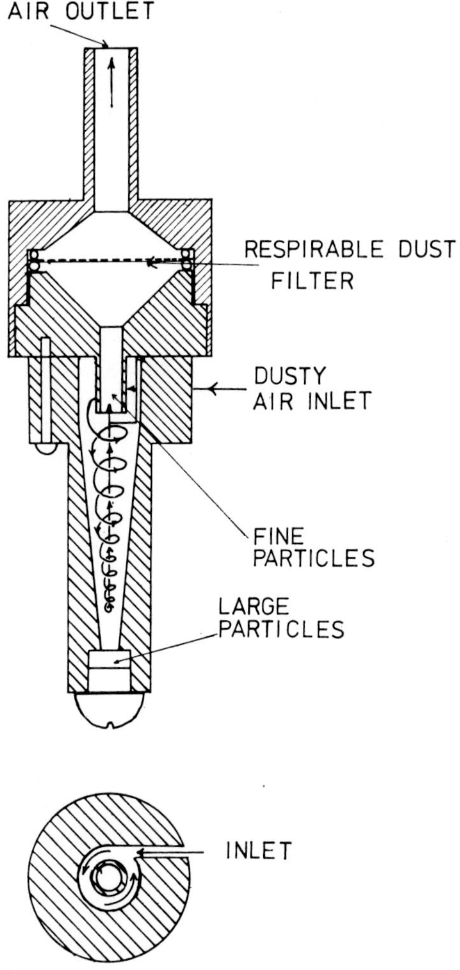

Fig. 8a. Diagram of a Cyclone Sampler.

Instrumental and evaluation errors begin with the problem of obtaining a representative sample of dust from a moving airstream. A sampling orifice, pointing into an airstream, will sample correctly only if the air speed into the orifice is equal to that outside (iso-kinetic sampling). If the sampling air speed is lower than the external airspeed, there will be some oversampling, and if higher some undersampling. A sampling orifice pointing across an airstream will always tend to undersample. Particles in the respirable size range, with very low falling speeds in air, are much less affected by these sampling errors than coarser dusts, but nevertheless great care must be taken if the external air speed is high (more than 4 m/s), particularly in gravimetric measurement.

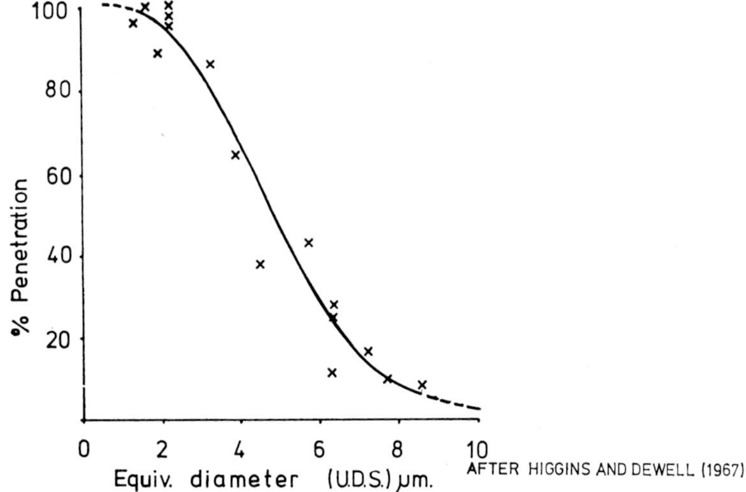

FIG. 8b. Selection curve for Cyclone Sampler.

The errors of particle sizing and counting by microscopy have already been discussed; experience with thermal precipitators suggests that a single dust sample has a standard deviation of no better than 20 per cent, and that unless great care is taken in training the observers, errors can be much greater than this. There is little doubt that gravimetric evaluation of dust concentration is far more accurate, provided the weight of sample collected and the accuracy of the balance used are compatible. For example, a sample weighing 1–5 mg may be measured easily with an accuracy of, say, 2 per cent, provided reasonable precautions are taken to avoid errors due to changes in the moisture content of the collecting filter. Glass fibre paper filters and polyvinyl chloride membrane filters are very little affected by changes in atmospheric humidity.

The problem of measuring the dust concentration to which the individual miner is exposed can be solved by the use of a 'personal' sampling instrument, with its dust inlet in the breathing zone; with this technique worker co-operation is essential.

The Duration and Frequency of Sampling

With the understanding that the hazard of dust is related to the product of concentration and time of exposure, there has been a move to longer sampling periods; dust is now most commonly measured over the working shift. The introduction of gravimetric sampling and in particular of personal sampling instruments has largely coincided with this development. The use of 'snap' sampling instruments such as the konimeter and tyndalloscope or short period samplers such as the thermal precipitator to measure the shift average concentrations, although often practised, is unduly laborious.

Periods of sampling shorter than the full working shift may be desirable in order to study the operation of dust control measures, and to investigate dust concentration patterns during the shift. The simultaneous deployment of a number of sampling instruments to examine the pattern of dust concentration is also a necessary feature of dust control work.

The frequency of dust sampling must be taken into account. In coal mines, for example, the day to day coefficient of variation of shift-mean concentration for a given coal face is about 30 per cent, so that it makes a marked difference whether a dust standard is intended as a value not to be exceeded on any day, or relates to the average over a number of days.

In conclusion, it will be clear that there is a great diversity of dust sampling techniques in use in different countries and mining industries which provide indices of varying merit of the dust hazard. The procedures and standards used in a number of countries have been summarised by Walton (1970).

For a variety of reasons of which perhaps the ability to make epidemiological comparisons is the most important, it is to be hoped that an increasing measure of uniformity will be attained in future.

References

Addingley, C. G. (1966), "Asbestos dust and its measurements." *The Annals of Occupational Hygiene*, **9**, 73.

American Conference of Governmental Industrial Hygienist (1970), "Threshold limit values for airborne contaminants." *American Conference of Governmental Industrial Hygienists, Cincinnati.*

Beadle, D. G. (1954), "A photo-electric apparatus for assessing dust samples." *Journal of the Chemical, Metallurgical and Mining Society of South Africa*, **55**, 30.

Bedford, T. and Warner, C. G. (1943), Medical Research Council Special Report Series No. 244. H.M.S.O., London

Breuer, H. (1961), "A filter device for selective sampling of respirable fine dust in coal mines." In *Inhaled Particles and Vapours*, II, p. 453, ed. C. N. Davies. Pergamon Press, Oxford.

Breuer, H. (1971), "Problems of gravimetric dust sampling." In *Inhaled Particles*, III, ed. W. H. Walton, p. 1031. Unwin, London.

Brown, J. H., Cook, K. M., Ney, F. G. and Hatch, T. (1950), "Influence of particle size upon the retention of particulate matter in the lung." *American Journal Public Health*, **40**, 450.

Chamberlain, E. A. C., Makower, A. A. and Walton, W. H. (1971), "New gravimetric dust standards and sampling procedures for British coalmines." In *Inhaled Particles*, III, ed. W. H. Walton, p. 1015. Unwin, London.

Collis, E. L. (1915), "Industrial pneumoconioses, with special reference to dust-phthisis." *Public Health*, August, 252–264, September, 292–305, October, 11–20, November, 37–41.

Crable, J. V. and Knott, M. J. (1966), "Application of X-ray diffraction to the determination of chrysotile in bulk on settled dust samples." *American Industrial Hygiene Association Journal*, **27**, 383.

Crossman, G. C. (1949), "Determination of free silica by dispersion staining microscopical methods." *Journal of Optical Society of America*, **38**, 417.

Dodge, N. B. (1948), "The dark-field color immersion method." *American Mineralogist*, **33**, 541.

Dodgson, J. (1963), "Use of interference microscopy for the mineralogical analysis of samples of airborne dust obtained with thermal precipitator." *Nature*, **199**, 245.

Dodgson, J., Hadden, G. G., Jones, C. O. and Walton, W. H. (1971), "Characteristics of the airborne dust in British coalmines." In *Inhaled Particles*, III, ed. W. H. Walton, p. 757. Unwin, London.

Dunmore, J. H., Hamilton, R. J. and Smith, D. S. G. (1964), "An instrument for the sampling of respirable dust for subsequent gravimetric assessment." *Journal of Scientific Instruments*, **41**, 669.

Gade, M. and Luft, K. F. (1963), "Die ultra rot spektroskopishe quartz bestimmung insbesondere von Grubenstäuben." *Staub*, **23**, 353.

Goldstein, B. and Webster, I. (1966), "Intratracheal injection into rats of size-graded silica particles." *British Journal of Industrial Medicine*, **23**, 71.

Gordon, R. L., Griffin, O. G. and Nagelschmidt, G. (1952), "The quantitative determination of quartz by X-ray diffraction." S.M.R.E. Research Report No. 52, Safety in Mines Research Establishment, Sheffield.

Green, H. L. and Watson, H. H. (1935), Medical Research Council Special Report Series No. 199. H.M.S.O., London.

Greenburg, L. and Smith, G. W. (1922), "A new instrument for sampling aerial dust." Reports of Investigations 2392, Bureau of Mines, U.S.A.

Hamilton, R. J. (1954), "The relation between free falling speed and particle size of airborne dust." *British Journal of Applied Physics*, Supplement No. 3, 90.

Hamilton, R. J. (1956), "A portable instrument for respirable dust sampling." *Journal of Scientific Instruments*, **33**, 395.

Hamilton, R. J., Wainwright, T. and Walton, W. H. (1951), "The effect of adhesive film thickness on the sampling efficiency of the konimeter." *British Journal of Industrial Medicine*, **8**, 14.

Hamilton, R. J. and Walton, W. H. (1961), "The selective sampling of respirable dust." In *Inhaled Particles and Vapours*, ed. C. N. Davies. p, 465. Pergamon Press, Oxford.

Harris, C. W. and Maguire, B. A. (1968), "A gravimetric dust sampling instrument (SIMPEDS): preliminary results." *The Annals of Occupational Hygiene*, II, 195.

Higgins, R. I. and Dewell, P. (1967), "A gravimetric size-selecting personal dust sampler." In *Inhaled Particles and Vapours*, II, ed. C. N. Davies, p. 575. Pergamon Press, Oxford.

Holdsworth, J. F., Price, F. H. and Tomlinson, R. C. (1954), "Inter-laboratory checks on the counting of coal dust particles on thermal precipitator slides." *British Journal of Applied Physics*, Supplement No. 3, 96.

Hunt, J. M., Wisherd, M. P. and Bonham, L. C. (1950), "Infra-red absorption spectra of minerals and other inorganic compounds." *Analytical Chemistry*, **22**, 1478.

Jacobsen, M., Rae, S., Walton, W. H. and Rogan, J. M. (1970), "New dust standards for British coal mines." *Nature*, **227**, 445.

Jacobsen, M., Rae, S., Walton, W. H. and Rogan, J. M. (1971), "The relation between pneumoconiosis and dust exposure in British coal mines." In *Inhaled Particles*, III, ed. W. H. Walton. p, 903. Unwin, London.

Kay, J. H. (1965), *Techniques for Electron Microscopy* (1965). 2nd Edition, ed. J. H. Kay. Oxford: Blackwell.

Keenan, R. G. and Lynch, R. J. (1970), "Techniques for the detection, identification and analysis of fibres." *American Industrial Hygiene Association Journal*, **31**, 587.

Klug, H. P. and Alexander, L. E. (1954), *X-ray Diffraction Procedures for Polycrystalline and Amorphous Materials*. John Wiley & Sons Inc. New York.

Kitson, G. H. J. and Winer, P. (1960), "Routine airborne dust sampling in collieries." *Journal of the Mine Ventilation Society of South Africa*, **13**, 153.

Kitto, P. H. and Beadle, D. G. (1952), "A modified form of thermal precipitator." *Journal of the Chemical Metallurgical and Mining Society of South Africa*, **52**, 284.

Kubālek, J. and Šimeček, J. (1968), "Dvoustupňovy prachoměr." *Pracovní Lékarství*, **20**, 349.

Landwehr, H. (1962), "Efrahrungen mit neuenwiskelten staubmessgeräten, die nach gravimetrischen prinzipien arbeiten." *Staub*, **22**, 112.

Littlefield, J. B., Feicht, F. L. and Schrenk, H. H. (1937), "The Bureau of Mines midget impinger for dust sampling." Report of Investigations No. 3360, Bureau of Mines, Washington.

Lippmann, M. and Harris, W. B. (1962), "Size-selecting samplers for estimating respirable dust concentrations." *Health Physics*, **8**, 155.

McCormick, P. Y., Lucas, R. L. and Wells, D. F. (1963), "Gas-solids separation." In *Chemical Engineer's Handbook*, Section 20, 62, ed. J. H. Perry, 4th Edition. McGraw-Hill, New York.

Mavrogordato, A. (1929), "The aetiology of silicosis." *IVe Reunion de la Commission Internationale Permanente pour les Maladies Professionnelles, Lyons*. A. Rey, Lyons.

Mavrogordato, A. (1939/40), "A grammar of Witwatersrand silicosis." *Journal of the Chemical Metallurgical and Mining Society of South Africa*, **40**, 326.

McCrae, J. (1913), *The Ash of Silicotic Lungs*. South African Instutite for Medical Research, Johannesburg.

Maguire, B. A., Barker, D. and Badel, D. A. (1971), "Simpeds 70: an improved version of the Simpeds personal gravimetric dust sampling instrument." In *Inhaled Particles*, III, ed. W. H. Walton, p. 1053. Unwin, London.

Morgan, A. and Holmes, A. (1969). "Neutron activation techniques in investigations in the composition and biological effects of asbestos." In *Pneumoconiosis, Proceedings of the International Conference, Johannesburg, 1969*, p. 52, ed. H. A. Shapiro, Oxford University Press, Capetown.

Orenstein, A. J. (1960), *Proceedings of the Pneumoconiosis Conference, Johannesburg, 1959*, J. & A. Churchill, London.

Owens, J. S. (1922), "Jet dust-counting apparatus." *Proceedings of the Royal Society*, series A, **101**, 18.

Pooley, F. D., Oldham, P. D., Chang-Hyun Um and Wagner, J. C. (1969), "The detection of asbestos in tissues." In *Pneumoconiosis, Proceedings of the International Conference, Johannesburg, 1969*, ed. H. A. Shapiro, p. 108. Oxford University Press, Capetown.

Roach, S. (1959), "Measuring dust exposure with the thermal precipitator in collieries and foundries." *British Journal of Industrial Medicine*, **16**, 104.

Robock, K. and Klosterkötter, W. (1971), "The cytotoxic action and the semi-conductor properties of mine dusts." In *Inhaled Particles*, III, ed. W. H. Walton, p. 453 Unwin, London.

Rossiter, C. E., Rivers, D., Bergman, I., Casswell, C. and Nagelschmidt, G. (1967), "Dust content, radiology and pathology in simple pneumoconiosis of coal-workers." In *Inhaled Particles and Vapours*, II, p. 419, ed. C. N. Davies. Pergamon Press, Oxford.

Schlick, D. P. (1971), "Respirable coal mine dust standards and their enforcement under the Federal Coal Mine Health and Safety Act of 1969." In *Inhaled Particles*, III, ed. W. H. Walton, p. 1007, Unwin, London.

Schlipköter, H.-W., Hilscher, W., Pott, F. and Beck, E. G. (1971), "Investigations into the aetiology of coal workers pneumoconiosis with the use of PVN-oxide." In *Inhaled Particles and Vapours*, III, in press, ed. W. H. Walton. Unwin, London.

Schmidt, K. G. (1955), "Die phasenkontrast milroskopic in der Staub technik." *Staub*, **41**, 436.

Talvitie, N. A. (1951), "Determination of quartz in presence of silicates using phosphoric acid." *Analytical Chemistry*, **23**, 62.

Talvitie, N. A. (1964), "Determination of free silica: gravimetric and spectrophotometric procedures applicable to airborne and settled dust." *American Industrial Hygiene Association Journal*, **25**, 169.

Talvitie, N. A. and Brewer, L. W. (1962), "Separation and analysis of dust in lung tissue." *American Industrial Hygiene Association Journal*, **23**, 58.

Timbrell, V. (1954), "The terminal velocity and size of airborne dust particles." *British Journal of Applied Physics*, Supplement No. 3, 86.

Timbrell, V. (1965), "The inhalation of fibrous dusts." *Annals of the New York Academy of Sciences*, **132**, 255.

Transvaal Chamber of Mines (1947), *Quality of Mine Air*. Transvaal Chamber of Mines, Johannesburg, 33.

Union of South Africa (1937), *The Prevention of Silicosis on the Mines of the Witwatersrand*. Government Printer, Pretoria, 273.

Walton W. H. (1947), "The application of electron microscopy to particle size measurement." Symposium on Particle Size Analysis. Supplement to *Transactions, Institution of Chemical Engineers*, **25**, 64.

Walton, W. H. (1954), "The theory of size classification of airborne dust clouds by elutriation." *British Journal of Applied Physics*, Supplement No. 3, 29.

Walton, W. H. (1970), "The measurement of respirable dust—the basis for gravimetric standards," In *Proceedings of the Symposium on Respirable Coal Mine Dust*, Washington, D.C., November 3–4, 1969. Bureau of Mines, Information Circular 84, U.S. Department of the Interior, Washington, D.C.

Weiss, B., Boettner, E. A., Stenning, M. and Arbor, A. (1970), "Determination of quartz: evaluation of the differential thermal analysis method." *Archives of Environmental Health*, **20**, 37.

World Health Organisation, (1968), *Pneumoconiosis: Report on a Symposium, Katowice, 1967*. World Health Organisation, Regional Office for Europe.

Wright, B. M. (1954), "A size-selecting sampler for airborne dust." *British Journal of Industrial Medicine*, II, 284.

Chapter 10

The Radiological Control of Dust Disease

Introduction

To control dust disease it is essential to know what kind of abnormality the dust produces and to diagnose its presence early enough to permit action to safeguard health.

Chest radiography has been the most commonly used diagnostic technique but for the purpose of pneumoconiosis control it is not equally effective in all mining industries. Its particular value is generally accepted where the airborne dust is either largely inert, such as in iron, barium and tin mining, or where it is only mildly fibrogenic, such as is produced by coal, china clay, graphite or diatomaceous earth mining. It is less effective in industries concerned with highly fibrogenic dusts, such as silica, talc and asbestos. These dusts may produce lesions which progress even in the absence of further exposure and thus the identification of abnormality on the radiograph cannot always be followed by effective action to protect the workman's wellbeing. The chest radiograph by itself is also inadequate where, as with asbestos and uranium dusts, the biological response to exposure may be neoplastic and may occur a considerable time after exposure has ceased. It is by no means certain, even if it were possible to identify the pathological changes at an earlier stage than can be revealed by the chest X-ray, that this would permit effective control of the lesions produced by these biologically active dusts. The use of modern respiratory function tests in the prophylaxis, diagnosis and management of the pneumoconioses has been advocated by the International Labour Organization (1966). It is in the further refinement of these, in combination with improvement in chest radiography and the development of cytological tests for pre-malignant change, that hope lies for the effective control of all types of dust disease.

It would, however, be unwise to rely only on biological controls where there are uncertainties about the relationship between exposure and response. Careful environmental monitoring must be considered as a necessary adjunct to the radiological examination of the mine-workers.

The Organization of the Examinations

To fulfil the objectives described in the introduction, arrangements must be made for the regular radiological examination of all mine-workers, including those who have newly joined the industry. Office staff working in the vicinity of asbestos mines should be included as airborne asbestos fibres may cause disease at a distance from where they were mined (Gilson, 1966).

New entrants should have their chest radiographs taken as part of the medical examination to determine their fitness for work. The film is used to assist in the overall assessment of health and to exclude those with serious clinical conditions, particularly sputum-positive tuberculosis. In addition, in young men it provides the normal "base line" against which subsequent change may be estimated and in those re-entering the industry may give evidence of previous exposure to dust.

The regular X-raying of all workers is the basis of the radiological control of dust disease. The primary purpose is to establish the prevalence of pneumoconiosis and to provide information on the extent to which the condition may be progressing. The temptation to examine only those exposed to airborne dust must be resisted. All workers must be examined; it is necessary to identify the presence of conditions other than pneumoconiosis, e.g. tuberculosis, bronchial carcinoma; these may, of course, occur in any mineworker. Secondly, abnormalities related to dust may appear in men whose exposure has ceased, e.g. progressive massive fibrosis in coal-workers (Rae, 1971) and, finally, it would be difficult, if not impossible, to examine only certain men when the examination of all was desired by the mineworkers and the organizations which represent them.

High attendance rates must be achieved at these examinations if reliable data on the prevalence of the disease and the effectiveness of dust suppression are to be produced. The target should be at least 85 per cent of all workers for a voluntary scheme. In most instances this will be achieved if its objects and aims are discussed in detail with management and trade unions before the examinations begin. Their co-operation is vitally important in making satisfactory local arrangements and in persuading the reluctant to come forward for examination. It seems doubtful, at least in the developed countries, whether such examinations should be made compulsory or a condition of continuing employment. Elsewhere it may be difficult to obtain the understanding and co-operation of the work force and thus the question of compulsion may have to be seriously considered.

The frequency of examination is largely determined by the degree of hazard: where this is high a substantial number of workers will develop the disease and its progression will be rapid. In these circumstances examinations should be held at short intervals until such time as the environmental hazard is reduced and brought under control. In mining industries where the dust is either inert or only mildly fibrogenic, e.g. coal, iron, tin, barium and kaolin the period between chest radiographs will normally be from two to six years. There is considerable doubt, however, as to the optimum time in those other industries, particularly asbestos, where the dust is more highly fibrogenic. Until more is known about the natural history of the changes produced by the inhalation of asbestos fibres, it would seem prudent to examine more, rather than less, often. A chest radiograph each year, or perhaps on alternate years, would appear to be a reasonable frequency for such workers.

The examinations can with advantage be carried out by teams whose management is undertaken by the industry itself. In this way quality control, so necessary in the production of consistently high quality radiographs, can be readily exercised.

It may be difficult to decide whether it is better to equip a mobile unit designed to visit the site of the mining operations or to set up a static centre to which the men can be brought. The decision should be made on the grounds of finance and logistics. It is certainly possible to produce high quality chest radiographs in a mobile unit. The cost of the vehicle is likely to be between one and three times the cost of the X-ray plant it accommodates. Against this expense must be off-set the cost of bringing the mineworkers to a central point and also the cost of the interference with normal working which this procedure entails. It is probably worthwhile equipping a mobile unit when more than 10,000 workers are to be examined annually in an area which can conveniently be visited by one unit.

Radiographic Technique

The pneumoconioses can be studied satisfactorily only on full-sized high quality chest radiographs. The earliest parenchymal and pleural changes are best identified by trained readers scrutinizing films in which the lung is shown in greatest detail. However good smaller films may be their use increases the difficulties of diagnosis and classification and the assessment of change between serial radiographs of the same subject. Although small films have advantages in terms of cost, speedy examination and lower storage space requirements these factors are of lesser importance than the additional information obtainable from full-size radiographs and the fact that the exposure required to produce a full-sized film entails a radiation dose approximately one-sixth of that required for the production of miniature films.

The most commonly used technique for chest radiography in the field or at screening clinics has been to use a kilo-voltage range of approximately 60–80 kV with an exposure time of 0·05–0·08 seconds (International Labour Organization, 1970). In conjunction with this some workers prefer to use grids to reduce secondary radiation and the associated loss of photographic detail.

A rotating anode tube with a focal spot no larger than 2 millimetres should be employed; the focal spot-film distance should be fixed at 1·8 metres.

Exposure control devices and automatic processing of the exposed film are helpful in maintaining consistency of technique.

It is most important that every attention be given to minimizing the radiation hazard to the patient. This is most conveniently done by confining the radiation to the chest area by means of a collimator. The finished film should show evidence of collimation by the presence of "cone cuts" at its edges. The hazard to the operator is eliminated by enclosing the tube, patient, and chest stand in a booth whose walls are impervious to radiation.

The advantages of using high kilo-voltages in the range 110–140 kV have recently been indicated (International Labour Organization, 1970). A reduction in the radiation dose to the patient and in the number of technically unsatisfactory films is claimed. Unfortunately this technique requires modern and costly equipment and an electrical supply of a quality not always available in the field. Whatever the respective merits of these two techniques, there is no doubt that meticulous attention to detail at every stage of the production of the film is all important. An adequate power supply must be arranged. Care must be taken with the exposure, the film cassettes, the intensifying screens and the films, while the manufacturer's instructions must be minutely observed in regard to the operation of automatic processing units. Providing due attention is given to all these factors, both techniques can produce radiographs of the high and consistent quality necessary for the study of the pneumoconioses.

The Interpretation of the Radiological Appearances

Radiological Classification

One of the most important advances in the epidemiology of the pneumoconioses has been the development of an international system for the classification of the radiological appearances. This classification standardizes the diagnostic criteria and permits the degree of abnormality to be recorded. Thus the prevalence of pneumoconiosis can be compared between countries and industries and any tendency to improvement or deterioration detected in the incidence of the disease as it affects a country, industry or particular mine.

Much of the credit for these advances goes to the International Labour Organization who published the original classification 20 years ago and who have done so much to encourage the improvements and refinements it has undergone since then.

This early system was intended primarily for coal-workers' pneumoconiosis and silicosis, the subsequent modifications being designed to cover a wider range of the pneumoconioses and to permit a finer and more sensitive grading of the amount of radiological abnormality.

The most recent version (International Labour Organization, 1970), contains two closely linked schemes, firstly, a short classification to be used principally for clinical purposes and for the types of pneumoconioses which were, with the exception of asbestosis, adequately described in the previous system (International Labour Organization, 1959), and secondly, an extended classification which incorporates both the elaborated scale of abnormality developed by workers of the National Coal Board in Great Britain (Liddell and Lindars, 1969) and also many features of the U.I.C.C./Cincinnati scheme (U.I.C.C., 1970) which was designed for the classification of the abnormalities produced by the inhalation of asbestos.

The short and extended classifications taken together can be used for all types of pneumoconioses and are suitable, both for clinicians concerned with the assessment of abnormalities in individuals and for epidemiologists concerned with the difference in the amount of abnormality between groups of workers and with the problem of defining the relationship between the inhalation of dust and the development of pneumoconiosis.

The essential features of the classification are shown in Tables 1 (*a*) and 1 (*b*). In both schemes the appearances are described in terms of small and large opacities. These are sub-divided into categories on a quantitative (profusion) and qualitative (type) basis. The short classification has four categories of profusion, 0 to 3, while the extended has twelve, 0/– to 3/4. Both have three sub-divisions of type. Apart from the extended scale of abnormality the principal differences between the two schemes are that the extended classification divides the appearances of the small opacities into "rounded" and "irregular" and grades both pleural abnormalities and alterations to the cardiac outline.

The validity of the classification has now been established by studies carried out in many different countries (U.I.C.C., 1970; Jacobsen, Rae, Walton and Rogan, 1971; Casswell, Bergman and Rossiter, 1971).

Representative examples of the various categories and sub-divisions are provided by the sets of standard films issued by the I.L.O. The international nature of the classification is demonstrated by the distribution of 900 sets of the 1958 standards to fifty-five countries.

Observer Variation

The use of standard films is strongly recommended for epidemiological studies. These investigations are concerned with comparing the prevalence of disease in groups of workers at different times and require large numbers of radiographs to be classified. The results will be valid only to the extent that similar standards of classification are used on all films. The level of classification adopted by one doctor may, however, differ from that of another and that of individual doctors may fluctuate

Table 1 (a)

International Classification of Radiographs of Pneumoconioses
(Revised, 1968)

Short Classification

Under Review—see Appendix

DESCRIPTION

No pneumo-coniosis	O:	No radiographic evidence of pneumoconiosis.
Suspect	Z:	Abnormal lung or hilar shadows the nature of which is uncertain and which may or may not represent a stage of pneumoconiosis.

PNEUMOCONIOSIS

Small opacities

Category (according to profusion)		*Symbols* (according to the greatest diameter of opacities)
1:	a small number of opacities	p: diameter up to about 1·5 mm
2:	opacities are more numerous	m (q): diameter exceeding 1·5 mm up to about 3 mm
3:	opacities are very numerous	n (r): diameter exceeding 3 mm up to about 10 mm

Large opacities

A: An opacity having a greatest diameter of between 1 and 5 cm, or several opacities each greater than 1 cm, the sum of whose greatest diameters does not exceed 5 cm.

B: One or more opacities, larger or more numerous than those in category A, whose combined area does not exceed one-third of the right lung field.

C: One or more large opacities, whose combined area exceeds one-third of the righ tlung field.

ADDITIONAL SYMBOLS

Obligatory

plc — calcified pleural plaques.
pl — significant pleural abnormalities.
co — abnormalities of the cardiac size and shape.
es — eggshell calcification of lymph nodes.
tba — opacities suggestive of active tuberculosis.
ca — suspect neoplasm.
od — other significant diseases not covered by one of the other obligatory or optional symbols. (In each case this should be described briefly under Remarks.)

Optional

ax — suspect coalescence of small rounded opacities.
cn — calcification in small rounded opacities.
cp — cor pulmonale.
cv — cavity.
di — significant displacement or distortion of the thoracic structure.
em — significant emphysema including large bullae.
hi — significant enlargement of the hilar shadows.
ho — honeycombing.
px — pneumothorax.
rl — pneumoconiosis modified by the rheumatoid process.
tb — opacities suggestive of inactive tuberculosis, excluding the calcified primary complex.
K — Kerley lines.

with time. It is of the greatest importance that every precaution should be taken to avoid mistakes arising from this source.

In an attempt to ensure uniformity of standards in the British coal industry groups of three to eight doctors have read the radiographs. All these doctors meet from time to time to discuss the use of the classification and its application to particularly difficult films (Rae, Ashford, Morgan, Pasqual and Pearson, 1963). These meetings also

Table 1 (b)

International Classification of Radiographs of Pneumoconioses
(Revised, 1968)

Extended Classification

Under Review—see Appendix

Feature	Categories and Symbols	
No pneumoconiosis	{Rounded	0/– 0/0 0/1
Suspect pneumoconiosis	{Irregular	
Pneumoconiosis		
SMALL OPACITIES		
Rounded		
Profusion	1/0, 1/1, 1/2; 2/1, 2/2, 2/3; 3/2, 3/3, 3/4	
Type	p, m(q), n(r).	
Extent	zones 1–6	
Irregular		
Profusion	1/0, 1/1, 1/2; 2/1, 2/2, 2/3; 3/2, 3/3, 3/4	
Type	s, t, u.*	
Extent	zones 1–6	
LARGE OPACITIES		
Size	A, B, C	
Type	wd (well defined) id (ill defined)	
SYMBOLS, OBLIGATORY		
	Site	*Grades*
Pleural calcification	diaph., wall, others	0, 1, 2, 3
Pleural thickening	{costophrenic	lower limit
(significant)	{other sites	0, 1, 2, 3
Cardiac outline	{co	—
	{ill defined	0, 1, 2, 3
Eggshell calcification	es	—
Active tuberculosis	tba	—
Carcinoma	ca	—
Other signif. disease	od	—

SYMBOLS, OPTIONAL†			
ax	cv	hi	rl
cn	di	ho	tb
cp	em	px	K

* The definitions of s, t, u, approximate to those of p, m, n, but refer, of course, to irregular opacities instead of rounded.

† For key see Table 1(*a*).

provide an opportunity for checks to be carried out on the doctors' reading standards. For this purpose films are specially selected to cover the range of abnormality and are re-read on the occasion of subsequent checks. Providing the batch is large enough, the results of the check will not be vitiated by a "memory" effect. Throughout such discussions and whenever films are to be classified regular reference should be made to the sets of standard films.

If opinions differ on the classification of a particular radiograph a decision is required on the category that is to be recorded. The choice lies between accepting one or other of the views expressed or making use of the different interpretations to provide more information. For example, if a film is classified as Category 1 by one doctor and Category 2 by another, it is more likely that the appearances lie on the border line between the categories rather than that the film is a "true" Category 1 or Category 2. One simple yet effective solution is to use the arithmetic mean of all available readings (Jacobsen, Rae, Walton and Rogan, 1970).

The difficulties introduced by alterations in reading standards with time can be overcome by reading old and recent films together in one batch.

Film Reading Technique

There remains the problem of how serial films from an individual should be read, for there is still no generally accepted answer to the apparently simple question of how serial radiographs should be handled in order to get unbiased estimates of the prevalence and progression of pneumoconiosis. Cochrane (1962) favours the procedure whereby all films are thoroughly mixed and then read singly in "random" order, whereas the writers consider that the films from each individual should be read together "side-by-side" on the viewing screen. It is probable that doctors accustomed to using the I.L.O. classification will produce very similar results by both methods but it is much less certain that this will be so for inexperienced observers. Further work is required on this problem.

Effect of Poor Radiographic Technique

The importance of consistently high quality radiographs has already been emphasized. It is difficult to classify poor films and survey results may be biased where there are large numbers of radiographs of inferior quality. The problem of how observers are affected by film quality is a complex one as it has been found that they may be affected in different ways at different times and may differ from each other in the type of effect produced, some doctors over-reading "white" films for example, while others under-read them (Wise and Oldham, 1964; Pearson, Ashford, Morgan, Pasqual and Rae, 1965). In view of the uncertainty about the amount and direction of the bias introduced by this factor every effort must be made to minimize the number of unsatisfactory films. In addition, it is wise to record the presence of poor film quality as the effect of including or excluding these films from the analysis can then be studied.

To summarize, the radiographs will have to be read on at least two occasions, first, at the time of surveys for clinical purposes to advise the individual and to tell him how the current film compares with any earlier one. It is necessary to provide this report speedily and therefore it is probable that film reading for this purpose will be undertaken by only one doctor who will be devoting his attention to the individual patient. The short I.L.O. Classification may be used at this stage. However, collective results from such readings may be biased by a number of factors and in consequence unsuitable for comparisons between mines or over time. For epidemiological purposes a second reading is therefore necessary. Here the extended classification should be used and to avoid the results being affected by the factors discussed above very careful consideration has to be given as to how and by whom the films are read.

Utilization of the Results

Clinical Results

Clinically the doctor's prime concern is with the individual. Each workman must be given a report on his X-ray and the opportunity to discuss it should he so desire. His personal physician, if known, must be kept informed of any significant findings and any further investigation that may be required should be arranged with his co-operation.

Advice must be offered on the question of social security benefits and the doctor should give what help he can to the workman who may be confused by the administrative procedures involved in making a claim.

As large numbers of reports will have to be sent out the advantage of using printed standard letters of notification should be considered. It is, in any event, important to keep an accurate record of the report that was sent to the workman and the advice that was given him if he was interviewed.

The confidential nature of the relationship between doctor and man must be respected and the results of the individual examination must on no account be divulged to management or trade unions except with the specific, and preferably written authority of the individual concerned.

The opportunity to see and talk with the individual mineworker provides an important mechanism for disease control.

The early appearance and rapid progression of radiographic abnormality will identify the individual who is hyper-susceptible to pneumoconiosis or who has been exposed to excessive dust concentrations.

These men should be interviewed and the situation explained. They should be advised to seek work in dust-free conditions and the doctor should enlist the co-operation of management in finding suitable employment.

The risk of developing the disabling form of pneumoconiosis, progressive massive fibrosis, is known to increase, certainly in coal miners, as the background category of simple pneumoconiosis increases (McLintock, Rae and Jacobsen, 1971). If men can be prevented from reaching the more advanced stages of simple pneumoconiosis the risk of their developing progressive massive fibrosis will therefore be low. When the radiographs reveal early pneumoconiosis in young men they should be advised of the real risk of subsequently developing disabling disease and should be advised to withdraw from work in dusty places.

Until more is known about the aetiology of progressive massive fibrosis the transfer from dusty working places of those hyper-susceptible to dust and the young men with early simple pneumoconiosis will be the most effective available measure of preventive medicine.

The relationship between exposure to asbestos and the development of bronchial carcinoma, pleural and peritoneal mesotheliomata is still obscure. It is probable, however, that their appearance will not be entirely prevented even if the men are removed from the dust at the earliest stages of radiographic pleural and parenchymal change. Effective prevention will be afforded only by strict limitation of the total exposure.

Clinical management of the pneumoconioses is discussed in detail in Chapter 6.

Epidemiological Results

The epidemiologist is concerned with group results. These may be used in a number of ways to achieve disease control.

First, from a consideration of how much disease there is at different mines places where the risk is high can be identified. Dust suppression measures can then be concentrated on these places and their effectiveness estimated from the amount of change revealed at subsequent radiological surveys.

Care must be taken to present the results to management in an intelligible form. The risks of drawing conclusions from statistics such as the overall prevalence and the number of cases receiving compensation in any given year should be indicated. These figures are liable to be greatly affected by factors not related to the dustiness of the working environment such as the number of men entering and leaving the industry, the local employment situation and the willingness of workmen to submit claims for compensation.

A better indicator of the pneumoconiosis levels in an industry is the "age specific prevalence rate", i.e. the number of men in a particular age group who have the disease. Prevalence statistics presented in this form may not be sensitive enough to indicate to management how the situation is changing over a short period of time. To overcome this difficulty National Coal Board workers evolved a "Progression Index" (McLintock, 1969). This is derived from the amount of radiological progression found over a five-year period in the men who worked at the coal-face at the time of the previous survey. The extended I.L.O. classification is used to read the films and a change from one category to another is regarded as one step of progression. The Progression Index for a particular colliery is the number of steps of progression per 100 men at that colliery over the five-year inter-survey period. Useful inter-colliery comparisons can be made using this index (McLintock, 1969). It should be borne in mind that the interpretation of such an index will be difficult if only small numbers of men are involved.

Another valuable index is the "Attack Rate", i.e. the number of men who develop the disease per 1,000 workers per year. This index may also be sub-divided by age group. Its main advantage is that it can be used where, as with asbestos or high quartz dusts, there is doubt about the relationship of disease progression to exposure. With these dusts radiological progression is likely to be more closely related to the total amount of past exposure rather than to the amount of exposure following the first radiograph. It follows that no indication can be obtained of the level of the current hazard by considering only radiological progression. The principal disadvantage associated with this index is that it is technically difficult to measure. Diagnostic difficulties are greatest where the abnormality is minimal and because of this the results may be difficult to interpret.

References

Casswell, C., Bergman, I. and Rossiter, C. E. (1971), "The relation of radiological appearance in simple pneumoconiosis of coal workers to the content and composition of the lung." In *Inhaled Particles and Vapours, III*, ed. W. H. Walton, p. 173, Unwin, London.

Cochrane, A. L. (1962), "The attack rate of progressive massive fibrosis." *British Journal of Industrial Medicine*, **19**, 52.

Gilson, J. C. (1966), "Wyers Memorial Lecture 1965: Health hazards of asbestos. Recent studies on its biological effects." *Transactions of the Society of Occupational Medicine*, **16**, 62.

International Labour Organization (1959), Meeting of experts on the international classification of radiographs of the pneumoconioses. 1958. Extract from *Occupational Safety and Health*, **9**, 63. International Labour Office, Geneva.

International Labour Organization (1966), "Respiratory function tests in pneumoconioses." *Occupational Safety and Health Series, No. 6*. International Labour Office, Geneva.

International Labour Organization (1970), "International classification of radiographs of pneumoconioses (revised 1968)." *Occupational Safety and Health Series, No. 22*. International Labour Office, Geneva.

Jacobsen, M., Rae, S., Walton, W. H. and Rogan, J. M. (1970), "New dust standards for British coal mines." *Nature*, **227**, 455.

Jacobsen, M., Rae, S., Walton, W. H. and Rogan, J. M. (1971), "The relationship between pneumoconiosis and dust exposure in British coal mines." In *Inhaled Particles and Vapours, III*, ed. W. H. Walton, p. 903. Unwin, London.

Liddell, F. D. K. and Lindars, D. C. (1969), "An elaboration of the I.L.O. classification of simple pneumoconiosis." *British Journal of Industrial Medicine*, **26**, 89.

McLintock, J. S. (1969), "The medical control of pneumoconiosis." *Transactions of the Society of Occupational Medicine*, **19**, 16.

McLintock, J. S., Rae, S. and Jacobsen, M. (1971), "The attack rate of progressive massive fibrosis in British coalminers." In *Inhaled Particles and Vapours, III*, ed. W. H. Walton, p. 933. Unwin, London.

Pearson, N. G., Ashford, J. R., Morgan, D. C., Pasqual, R. S. H. and Rae, S. (1965), "Effect of quality of chest radiographs on the categorization of coal-workers' pneumoconiosis." *British Journal of Industrial Medicine*, **22**, 81.

Rae, S., Ashford, J. R., Morgan, D. C., Pasqual, R. S. H. and Pearson, N. G. (1963), "A comparison of some alternative procedures in the classification of chest radiographs for coal-workers' pneumoconiosis." *British Journal of Industrial Medicine*, **20**, 293.

Rae, S. (1971), "Pneumoconiosis and coal dust exposure." *British Medical Bulletin*, **27**, 53.

U.I.C.C. (1970), "UICC/Cincinnati classification of the radiographic appearances of pneumoconioses." A co-operative study by the U.I.C.C. committee. *Chest*, **58**, 57.

Wise, M. E. and Oldham, P. D. (1963), "Effect of radiographic technique on readings of categories of simple pneumoconiosis." *British Journal of Industrial Medicine*, **20**, 145.

Appendix

At the IVth International Pneumoconiosis Conference, held by the International Labour Office in Bucharest in September, 1971, the following recommendations were announced at the plenary session.

1. There should be a synthesis between the I.L.O. 1968 Classification and the U.I.C.C./Cincinnati scheme. This synthesis should be known as the "I.L.O. U./C. Classification of the radiographic appearances of the pneumoconioses; 1971." (The synthesis is defined in paragraph 2, below.)

2. The short and extended classification of the I.L.O. (Revised 1968) Classification should be retained but with the following changes:

(*a*) in the short classification Category Z would be omitted and small irregular opacities would be classified into types s, t and u, each type having a category of profusion 1, 2 or 3.

(*b*) the extended classification would be similar to that given in the Revised 1968 scheme but modified in that the distinction between "obligatory" and "optional" additional symbols would be abolished and the classification of pleural thickening would be more detailed.

3. A new set of standard films illustrating the different types and categories should be issued as soon as possible.

Chapter 11
Occupational Dermatitis in Miners

General

Occupational dermatitis is a major cause of disability in mining. Although we consider the terms eczema and dermatitis as being synonymous, dermatitis is used here to denote an inflammatory reaction of the skin to some external agent acting either as a primary irritant or as an allergic sensitizer. Furthermore, it is important to realize that, histologically, there is no essential difference between dermatitis and eczema, the former simply implying a specific aetiology, whereas the latter, without qualification, implies an endogenous cause.

In mining processes in Great Britain by far the greatest number of men are employed in coal mining with much smaller numbers employed in the mining of haematite, lead, tin, clay, slate and salt. In other parts of the world deep mining is undertaken for gold, copper, diamonds, asbestos and many other minerals. The conditions vary enormously from one type of mining operation to another, showing variation in geography, depth, temperature, humidity, ventilation and the type of mineral involved, together with its specific physical and chemical characteristics; each factor has some bearing on the aetiology of the dermatitis occurring in that particular occupation.

In mining the frequency of trauma and respiratory disease tends to overshadow the problems of occupational dermatitis. Many workmen with dermatitis may continue in their employment while under treatment provided that the lesions are not too extensive. Matthews (1959) in a survey involving two collieries in South Wales showed that there was an almost equal prevalence of occupational and non-occupational dermatitis, tinea pedis being excluded.

Dermatitis in the miner, whatever its precise causation, is often protracted and may be a severe handicap to the patient, making it difficult or impossible to carry out the more productive and remunerative jobs.

Reaction of the Skin to External Irritants

The skin provides some protection against noxious agents from outside, this being one of its primary physiological functions. This defence is far from perfect, however, as many substances penetrate readily into the epidermis, even when it is intact.

The first line of defence is a surface film of sebum emulsified with sweat and breakdown products from the horny layer. This lipid film protects, to some extent, the horny layer from loss of its normal water content as do lipids deeper in the stratum corneum. It has a negligible effect in preventing the penetration of certain substances. The surface film, also known as the "acid mantle", is slightly acidic (pH 4·2–5·6) and will normally withstand the action of moderately strong acids but is more easily damaged by alkaline substances. Beneath the mantle is the stratum corneum or horny layer which is the most protective layer of the skin. Breach or maceration of the stratum corneum may be produced by friction, heat, trauma and excessive sweating, all of which may predispose to the development of dermatitis. In certain sites the openings of the hair follicles, sweat and sebacous glands may provide a portal of entry into the epidermis, especially if the irritant or sensitizer is fat soluble. Excessive moisture promotes cutaneous absorption and it is of practical importance that plastic and rubber gloves, shoes, boots and overalls may provide a measure of occlusion sufficient for this to be significant in some occupations.

The resistance of the skin to external irritants also varies with:

(i) Race: The dark skin is generally considered to be more resistant than the fair—the African and Indian races being less disposed to eczema and dermatitis than the white. Conversely, the Mongolian races are more likely to develop these conditions.

(ii) Age: This appears to have some influence on the development of industrial dermatitis. Surveys of industrial plants have shown striking evidence of the susceptibility of the young and inexperienced worker, although children generally exhibit less contact dermatitis than other age groups, possibly due to their more protected environment. A new worker may regard a known hazard lightly and may not use the protection provided. Furthermore, he may not have the opportunity of becoming "hardened" —a phenomenon which involves adaptation of the skin to primary irritants together with a hypo-sensitization which develops in some workers on continued exposure.

With increasing age the risk of primary irritant dermatitis increases, the skin of the elderly recovering slowly from chemical trauma.

In contrast to the early appearance of dermatitis in many industries, in coal mining it has been found to occur mainly in the 30 to 50 age group after a latent period of many years (Williamson, 1962).

(iii) Psychological factors: Emotional factors may alter the resistance of the skin, possibly by producing hyperhidrosis, and may "trigger off" a dermatitis.

(iv) Constitutional factors: Atopic subjects, i.e. those with a strong family history of bronchial asthma, eczema, hay fever and urticaria with xerotic (dry) skin are more liable to primary irritant dermatitis. Seborrhoeic subjects may also be more susceptible, as may the patient with xeroderma. Previous sensitization with one allergen involves a liability to subsequent sensitization with chemically related substances.

Patients with pre-existing eczema engaged in an unsuitable occupation may experience an aggravation of their eczema from working conditions. It is important to recognize this factor so as to avoid confusion with cases arising primarily from external irritants.

(v) Environment: It is obvious that environment in its complete sense will influence the genesis and progress of the dermatitis.

Classification of Occupational Dermatitis

The various agents which can cause an occupational dermatitis may exist in solid, liquid or gaseous form. They may be grouped under the following general headings:

Primary Irritants

A primary irritant is a substance which in most people is capable, even at first exposure, of causing a dermatitis if applied in sufficient concentration for a sufficient length of time. This condition has more recently been sub-divided into (*a*) a primary toxic dermatitis which is caused by strong irritants after one or two brief applications, and (*b*) a cumulative "insult" dermatitis where a dermatitis develops after repeated insults by weak primary irritants over long periods, e.g. soap, detergents, oils and solvents (Fig. 1).

The hands are particularly liable to be involved and the distribution of the dermatitis is characteristically over the dorsal rather than the palmar surfaces, usually starting on the interdigital webs and spreading over the dorsal aspects of the hands and wrists. A nummular (coin-shaped) pattern may be indistinguishable from a nummular eczema except by the history and distribution of the lesions.

In industry other than mining, primary irritants are often dusts, acids or alkaline substances and in engineering workshops common causes of primary irritant dermatitis are degreasing agents and solvents, together with harsh abrasive substances which may be used for cleansing the skin after work. Apart from the more usual type of occupational dermatitis which occurs in mining and is described later, primary irritant dermatitis occurring in response to the following substances is occasionally seen:

Sulphuric acid from cap lamp batteries.
Alkalis—sodium hydroxide in lamp batteries.
Certain oils and greases.

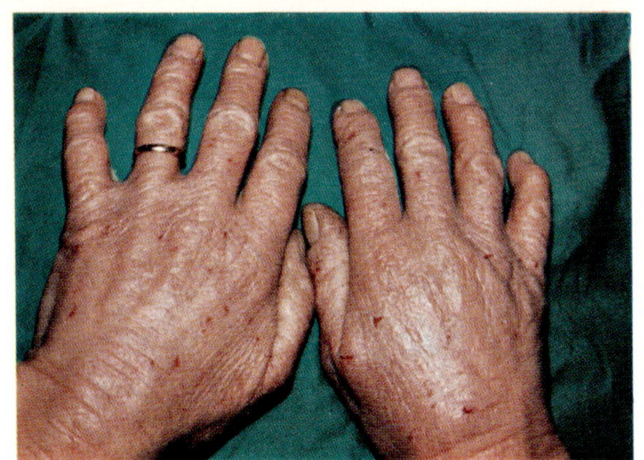

Fig. 1

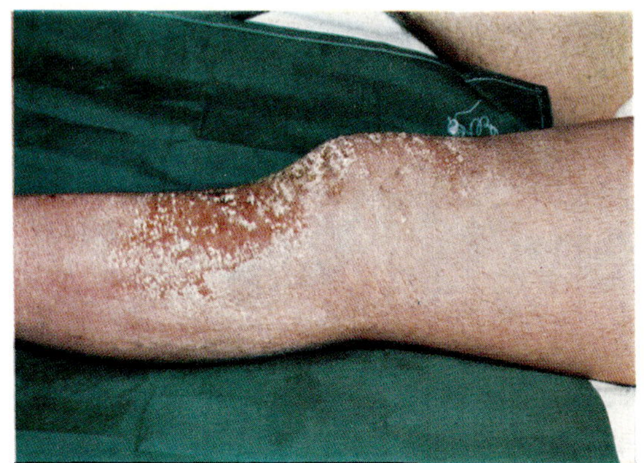

Fig. 2

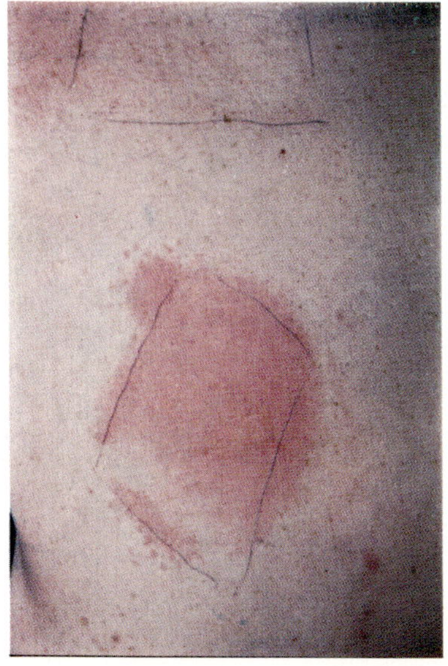

Fig. 3

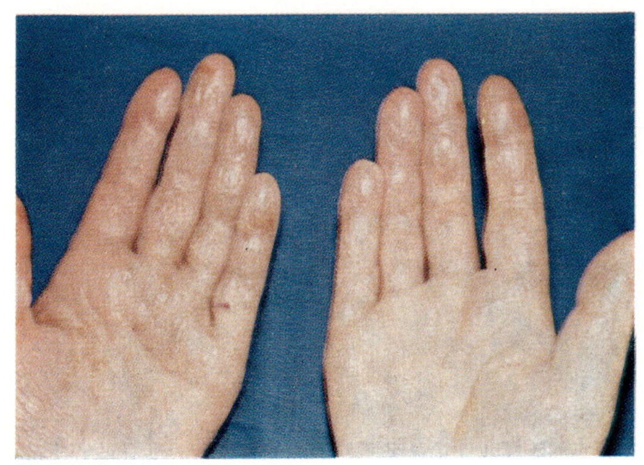

Fig. 4

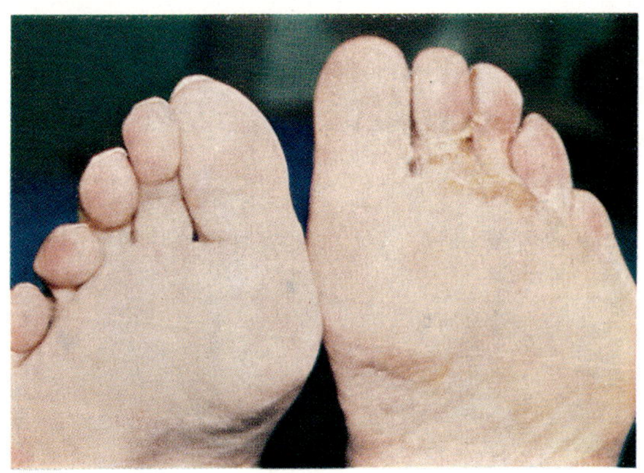

Fig. 5

Cement and lime.

Degreasing agents, solvents such as trichlorethylene.

Mineral salts in high concentration in underground water, e.g. sodium, magnesium and calcium chlorides.

Sensitizers

A sensitizer is an agent which does not cause any perceptible effect on first exposure and, in the majority of cases in industry, visible effects will not develop until there has been long continued exposure to it. Again, the agent itself may be in a liquid, solid, or volatile form. In some cases a reaction may develop after a very short exposure, as for example, in the local application of sulphonamide and penicillin preparations (Fig. 2). Only a small proportion of individuals exposed become sensitized.

Once the skin becomes sensitized it usually remains so, although the sensitivity may slowly decline if further exposure is avoided. It may also become sensitive to substances of a similar chemical structure—the phenomenon of cross sensitization. When an area of a patient's skin becomes sensitized to some agent the whole of the skin also becomes sensitive; the use of the patch test* as a diagnostic agent rests upon this fact (Fig. 3). Many industrial sensitizers are non-protein substances, and are, therefore, unable to stimulate cellular mediated hyper-sensitivity by themselves. They are believed to act as haptens or partial antigens by combining with protein in the skin to form complexes, which then induce a sensitivity reaction of the delayed type.

In factories and workshops sensitization dermatitis is not uncommon but in mining it is rare. However, materials occasionally causing sensitization in mining are:

Explosives and their sheaths.

Hydraulic and flushing oils leaking from hydraulic chocks and props, drills, hammers or picks.

Rubber lamp cables.

Rubber boots, rubber gloves and protective footwear. Sensitization here arises from anti-oxidants and accelerators used in the manufacture of rubber. In footwear the main sensitizing agents include dyes, chromium salts, rubber accelerators and formaldehyde.

Chemicals in leather. Chromate sensitivity may be produced by hat bands, leather gloves and footwear.

Resins, plastics, e.g. protective gloves.

Chemicals used in the treatment of timber, e.g. creosote, fire proofing chemicals.

Chromate as a contaminant of cement.

Chemicals used in the fire proofing of brattice cloths.

Antiseptic substances, such as flavine and balsam of Peru or other

* See Appendix 1.

local applications such as antihistamines and local anaesthetics have been responsible for sensitization dermatitis arising as a result of treatment of wounds in First Aid and Casualty Departments. Medical Departments in most industries are now aware of the hazards associated with these substances and no longer use them.

To emphasize the difference between these two types of dermatitis, the main features of each are given below in tabular form:

Primary Irritant	*Sensitization*
Would affect normal skin in all exposed persons if applied in a sufficiently concentrated form for a sufficient length of time.	Affects only a limited number of those exposed.
Only the exposed area affected.	Whole of the skin may be affected.
Effect is variable according to concentration of irritant and duration of exposure.	Reaction varies more in relation to frequency of application, degree of exposure and potency of the sensitizer.
Reaction may be immediate or delayed.	Reaction does not occur until sensitization of the skin is established. After that it is immediate.
Patch test gives negative result when the irritant is applied in low dilution; if applied undiluted, may give a positive reaction.	Patch tests with suspected allergens in low dilution are likely to give positive results.
Occurs directly on the exposed site and consists of an erythema, vesication and oedema varying in degree according to the potency of the irritant substance.	Onset is rapid, sometimes explosive and consists of erythema, vesication and oedema together with marked itching on the exposed site with often secondary sensitization spreading to other areas of the body.

Despite the apparently clear-cut differentiation, there is often some overlap between the two types; a primary irritant may at times act as a sensitizer and vice versa. One further aetiological factor must always be considered, wear and tear.

Wear and Tear

This is certainly the most important factor in mining. It has been shown that out of 41 cases of occupational dermatitis, 68 per cent of cases were of this type and 29 per cent were eczematous dermatitis of constitutional origin aggravated by the working environment. Furthermore, there is a long latent period of many years before the eruption develops, usually in middle life, the highest prevalence being in the 36–45 year group (Williamson, 1962).

The condition appears to be a consequence of long continued exposure to an inert dust which produces an eventual breakdown of the skin with the development of an eczematous dermatitis. The dust acts as a weak primary irritant of a cumulative type which, while not producing a lesion under normal circumstances, does so when the protective mechanism of the skin becomes exhausted. Exhaustion arises from prolonged contact, along with friction and sweating which, together with increasing age, render the skin more vulnerable to breakdown. Chromate contamination has been thought to be a factor in the production of miners' dermatitis but this is unlikely.

Once it has appeared, the condition is often of a protracted nature, in this particular series showing an average duration of four years, with 71 per cent of cases lasting over one year and only 2 per cent less than one month; there was a fairly marked tendency towards relapse.

Generally, there is a predilection for the condition to occur on the legs, ankles and feet, together with lesions on the dorsal surfaces of the hands and forearms. In parts of the mine not immediately involved in mineral extraction the preponderance of the lesions would seem to be on the hands and forearms.

In all the foregoing varieties secondary eruptions may occur on other parts of the body due to auto-sensitization.

Reasons for Chronicity

In theory an occupational dermatitis should clear rapidly when the cause is removed. Unfortunately, this may not occur in practice for a number of reasons, which may include:

   (i) Chronic irritation of the skin by overwashing or by the application of an antiseptic solution in the mistaken belief that the condition is due to infection.

  (ii) Treatment with unsuitable preparations, producing a super-added primary irritant or contact dermatitis.

 (iii) Lack of sedation to relieve itching and to break the vicious circle of irritation, scratching, skin damage and further irritation.

  (iv) The presence of polyvalent sensitivities.

   (v) Hot conditions at work inducing excessive sweating, coupled with dusty conditions producing friction between the clothing and the lesion.

  (vi) Secondary infection of the lesions.

 (vii) Continued exposure to irritants.

(viii) The presence of an underlying constitutional element, the main factors to consider here being:
    (*a*) the seborrhoeic skin
    (*b*) the dry skin—xeroderma and ichthyosis
    (*c*) the senile skin
                    which have a low resistance to damage.

(ix) Psychological factors; these are important and should always be assessed in the overall picture.

(x) Possible diagnostic errors.

The Diagnosis of Occupational Dermatitis

Apart from the appearance of the eruption, a careful history is the most important step in reaching an accurate diagnosis. The physician must be something of a dermatologist, an engineer and a chemist. Points to establish in the history are:

(i) The patient's occupation—an exact description of this in simple terms should be noted including all possible substances with which he comes in contact. It should also be recorded whether other workmen have been affected similarly.

(ii) The primary site of onset of the eruption.

(iii) Local treatment given and whether any exacerbation was produced by this.

(iv) Previous drug therapy should be noted: the question of improvement of the eruption when the patient is on holiday or off work is important.

(v) Previous asthma, eczema/dermatitis or allergic conditions; in addition, note should be taken of previous nervous conditions, such as anxiety and depression.

(vi) Family history—a strong history of eczema or atopy should be given due consideration.

(vii) Washing facilities used: barrier creams and hand cleansers available.

(viii) Domestic, financial and social aspects; whether there have been domestic crises, housing problems, dissatisfaction with working conditions, fear of unemployment or disability, whether the patient has too much or too little intelligence for the job.

(ix) Any hobbies such as gardening, painting, photography and car maintenance—contact with cement, glue, oil or epoxy resins.

Examination

As in the solution of any general medical problem, a careful examination should follow, at which the whole of the skin surface should be inspected in a good light, together with the appropriate physical examination. Urine examination should always be performed to exclude glycosuria.

The distribution and character of the lesions should be considered but too rigid an attitude should be avoided, for example, lesions may assume a nummular pattern but if the distribution is consistent and the changes occur with work and remit when the patient is off work, occupational dermatitis must be considered to be highly likely. This waxing and waning in response to work is very important.

In suspected cases of sensitization, dermatitis patch testing with the suspected substances will often be helpful. In view of the occasional "flare-up" produced by this procedure, a patch test should not be done in the acute phase. The patch test, if negative, usually excludes a sensitizer. In some centres battery patch testing to as many as 20 common contactants is undertaken.

Differential Diagnosis

Other conditions which should be considered in reaching a diagnosis are:

(i) *Contact Dermatitis of Non-occupational Origin*

One must not forget that a patient's exogenic dermatitis may be of non-occupational origin and be caused by some agent unconnected with his work, for example, plants, detergents, materials used in home decorating, car maintenance or even the material of a garment.

(ii) *Pompholyx*

Here the eruption is symmetrical, primarily affecting the sides of the digits and is usually of a "sago grain" pattern showing microvesicles which break down, weep and eventually scale. Non-inflammatory vesication of the palms or soles is almost unknown in an occupational dermatitis. Patients with pompholyx often have hyperidrosis of the palms and a fine tremor of the outstretched fingers. The condition tends to be worse in the warm weather. It may also be associated with a tinea pedis, when a pompholyx occurs as an "ide" (sympathetic) eruption which resolves when the lesion on the feet is treated (Fig. 4). Not uncommonly, pompholyx of the hands occurs as a psychosomatic disorder at times of stress.

(iii) *Scabies*

Secondarily infected scabies may cause confusion in a patient who has not had a complete examination. Burrows should be sought in the creases of the fingers, palms, ulnar border of the hands, wrists, elbows, axillae, buttocks and soles, around the umbilicus and genitals. With experience, the acarus can be picked out from the head of the burrow with a needle or microscopical examination of a scraping from a suspected burrow may often reveal an acarus or ovum.

(iv) *Dermatophyte Infection*

A chronic scaling lesion of the palm and palmar surface of the fingers, particularly if unilateral with little inflammatory action, may be due to ringworm. The final diagnosis rests upon microscopical examination of a scraping from the lesion. It is important to remember that treatment with one of the fluorinated cortico-steroid preparations greatly alters the classical appearance of ringworm infection.

(v) *Nummular Eczema*

Here the lesions consist of discrete, coin-sized area of redness, weeping and crusting on the dorsum of the feet, hands, arms and forearms, running a chronic course. This condition is normally endogenous in origin but a similar pattern due to chromate and nickel sensitivity may occur.

(vi) *Lichen Simplex Chronicus*

This occurs as localized area of thickened, lined and pigmented skin occurring on the forearms, nape of neck, thighs and lower legs, and is produced by prolonged rubbing and scratching.

Rarer conditions which may cause difficulty and should be considered in the appropriate case are:
(*a*) Psoriasis of the hands.
(*b*) Acrodermatitis perstans (persistent pustular pompholyx).
(*c*) Seborrhoeic eczema.
(*d*) Atopic Eczema (including Besnier's prurigo).
(*e*) Lichen planus.
(*f*) Syphilis: secondary and tertiary lesions.

Cutaneous Hazards of Mining

The main irritant affecting the miner's skin is mineral dust. In certain situations there may be much sweating associated with hard physical work in a warm environment. The workings may be wet with water from either natural sources or water sprays used for dust suppression. Sometimes the mineral content of natural waters may show a high concentration of sodium chloride, magnesium chloride and calcium chloride, which causes the mineworker to complain of stinging and smarting of the skin. These waters will occasionally produce a burning erythematous eruption at the site of contact.

Mineral dust is sometimes abrasive when applied to the skin, coal dust is not. Most dusts when implanted in a wound do not give rise to irritation but produce superficial tattooing. It is possible that any irritant properties a dust may have is related to particle size and composition; for example, anthracite is more abrasive than bituminous coal, with steam coal occupying an intermediate position. Stone dust is definitely more abrasive; this effect increases through the range of the fine clays, clays, shales, silts and sandstones.

With the advent of communal baths, miners may wear the same clothing for work for far too long without having it washed and cleaned and it seems likely that these garments becoming impregnated with a mixture of mineral dust, sweat, mine water and oil eventually act as a mild surface abrasive.

Opposed skin surfaces are often rubbed together in heavy occupations but the unusual working environment of the miner may compel him to work for longer periods in cramped and awkward positions which bring into close apposition the surfaces of the calves with the posterior aspects of the thighs and also the forearms and sides of the trunk. Eruptions may be produced in a similar way on the forehead under the hat band of a protective helmet, beneath the trouser belt and under the knee pads and straps, beneath the lamp battery and over the sacrum and round the top of boots.

Mention has been made of other types of occupational dermatitis occurring in the mineworker. These are small in number compared with the "wear and tear" group. As mechanization proceeds, there will inevitably be greater contact with oils and greases to which the occasional miner may become sensitive.*

Tinea pedis,† though not directly a skin hazard of mining, is a problem in the heated communal baths and its spread has been investigated extensively in coal miners by Gentles and Holmes (1957).

The Prevention of Occupational Dermatitis in Mining

This problem can be sub-divided as follows:

Control of the Environment

The factors concerned in dermatitis are mineral dust, temperature, ventilation, humidity and wet working conditions. Control, where possible, of this environment is mainly the concern of the mining and dust suppression engineers, together with advice, where necessary, from the doctor. The control of dust hinges on the adequacy of wet methods of dust suppression, together with vacuum extraction in appropriate cases and good general ventilation. Temperature is difficult to control in a mine, although adequate ventilation will help and in hot, deep mines the use of cooling apparatus in the intake air may reduce temperature and sweating and make working conditions more bearable.

In order to reduce the frictional component of dust in the clothes of the mine worker, it is essential that all working garments should be washed frequently and kept in a state of good repair. A one piece, light-weight and fire proof overall with central laundering facilities at work would have obvious advantages.

The Medical Aspects

The doctor in the mining industry may reduce the incidence of industrial dermatitis by paying careful attention to existing dermatitis when carrying out medical examination of new entrants. It is desirable that he should have a good working knowledge of the processes involved, together with their associated dermatological hazards.

---

* See Appendixes 2 and 3.
† See Appendix 4.

A past history of eczema, occupational dermatitis, Besnier's prurigo, xeroderma, ichthyosis or "the seborrhoeic diathesis" renders the skin more likely to subsequent breakdown.

The presence of a skin lesion may, at first sight, seem to exclude a new entrant but this should depend upon the diagnosis of the lesion and the site involved, coupled with the particular occupational hazards of the work contemplated; for example, a patient with severe acne vulgaris would be unsuitable for work with pitch, tar or oil; the man with extensive psoriasis is better excluded as even with treatment, relapse is likely, although a mild, discoid psoriasis may do quite well provided that there are no lesions over the prepatellar region, if kneeling is anticipated. On the other hand, ichthyosis does not do well where there is a good deal of dust present and where scrubbing in the bath is necessary for its removal.

A suggested scheme for the assessment of the new entrant to mining might be as follows:

Eczema

Patients with constitutional, seborrhoeic, gravitational eczema or pompholyx should not be allowed to work underground unless it is slight and even then should not work in dusty conditions.

Occupational Dermatitis

Unless it is mild and due to specific conditions not likely to be met with within the particular mining industry, cases should not work underground and should be graded for surface work only. Those with a past history of severe, recurring dermatitis would not be suitable for employment in mining.

Psoriasis

Isolated patches which have not caused any trouble should not debar the entrant from work underground. If, however, the condition is more generalized, it is unlikely that such a case would be suitable for work in the environmental conditions of coal mining.

Ichthyosis

The new entrant suffering from the more severe forms of this condition is unsuitable for employment in the mining industry.

General

Entrants showing chronic and widespread or frequently relapsing skin conditions will be unsuitable for mining, for example:

    (*a*) Chronic inflammatory dermatoses, e.g. recurrent folliculitis.
    (*b*) Other chronic diseases, e.g. dermatitis herpetiformis, parapsoriasis. Many of these will already be under specialist supervision.

(*c*) Cysts, tumours and other diseases of the skin of such extent and position as to interfere with the normal wearing of clothes and equipment.

Education

In his preliminary training the new entrant should have some of the principles of prevention instilled into him. Instruction should include a description of the hazard involved in the various jobs, and should emphasize the importance of careful washing and drying of the skin, the necessity for regular and frequent change of working clothing, avoidance of harsh abrasives and soaps, paraffin and other unsuitable substances for cleansing purposes. The causes and effects of occupational dermatitis and its non-contagious nature should be explained. Further, should skin trouble arise, the importance of early treatment to prevent chronicity should be emphasized. Ignorance and fear are important causes of prolongation and often an early diagnosis and prompt treatment will allay this anxiety.

Minimal Contact

This is self-explanatory but it is easier to obtain in a surface plant, fitting shop or engineering workshop than it is underground in a mine. If it is not possible to reduce external contact to an absolute minimum, the question then arises of providing suitable protective clothing. In the main, this is confined to the provision of gloves usually made from leather or plastic. However, dust may get inside these during work, and this, together with sweating, produces frictional lesions. In some cases, a sensitization dermatitis may develop in reaction to the material of the glove itself.

Avoidance of Sensitizing Preparations in the Treatment of Injuries and Skin Lesions

In the Medical Department primary irritant and potential sensitizers should be avoided for topical application in treatment. Flavine, balsam of Peru, antihistamine creams, sulphonamides, certain antibiotic preparations such as penicillin, chloramphenicol, neomycin ointment and local anaesthetics are the common offenders and should not be used in local treatment. It is also wise not to use drugs topically which, if sensitization is established, would then preclude their use systemically on some future occasion. Sodium fucidate 2 per cent and chlortetracycline 3 per cent in an ointment or cream base are useful topical antibiotic preparations. Certain non-antibiotic antiseptics such as iodochlorhydroxyquinoline and dichlorohydroxyquinaldine (British proprietary preparations Vioform and Steroxin) are also of value.

Regular Inspection of the Skin

This is again easier to carry out in the factory or workshop than in the mine but nurses and medical orderlies should be trained to pick out the early lesion in their patients.

Barrier Creams

At the present time there is considerable doubt as to the efficiency of these preparations and it seems likely that their greatest benefit is in helping to remove dust and dirt after a day's work. They may also be useful for training the workman in a prophylactic routine, the use of a suitable barrier cream being only a part of a preventive programme. In wet conditions underground it may be helpful for the worker to apply a water resistant barrier cream before work and in workshops an oil resistant type should be provided in dispensers. Hand cleansing agents are certainly or some value for use after work, if only to prevent petrol, paraffin and harsh abrasives being used as cleansing agents.

Treatment of Occupational Dermatitis

Generally the mine doctor should consider that it is within his province to treat patients with occupational dermatitis and other skin conditions whilst the patient remains at work. In many countries the mine's medical centre is not only responsible for the treatment of the patient but also of his family and will often include full hospital facilities. Where treatment is undertaken, it is advisable that this should be done by agreement with the patient's personal physician, if he has one, and any change in the treatment should be notified. In all cases, careful records should be kept. The saving of working time when daily dressing is needed is enormous where this can be done efficiently in medical departments.

With these points in mind, a scheme for the treatment of occupational dermatitis is given below:

Treatment—General

Patients should be advised about the cause of their trouble and about the precautions they should take to avoid contact with further non-specific irritants, sensitizers or cross sensitizing substances.

The Acute Widespread Eruption

In the acute stage, especially if widespread, physical and mental rest is required and the patient is better treated off work, either under the care of his personal physician or in a hospital ward. Sedation is valuable to relieve itching and to ensure adequate sleep. Useful drugs are amylobarbitone 30 mg two or three times daily; diazepam 2 or 5 mg two or three times daily with further hypnotics at night if required such as nitrazepam 5 to 10 mg. Antihistamine drugs, e.g. promethazine hydrochloride or trimeprazine tartrate may also be used for the sedative and anti-puritic effect. Sedation should be continued in a reduced dose for several weeks after the condition has settled.

Affected areas should not be washed with soap and water but cleansed with arachis oil.

When the patient returns to work it is likely that the skin will still be in a reactive stage and irritated by non-specific irritants. It is useful, therefore, to arrange suitable alternative and relatively dust-free work for three or four weeks in appropriate cases before a trial return is made to their previous occupation.

Sub-acute and Chronic Cases

Management of these phases is less restrictive and is based on the following principles:

(i) To remove the patient from the primary irritant or sensitizer, if known, and to continue with necessary surveillance.

(ii) To provide alternative work where necessary. Many of these patients are better off, both financially and mentally, in continuing employment and should be encouraged to work whenever a reasonable job can be offered. The alternative employment provided should be reasonably clean and not in warm, humid or wet conditions. The patient should cleanse his skin, using a minimum of soap and water on the affected area, with arachis oil on cotton wool. This type of case can often be supervised by the mine doctor and the nursing staff.

Local Treatment

Often the simplest of treatments with some soothing application and protection from further noxious agents is required. In the "weeping" stage calamine lotion, or if the skin is too dry, oily calamine lotion, is useful but topical corticosteroids, for example, hydrocortisone 1 per cent in an ointment or cream base or the more powerful fluorinated corticosteroids, such as flucinolone acetonide 0·025 per cent, betamethasone valerate 0·1 per cent ointment or cream may produce more rapid improvement. Later these preparations can be diluted with oily cream or cetomacrogol in up to 1 in 8 dilution. Half strength Lassar's paste (salicylic acid 1 per cent, starch 12·5 per cent, zinc oxide 12·5 per cent, soft paraffin to 100 per cent) which is softer and easier to spread than the full strength paste, is useful in the sub-acute stage, as is coal tar solution paste (coal tar solution 5 per cent, zinc oxide 25 per cent, soft paraffin to 100 per cent). When redressing with a paste preparation it should be applied to areas where it has previously come off, removing the used paste with arachis oil. Covering with the appropriate size of tubular gauze dressing or stockinet forms a light protective dressing.

When secondary infection is present, potassium permanganate soaks or baths in a strength of 1 in 4,000 to 1 in 8,000 twice daily followed by the application of oily calamine lotion or a corticosteroid anti-bacterial preparation, for example, betamethasone valerate and clin-quinol are useful. Systemic antibiotic therapy may also be required.

In chronic dermatitis of the hands corticosteroid ointment is more effective if applied daily and occluded with polyethylene film gloves and sealed at the wrist with cellophane tape. In resistant cases superficial radiotherapy is often helpful. Mention should be made of other pro-tective occlusive dressings which can be applied by a nurse to prevent further itching and self-inflicted trauma; a useful form of these is ichthyol or coal tar impregnated bandages which may be used in either weeping eczema, sub-acute eczema with slight scaling, or in chronic lichenified eczema.

Prognosis

Many early cases of occupational dermatitis will settle quickly on the foregoing regimes. For reasons mentioned elsewhere, some may become resistant to treatment and form a hard core of patients attending dermatological clinics. In these cases there are often superimposed psychosomatic factors. Absence from work is likely to increase anxiety and adversely affect the course of the skin lesion; the longer the absence, the greater the anxiety produced.

At times relapse is found to be due to the patient having been put into some unsuitable job. Each case should be decided on its merits for there are considerable variations in the capacity to work or to accept disability.

It is generally accepted that once a patient develops a sensitization he will never be able to handle that substance at work again. In these cases the usual plan is for the patient to avoid the offending agent or, if this is impossible, a change of occupation is indicated. The patient with a primary irritant dermatitis is likely to meet with further irritants in whatever job he undertakes and will probably fare just as well by continuing in his previous occupation but taking suitable protective measures.

In the type of occupational dermatitis which occurs most commonly in mine workers, the "wear and tear" variety, it was found (Williamson, 1962) that slightly more than two-thirds of the patients affected, having been off work, returned to their previous occupation, the remainder being settled in alternative work underground or on the surface. It seemed that some of the more severe cases were remaining in unsuitable employment rather than suffer a fall in earnings. This agreed closely with previous findings by Matthews (1959) and Morgan and Davies (1956). In those patients who returned to their previous employment underground, it appeared that there was a greater risk of relapse than in those who were placed in alternative work. This may be because a change to alternative work usually involves a reduction in surrounding dust concentration, less physical exertion, often improved ventilation and consequently less sweating.

Appendix 1

A Method of Patch Testing

A patch test should not be undertaken in the acute stage.

A small portion of the suspected substance is applied to the unaffected skin usually on the upper back or inner aspect of the upper arm. If this is a powder it should be moistened with water and covered with a small square of gauze which is then fixed in position by adhesive strapping. Scrapings or shavings from solid substances to be tested can be applied in a similar manner. If the substance is in solution, a small piece of gauze or lint 15 mm square may be saturated with the solution and applied similarly. The strength of the solution needs to be dilute and reference should be made to a standard dermatological textbook for the required concentration for that particular substance. Special patch test dressings are now manufactured consisting of an aluminium foil backing with a small central pad to which the suspected agent is applied.

A control test with the covering material, but without the suspected sensitizer, should also be applied to another area. Both sites are then examined at 48 and 96 hour intervals, the reading being taken 20 minutes after removing the covering dressing. If, at any time, itching beneath the patch test becomes intolerable, the patient should remove it himself and report his findings.

If the offending substance is thought to be a photo-sensitizer the patch test may require exposure to sunlight before reading.

If the patch test is positive there will be, at the minimum, an erythematous eruption corresponding to the shape and size of the sensitizing agent or of the saturated gauze or lint applied; but there will be no corresponding reaction at the control site. All grades of reaction to the sensitizer may be seen and, at times, the lesions may be severe enough to produce a recrudescence of the original eruption.

Where a severe reaction may be expected an open patch test is used first. This involves application of the substance to the skin with no covering dressing.

Appendix 2

Furunculosis

Furunculosis is a common cause of skin disability in miners—one furuncle in an awkward situation can make work impossible. Outbreaks tend to occur in hot wet mines sometimes where the saline concentration of the water is high. Infection is due to the staphylococcus aureus and the site of the lesion is usually that which is subject to most friction—e.g. the neck, around the knees, the belt area and beneath knee pads. In all cases the urine should be tested to exclude glycosuria, a full blood count is advisable, and a swab taken from a lesion for culture and sensitivity testing of the organism.

Treatment

(*a*) *General*

It is important to ensure that working clothing is kept clean and changed frequently. When there are multiple lesions or if the patient has systemic effects, a course of the appropriate antibiotic is indicated. In severe and intractable cases a course of ultra violet light treatment to the whole body is often effective. In certain cases, a course of superficial X-ray therapy to the affected area is helpful.

(*b*) *Local*

The lesions should be kept as dry as possible and should be painted around with brilliant green 1 per cent or gentian violet 1 per cent in spirit. Local dressings of paste mag. sulph. or ung. ichthammol are useful; sodium fucidate 2 per cent ointment may abort an early lesion. In most cases of furunculosis it is thought that the organism is repeatedly spread over the skin surface from certain reservoir sites, such as the external nares and perianal and genital regions. Where the lesions are on the upper limbs and the upper part of the trunk and face, it is useful, therefore, to apply an antibiotic, usually neomycin, to the external nares daily and where lesions are mainly on the lower limbs and lower part of the trunk, to dust the perineum and perianal areas with a powder containing hexachlorophene. To reduce skin contamination further it is advisable for the patient to use a soap containing hexachlorophene.

Appendix 3

Skin Hazards From Oil and Grease in the Mining Industry

Fitters, welders and workers in engineering workshops are more liable to be affected by oils and greases, which are not a very important cause of skin trouble in underground workers. Further mechanization will, however, increase the miner's exposure to such substances.

Oils and greases can produce:

(*a*) Folliculitis.

(*b*) Sensitization dermatitis—which may be due also to the additives or antiseptics in the oil itself.

(*c*) Primary irritant dermatitis.

(*d*) Keratosis and carcinoma after long continued exposure, e.g. carcinoma of the scrotum.

It should be remembered that the condition of grease gun injury may occur in garage and maintenance workers where grease is injected accidentally under high pressure into the tissue planes, usually in the hand. Unless relieved by widespread decompression, the injury will give rise to sloughing of the tissues.

Dermatitis, often attributed to oil, may occur as a result of faulty hand cleansing after work with solvents or hard abrasive substances Further, there is an abrasive effect of metal swarf, often present in waste soluble oil, upon the skin itself.

Types of Oil Used

Industrial lubricating oils are generally mineral oils derived from crude petroleum by distillation. The skin effects are determined mainly by the temperature of distillation. Those which distil at low temperatures tend to have greater primary irritant and solvent effect than the higher temperature distillation residues which tend to cause oil acne and folliculitis or long-term effects on the skin such as keratosis and carcinoma. Common oils in use are:

(i) Straight oils without additives for hydraulic props and pneumatic picks.

(ii) Complex, additive oils for lubrication of locomotives and haulage engines.

(iii) Engineering cutting oils, often mixtures of oil, soap, phenol, creosote and antioxidants.

(iv) Straight cutting oils.

(v) Mineral oils with additives such as sulphur and chlorinated agents for cutting hard metals.

(vi) Greases—oils without additives but solidified with lime or soda and an inert filler such as chalk or graphite.

Appendix 4

Tinea Pedis

Tinea pedis (athlete's foot) is caused by a parasitic fungus (ringworm) which grows in the horny layer of the skin and which can also infect the nails. Infection can be spread by the bathroom floor at home, in hotels, in changing rooms and pithead baths. Investigations (Gentles and Holmes, 1957) of some 2,000 men at coal mines and power houses showed that 21 per cent of persons were infected in some degree with tinea pedis.

Type of Fungi
   (i) Trichophyton mentagrophytes
  (ii) Trichophyton rubrum
 (iii) Epidermophyton floccosum
Trichophyton mentagrophytes is the commonest organism, but the incidence of trichophyton rubrum is increasing. The latter may be extremely resistant to treatment at times.

Clinical Signs
Peeling, redness, maceration, raw areas, fissures, vesicles (small blisters) and secondary dermatitis.

Clinical Types
   (*a*) Interdigital: usually between 4th and 5th toes, maceration, peeling, scaling, fissuring.
   (*b*) Acute Vesicular: groups of itchy vesicles with scaling and peeling on raw areas on sole of foot, between or under toes—common in a hot summer (Fig. 5).
   (*c*) Dry, scaly: sharply defined, dull red, scaling areas on sole which commonly spread to dorsum and sides of foot, leg and hand.
   (*d*) Nails: yellow, brown and black in colour, thickened, distorted and friable nail plates, the lesions often commencing at the side.

Skin inflammations of the feet and toes should not immediately be labelled tinea pedis. Similar appearances may result from simple sweating and maceration of feet, pompholyx, eczema, and dermatitis of traumatic or contact type. A scraping of the lesion or a blister top should be taken and examined microscopically, after soaking in 10 per cent potassium hydroxide and gently warming the slide. This substance clears the keratin revealing the characteristic mycelia showing through the cleared scales. Culture and identification of the fungus from another scraping can be useful and are certainly called for in resistant cases.

Complications
   (*a*) Dermatitis from over treatment or from friction of shoes.
   (*b*) Secondary infection, e.g. cellulitis, infective dermatitis.
   (*c*) Toxic-ides, vesicular pompholyx of hands (Fig. 4), erythema of body, secondary sensitization spread.
   (*d*) Tinea cruris ("Dhobi's itch") in groins or buttocks.
   (*e*) Spread to legs, hands, body and other areas of the body.

Treatment

General

    (i) When in doubt as to the diagnosis, treat as for acute dermatitis rather than risk aggravation by treatment. Many acute cases will clear with such treatment without the use of fungicides. Normal peeling of the skin after dermatitis removes the keratin in which the fungus lives.

   (ii) Even in accepted cases avoid over treatment and supervise chronic cases.

Interdigital Tinea

    (i) Acute vesicular moist raw areas paint with pig. magent. or gentian violet 1 per cent aqueous solution.

   (ii) If chronic and scaling treat with ung. acid benz. co., alternative preparations being zinc undecenoate acid ointment or tolnaftate cream. Zinc undecenoate powder or tolnaftate powder should be used as a prophylactic.

Acute Vesicular Tinea

    (i) Rest.

   (ii) Foot baths of potassium permanganate 1/8,000 in water followed by the application of oily calamine lotion.

  (iii) Following the acute stage pig. magent. Alternative preparations which may be used are ung. acid. benz. co. or tolnaftate cream.

Dry, Scaly Tinea

Ung. acid benz. co. or tolnaftate cream.
Dithranol ointment (under medical supervision only).

Nails

Fungus infection of the nails was virtually incurable until the introduction of griseofulvin, and even now requires prolonged treatment as there is a high relapse rate.

Griseofulvin

The use of this drug in fungus disease of the skin, hair and nails is an important advance. However, accurate diagnosis and selection of cases are important; minor fungus infections can be treated successfully with topical remedies.

    Griseofulvin given orally is taken up by the newly formed keratin which does not then support the growth of the fungus. It should, therefore, be given until the whole of the affected keratin is shed. This varies with the tissue affected and with tinea of the nails this may take several months.

It has no antibacterial effect and is not active against candida albicans (monilia).

Fine particle griseofulvin is used for greater absorption (tab. griseo-fulvin F.P. 125 mg and 500 mg) the usual adult dose being 4–9 tablets each of 125 mg taken daily with food. Side effects are infrequent, usually mild and transient, e.g. headache and gastric discomfort. It is not normally indicated in tinea affections of the toe clefts but is indicated when palms and soles may be involved.

References

Gentles, J. C., and Holmes, J. G. (1957), "Foot ringworm in coal miners." *British Journal of Industrial Medicine*, **14,** 22.

Matthews, B. F. (1959), "Dermatitis in the South Wales mining industry. A report of a survey of two collieries." *British Journal of Industrial Medicine*, **16,** 200.

Morgan, J. K. and Davies, J. H. T. (1956), "The influence of attitudes in rehabilitation of industrial cases". *British Journal of Dermatology*, **68,** 41.

Williamson, D. M. (1962), M.D. Thesis, Leeds University. "The Problem of Dermatitis in the Coal Miner."

Chapter 12

Beat Diseases

Introduction

This term, which refers broadly to occupational bursitis and cellulitis occurring in miners, is a colloquial expression and may have originated from the throbbing pain so often associated with the acute stage of these conditions.

Bursitis is one of the oldest occupational disabilities recorded and occurs in any occupation which involves pressure or friction or repeated minor trauma over a subcutaneous bursa. Apart from mining, the olecranon bursa may be affected, for example, in students and bricklayers and the pre-patellar bursa in housemaids, clergymen and nuns. Adventitious bursae may arise due to repeated local trauma as, for example, on the vertex of the skull in market garden porters, over the 7th cervical spinous process in fish porters and over the upper part of the shoulder and clavicle in bricklayers, dustmen and timber porters. Tailors used to develop adventitious bursae over the lateral malleoli due to working in a cross legged position.

The greatest sufferer now from the beat disorders is the coal miner. These conditions are associated with work in confined places, in low coal seams and headings where standing work is difficult or impossible. Wet conditions may also be an associated factor increasing the traumatic effect of coal and rock particles and predisposing to maceration of the overlying skin.

Classification of Beat Disorders

The beat diseases comprise:

(i) Subcutaneous cellulitis of the hand—beat hand.

(ii) Subcutaneous cellulitis or acute bursitis over the elbow—beat elbow.

(iii) Subcutaneous cellulitis or acute bursitis arising at or about the knee—beat knee.

(iv) Inflammation of the synovial lining of the wrist joint and tendon sheaths—tenosynovitis.

Beat Hand

This is essentially an acute cellulitis affecting the subcutaneous tissues of the palms due to infection with either a streptococcus or a staphylococcus. It occurs in miners handling shovels or picks, the portal of entry

14

of infection being a small abrasion or fissure resulting from repeated jarring of the palm by the handle of the tool. Hyperkeratosis of the palm and callosity formation with subsequent fissuring is probably an important antecedent factor.

The symptoms are pain, initially of an aching character, becoming throbbing if pus is present under tension, together with erythema and swelling. There may be loss of function as shown by limitation of movements of the fingers and wrist with local tenderness on palpation. Lymphangitis, epitrochlear and axillary lymphadenitis may follow if treatment is not started early with an appropriate antibiotic. Usually the condition resolves with antibiotic therapy but, if neglected, surgical incision and drainage may be required. Furthermore, if delay occurs, extension of the infection may occur to the palmar tendon sheaths and fascial spaces with the possibility of subsequent contracture of the fingers. This condition is not confined to miners and may similarly affect boiler stokers.

Prevention

This consists in ensuring that the handles of all tools are smooth and have no projecting splinters. Well fitting protective gloves with an elastic wrist cuff may be helpful but whilst reducing the tendency to callosity formation, may sometimes predispose to direct trauma if coal or stone particles become lodged within the glove. Early treatment is essential and may be undertaken in the mine's medical centre.

Beat Elbow

This is an acute inflammation affecting the olecranon bursa and the surrounding subcutaneous tissues. There are two types:

(a) Acute Simple or Traumatic Bursitis

This results from either a single blow to the unprotected elbow, for example, while swinging a heavy tool in a confined space or crawling along a mechanized coal face. The condition presents with severe acute localized pain settling as a fluctuant swelling develops rapidly over the olecranon. A similar condition may arise where a miner working in a very low coal seam has to pivot on one elbow repeatedly while using a shovel. Aspiration of the swelling reveals a serosanguinous fluid or often pure blood, indicating that a haemobursa is present. This may resolve slowly with conservative therapy or become chronic and asymptomatic. Aspiration, which may need to be repeated and followed by a firm pressure dressing, offers the best chance of recovery. In chronic cases where the bursa wall is hypertrophic and fibrin bodies are present, excision of the bursa is indicated.

(*b*) Infective Bursitis

This may follow extension from a local infective lesion on the forearm or elbow, usually a superficial folliculitis, or may arise from direct entry of infection through an abrasion in the region of the elbow.

Prevention

Apart from the acute traumatic bursitis, beat elbow is not seen in higher coal seams. Where it is necessary for a miner to work in particularly low seams, an elbow pad is helpful, although these are not often acceptable to the workmen because of the difficulty of keeping them in position.

Beat Knee

This is by far the most important and commonest of this group of disorders. It is a persistent, though decreasing, problem of narrow seam mining, occurring in seams of between 0·75 and 1·4 metres. In Great Britain the incidence in 1969 was 5·5 per thousand workers, having decreased gradually from 12 per thousand in 1962. This reduction is multifactorial, resulting from exhaustion of the more unprofitable and narrower seams and from improved preventive measures and early treatment.

Aetiological Factors

During the past twenty years, as coal seams were worked out, many became narrower and more difficult to work. With seams of about one metre in height the workman may have to spend anything from a quarter to the whole of a working shift on his knees performing hard manual work (Roantree, 1957). Only the introduction of automatic mining in these thin seams will further reduce the incidence.

The Kneeling Posture

Kneeling and squatting positions become so much a matter of habit and comfort in narrow seam miners that they will adopt this position for relaxation. Sharrard (1965) points out that there is nothing more striking than to see a group of miners clearing snow by shovelling on their knees. The main pressure area in both kneeling positions is a triangular area bounded by the inferior part of the patella, the tibial tubercle, and the condyles of the femur.

The Skin

The skin responds to intermittent pressure and friction with hyper-keratosis, a feature of the pre-patellar area of most miners, which becomes rugose and thickened. Maceration of this area may result from sweating associated with high temperature and humidity in deep seams. The type of floor in the seam or hardness of coal particles does not seem to play a significant part in the incidence of beat knee, nor does, apparently, the wetness, temperature or humidity, although these factors may have a tendency to produce maceration of the skin (Sharrard, 1963).

Occupations Affected

The greatest proportion of miners with beat knee are colliers, who have to kneel mainly in one place over a whole shift. Other workers at risk are packers, rippers and maintenance men who kneel and crawl intermittently.

Individual Susceptibility

Among miners working in identical conditions some will never develop beat knee. Indeed certain individuals never wear protective knee pads at all on the coal face. Watkins, Fernandez and Edmonds (1968) suggest that the incidence of beat knee decreases with increasing age, the younger men showing the higher incidence. There are a number of reasons for this finding, including non-adaptation of the skin and bursae to pressure, and inability of the cruciate ligaments of the knee to stretch adequately so as to allow the subject to rest back on his heels. A further factor may be that the younger miner tends to work harder and faster and undertakes more overtime work.

It has been shown (Sharrard, 1963) that no correlation exists between a prominent tibial tubercle and the incidence of beat knee. Height of the subject may affect stresses on the knees but weight does not appear to be a factor. Short men wear out protective knee pads more rapidly than tall men because of the greater frequency of leaning forwards and backwards when shovelling. Beat knee often develops after restarting work in the coal face following a period of absence.

Classification

In an intensive clinical survey of the aetiology of beat knee, Sharrard (1963) investigated 579 coal face workers, of whom 233 showed evidence of either past or present beat knee at the time of examination. These were classified into three groups:
  (i) Inflammatory lesions (28)
  (ii) Acute simple bursitis (109)
  (iii) Chronic simple bursitis (96).

This classification can be compared with that of Roantree (1957) who reviewed 102 cases of beat conditions of the knee in which he found it possible to classify all cases into one of three groups, namely inflammatory, pressure lesions and other conditions. Roantree's second group compares closely with Sharrard's group two and three. The prepatellar bursa was affected in each case more than twice as often as the infra-patellar or compound bursae involving both regions.

Inflammatory Lesions

These usually start with an infected hair follicle, a superficial folliculitis, over the anterior aspect of the knee. This may heal spontaneously with no loss of working time if situated in an area which is not subject to pressure. Roantree (1957) is of the opinion that transmission of weight through infective foci exercises an unfavourable effect upon natural attempts at localization of the infection leading to development of follicular abscesses with a circumscribed zone of cellulitis (Fig. 1). The infecting organism is usually a staphylococcus aureus, coagulase positive, but occasionally a haemolytic streptococcus is isolated where there is a diffuse cellulitis. Coal particles may occasionally be discharged from localized abscesses, indicating that some of the lesions may arise as a result of penetration by a spicule of coal or stone into the skin.

Effusions which may arise in the underlying bursae are only very rarely infected, being usually sympathetic and such as may occur in the knee joint in association with an acute osteomyelitis at the lower end of the femur. These effusions resolve rapidly with the disappearance of the adjacent infective lesion. Over the years there has been a diminished incidence of infective lesions as compared with earlier reports (Collis and Llewellyn, 1924). This may be due to improved personal hygiene engendered by the introduction of pit head baths and improved protection for the knee.

Treatment of Inflammatory Lesions

Wherever possible a swab should be taken from the lesion for bacteriological examination, including assessment of sensitivity of the organism to antibiotics, but this should not delay early treatment, preferably with an initial intramuscular injection of penicillin. Fucidic acid 2 per cent ointment locally may help to abort an early folliculitis and an antibacterial dusting powder containing hexachlorophane applied to the skin surface daily after bathing will help to reduce bacterial flora. The urine should be tested routinely for glycosuria. Cessation of work with rest, elevation of the limb and quadriceps exercises are important, as is a period of alternative work before kneeling is recommenced.

Acute Simple Bursitis

This is the most important lesion arising as a result of kneeling. In a few instances, as in beat elbow, there is a history of acute trauma in the form of a direct blow upon the knee followed by immediate swelling and tenderness. Most cases, however, develop spontaneously while kneeling at work or after returning home. The appearance is easily confused with an infective bursitis, the bursa being hot and tender with discoloration of the overlying skin. Aspiration of the bursa almost always produces a sterile fluid which is often pure blood (Fig. 2).

Where an acute episode is superimposed on a chronic simple bursitis, the fluid is usually blood-stained.

The immediate cause of acute simple bursitis appears to be a haemo-bursa due to rupture of small blood vessels in the wall of the bursa

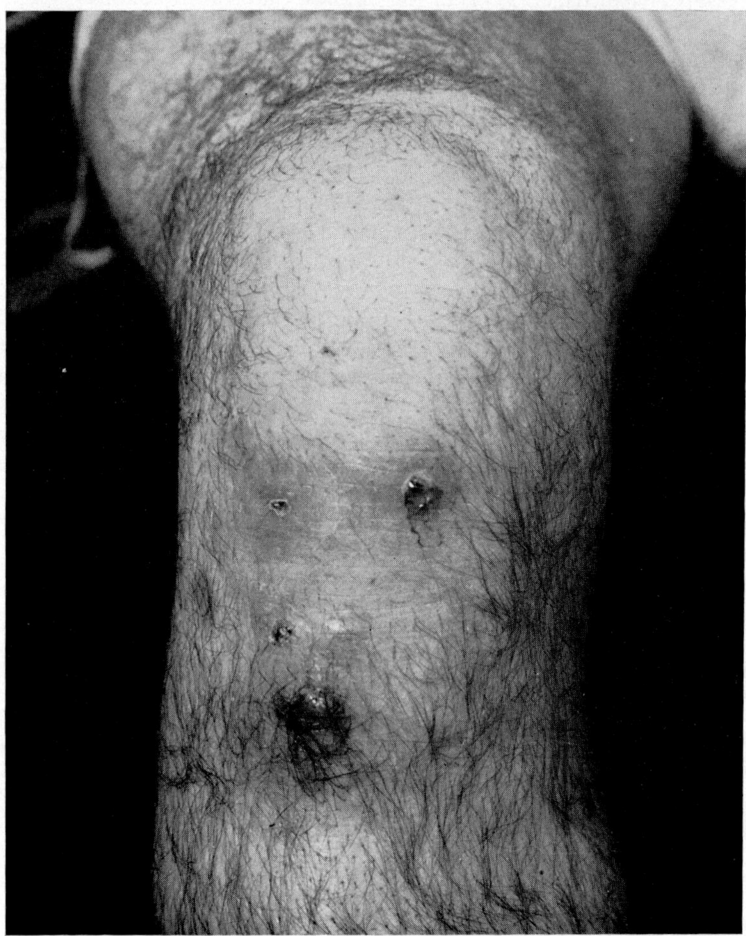

Fig. 1. Beat knee, inflammatory type: follicular abscesses with staphylococcal cellulitis.

Sharrard (1965) has found, by a series of experiments designed to discover forces and pressures exerted upon miners' knees in the course of kneeling, that immense shearing strains and loads are set up in alternate knees during shovelling movements. These fluctuations are extensive and pressures may rise to as high as $14\cdot06\,\mathrm{kg\,cm^{-2}}$ during

every movement, an average miner moving his shovel once every two
to five seconds.

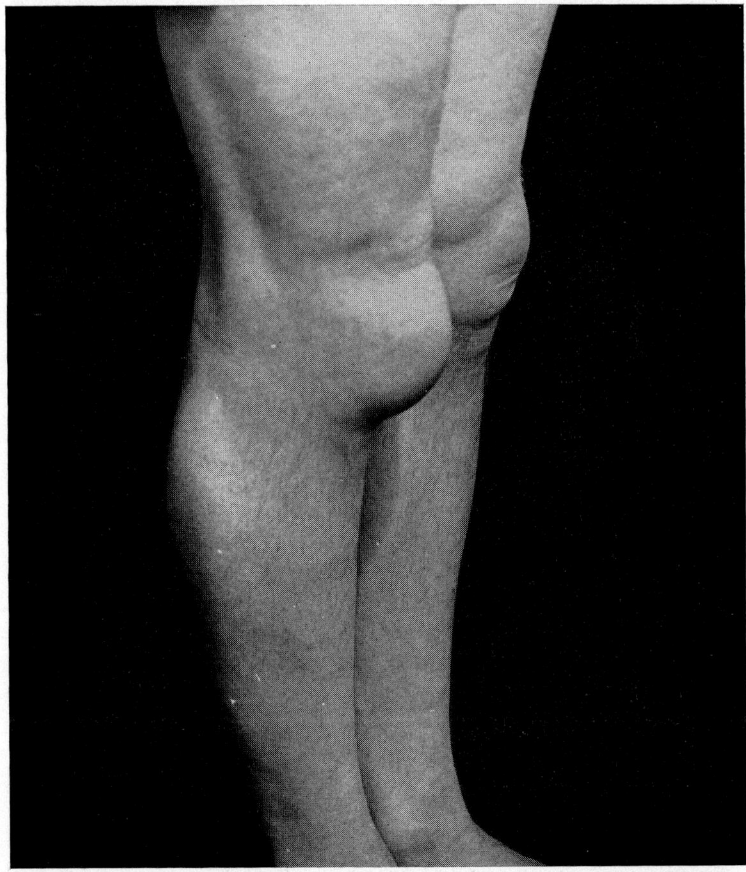

FIG. 2. Right acute simple pre-patellar bursitis: haemobursa on aspiration.

Chronic Simple Bursitis

This is the commonest form of bursitis in miners presenting with a
"cold" and persistent fluctuant swelling often with a previous history
of an acute episode that has not resolved (Fig. 3). In these cases
aspiration reveals a yellow fluid except where there has been a recent
exacerbation, when it is usually blood-stained. Histological sections
show marked fibrosis in the wall of the bursa and obliteration of many

of the large vessels. Long-standing cases may show deposits of haemosiderin in the wall. It has been suggested (Sharrard, 1963) that the

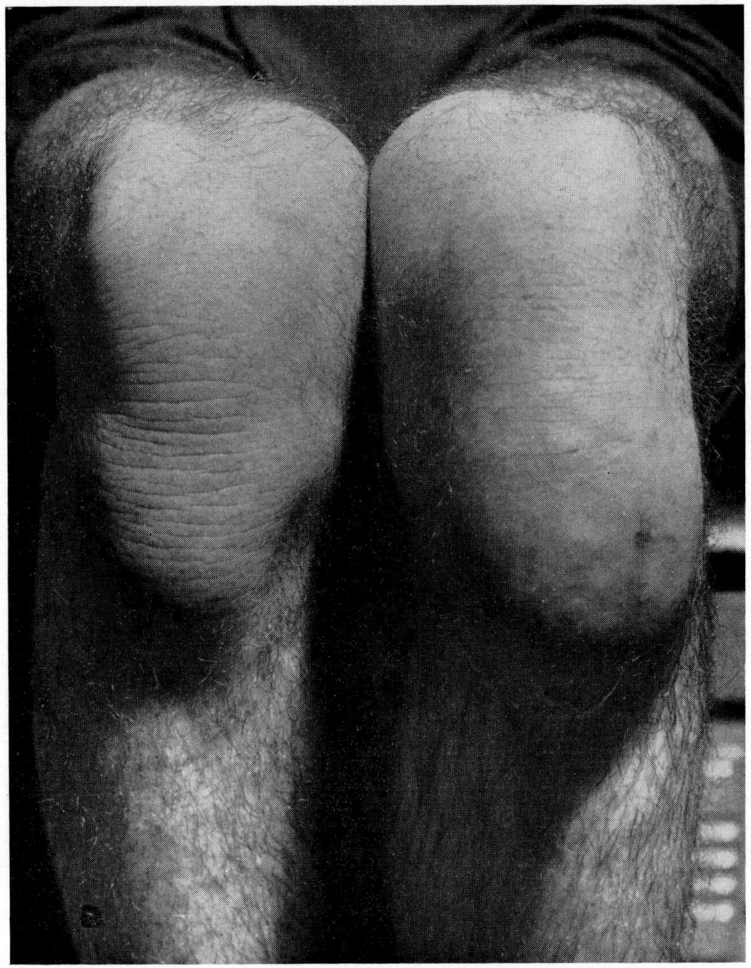

Fig. 3. Chronic simple bursitis affecting both infrapatellar bursae: haemobursa on aspiration.

normal mechanism for absorption of bursal fluid is faulty, the breakdown products of blood being slow in diffusing away, haemosiderin being trapped in the synovial membrane for long periods following injury. Larger particles are removed by phagocytosis and may then tend to block the lymphatics. Absorption of fluid is thus slowed accounting for the chronicity of the lesion.

Treatment of Simple Bursitis

Acute Simple Bursitis

Immediate aspiration of the bursa with a wide bore needle under local anaesthesia before organization has taken place followed by the application of a firm padded pressure bandage, gives the best results. A few cases will require further aspiration and improvement may be enhanced by the instillation of 1 ml of hyaluronidase after aspiration.

Chronic Simple Bursitis

Aspiration is seldom of value in the chronic form but may be helpful in an acute exacerbation. If a suitable knee pad cannot be obtained to accommodate the contour of the swelling without discomfort (McKenzie, 1966), excision of the bursa is indicated. Sharrard (1965) advocates a generous incision skirting the lateral margin of the bursa to avoid any weight-bearing area, the cutaneous nerves being avoided as far as possible. Healing is usually uneventful.

Prevention of Beat Knee

Wherever miners have to kneel in confined spaces the development of beat knee in some will be unavoidable. The incidence of the inflammatory lesions can be reduced by the adoption of regular washing of the skin with active antibacterial agents and by the use of antibacterial dusting powders in chronic staphylococcal carriers.

Any attempt to minimize the incidence of beat knee must be directed towards distribution of the acute pressure ensuing from pivoting on the knee over a wider area. That this is an important factor has been shown by Fernandez (1968), who described how men with beat knee could often continue to work provided that a large dressing was placed between the affected knee and a normal knee pad. McKenzie (1966) has shown how a much larger knee pad composed of sorbo rubber and extending half-way down the anterior tibial surface with a cup-shaped concavity for the distended bursa can enable a miner to continue working at the coal face. The disadvantage of these knee pads is their size and instability. Some form of knee protection would appear to be essential but many of the previous knee pads have not been very effective in cushioning the extremes of pressure fluctuations on the knee. Pads lined by felt and made from conveyor belting or leather prevent direct trauma to the knee by spicules of coal or stone but have no cushioning or absorbing effect and at times may become so hard as to predispose to bursitis themselves.

The National Coal Board of Great Britain, following an extensive investigation into the design of knee pads, together with experimental testing, have produced a comprehensive specification. The aims were (*a*) to provide adequate cushioning without making the kneeling surface unstable, (*b*) to allow free escape of sweat, pit water and coal grit on the kneeling surface, and (*c*) to be comfortable to work in, not only when kneeling, but also when crawling and walking. The outer cover is designed to be durable yet sufficiently pliable to allow reasonable flexion at the angle of the pad when the worker is walking and the knee extended. The casing should not be so soft that the straps cut through too readily or tear loose from it. The inner lining must be thick enough to cushion the knee adequately but there must be no marked movement of the inner pad on the outer cover producing instability. This specification for knee protection together with instruction of the miners in early self-diagnosis and the provision of effective treatment should maintain the reduction in the incidence of this condition which has occurred in recent years.

References

Collis, E. L. and Llewellyn, T. L. (1924), Special Report, No. 89. Medical Research Council, London.

Fernandez, R. H. P. (1958), "A paradox in the treatment of beat knee." *British Journal of Industrial Medicine*, **15**, 110.

McKenzie, G. F. (1966), Personal communication.

Roantree, W. B. (1957), "A review of 102 cases of beat conditions of the knee." *British Journal of Industrial Medicine*, **14**, 253.

Sharrard, W. J. W. (1965), "Pressure effects on the knee in kneeling miners." *Annals of the Royal College of Surgeons of England*, **36**, 309.

Sharrard, W. J. W. (1963), "Aetiology and pathology of beat knee." *British Journal of Industrial Medicine*, **20**, 24.

Watkins, J. T., Fernandez, R. H. P. and Edmonds, O. P. (1958), "A clinical survey of beat knee." *British Journal of Industrial Medicine*, **15**, 105.

Chapter 13

Extremes of Temperature

Introduction

The inescapable need to provide adequate ventilation in mine workings has faced the engineer in antiquity and doubtless in prehistoric times. In the modern industrial era the hazards to health and the limitations of work imposed by extremely hot environments have become increasingly serious as mines have gone deeper and when, as is often the case, they have been sunk in hot countries. Mines where the problems of heat stress are of very great concern include certain deep coal mines in Continental Europe, opencast and deep mines in tropical Africa, tropical Australia, tropical India and Japan. The problem is above all of crucial significance to the South African gold mining industry.

Systematic studies of physiological responses to heat under mining conditions were inaugurated in Britain at the turn of the century by J. S. Haldane, whose studies encompassed both tin and coal mining. His pioneering investigations have been greatly extended in many countries in response not only to the needs of industry, but also to hose arising from military activity in tropical environments, particularly during the two world wars. Perhaps the major advance arising from all this research over the last thirty years or so lies in the deeper understanding of both the processes and the limitations of physiological adaptability to hot conditions, so that appropriate control measures in the interest of working efficiency can take account of both the characteristics of the mine worker and the thermal properties of the mining habitat. In addition, a substantial understanding has been achieved with regard to the pathogenesis of heat illness, including those syndromes encountered in mining conditions—heatstroke, heat syncope, salt and water deficiency. Improved measures both of treatment and prevention are now available.

Cold conditions present a much smaller problem. They are discussed briefly at the end of the chapter.

Assessment of the Heat Stress of Mining Conditions

Factors

All the factors contributing to a high heat load (and thereby to a reduced working capacity) are apt to be present in many mining situations. The environmental factors involved are: high air temperatures, high mean radiant temperatures (i.e. surface temperatures in excess of air temperature), high atmospheric humidity and relatively low air movement. In addition to these, the metabolic heat generated by mining work is usually at a high or moderately high level. The amount of clothing (i.e. its insulation value) is also to be taken into account as it is not always the case that only a minimum is worn underground. Protective clothing and equipment may need to be used, as for example in rescue operations.

The mining situations we are concerned with relate to conditions more severe than the upper limit of the "comfort zone"—conditions which would be described as "warm", "too warm", "hot" or "too hot". Although the comfort zone represents the optimum in subjective terms as well as for the performance of many "mental" tasks, the physical activities of mining and some psychomotor tasks (e.g. drilling) can certainly be performed satisfactorily in conditions which are subjectively unpleasant. The body can do this because of its ability to regulate its internal temperature at steady state levels in response to heat loads beyond the comfort zone, though this entails a physiological cost or strain. The quantitative assessment of the severity of such conditions (and thereby the setting of permissible limits) must be done by taking into account the severity of the physiological effort involved in making adjustments to the heat stress of mining conditions.

Clearly, we need to know in quantitative terms how the various factors, environmental and metabolic, combine to influence the heat balance of the body. The basic physiological principle here is that over a fairly wide range of increasing heat loads the temperature regulatory system can respond so as to restore a balance between heat gain and heat loss and thereby re-establish a new steady state temperature at a somewhat higher level. This homeothermic response depends on the capacity of the compensatory systems, particularly the peripheral circulation and the sweat glands, to increase heat loss to the required extent. When the limit to heat transfer is reached the internal or "core" temperature will no longer achieve a steady state; instead, there will ensue an uncontrolled rise of body temperature which may reach dangerous values. Beyond these steady-state limits only short exposures can be endured. At rectal temperatures above 39°C many men will find conditions unendurable. Where tolerance times are very short the rise of body temperature will be so rapid that fainting or other signs of distress may occur even before this temperature is reached.

The body's adaptive capacity can be much enhanced by the process of physiological acclimatization, that is, by repeated exposure to the hot conditions as was noted amongst miners by Moss (1923), Vernon (1923) and Dreosti (1935). The physiological changes have been studied and described in great detail in many publications. A sufficient description is that given in a recent WHO report (1969), "essentially, during the first exposure to heat an unacclimatized man displays a high rectal temperature and pulse rate and a low sweat loss; he experiences discomfort and even distress which under certain conditions may be so severe that further exposure has to be avoided. Acclimatization results in a reduction of the discomfort and distress and the rectal temperature and heart rate fall, while sweat loss increases. There is good reason to believe that the benefits of acclimatization are due to an increased sweat production and a lower skin temperature. The process of acclimatization largely occurs within the first 4–6 days of repeated or continuous daily exposure and is complete, or nearly so, within two weeks. Acclimatization is relative, in the sense that men who have become fully acclimatized to their conditions of work are not fully acclimatized to conditions in which the heat load is higher. Since the total heat load includes a metabolic component, it follows, for example, that a sedentary worker in a hot climate is not acclimatized to hard work in that climate, and if he does attempt hard work he will suffer discomfort or distress. The benefits of acclimatization seem to decay quickly at first, although they may not be entirely lost for about three to four weeks." In mining situations the state of heat acclimatization is of profound significance in setting permissible working limits. Deliberate acclimatization of new entrants is practised on the Witwatersrand (Wyndham, Strydom, Morrison, du Toit and Kraan, 1954).

Factors such as age differences within the range found in mining populations, say up to 45 years, or ethnic or racial differences, would appear to have very little if any influence on practical limits of thermal tolerance. Body build, i.e. weight and musculature, is clearly of importance, since moderate or hard mining work calls for a work capacity commensurate with the fairly high energy requirements; obesity is known to reduce heat tolerance and even to predispose to heat-stroke.

Indices of Heat Stress

A large number of scales or indices have been devised to provide quantitative ratings either of the subjective feelings of "warmth" or of the extent of physiological adjustments experienced under different combinations of environmental factors, work load and clothing. Of these indices two in particular have found wide application in mining and other hot industries—the (Corrected) Effective Temperature Scale (C.E.T.) and the Predicted 4-Hourly Sweat Rate (P4SR). Detailed descriptions of these are available in many publications (Bedford, 1940; Leithead and Lind, 1964; Smith, 1955; Macpherson, 1960; W.H.O., 1969).

The Effective Temperature Scale is essentially a scale of warmth or subjective comfort. The C.E.T. combines the temperature, humidity and rate of movement of the air and radiant temperature in a single value expressed as the temperature of still air, saturated with water vapour which has the same subjective effect as the conditions under test. Two scales are available—the basic scale for persons stripped to the waist and the "normal" scale for persons wearing light indoor clothing. In the mining applications discussed below the "basic scale" will be referred to. The E.T. scale has a number of limitations: it does not incorporate the work factor; above E.T. 32°C it overweights the dry-bulb; its scale units do not indicate equivalent movements of physiological stress—though fairly high and useful correlations (parabolic regressions) with sweat rate and body temperature are found (Smith, 1955). In using the E.T. scale to lay down conditions which are physiologically acceptable or not it is necessary to specify precisely the work level and the physiological criteria used.

The P4SR is succinctly described in the W.H.O. (1969) report. It was devised empirically (McArdle, Dunham, Holling, Ladell, Scott, Thomson and Weiner, 1947) from the results of a large series of observations of the sweat losses of men exposed in the laboratory to a variety of climates, different levels of energy expenditure, and wearing shorts or overalls. Within wide ranges, the heat stress of any combination of dry- and wet-bulb temperatures, globe temperature, air movement, the level of clothing worn, and the rate of work can be assessed from the nomogram. The assessment is in terms of the average amount of sweat loss to be expected, within the limits of sampling error, in a group of young, fit, acclimatized men exposed to the conditions in question for 4 hours. The scale can also be used to specify conditions for unacclimatized subjects, provided the P4SR is regarded as a conventionally agreed reference scale. On this basis the nomogram may be and has been extrapolated to values well outside the range of the original conditions though it is known that when the P4SR exceeds 5 litres the observed sweat rate falls increasingly below the predicted value.

As a rough guide, a 32°C C.E.T. with medium work loads (125 $kcal/m^2/h$) is equivalent to a P4SR of 4, with heavy work about 5 (Smith, 1955). The relationship of P4SR to body temperature yields a fairly high correlation (Smith, 1955; Wyndham, Allan, Bredell and Andrew, 1967) and this can be used in specifying limits for work in hot conditions.

Other indices, much simpler than the E.T. or P4SR, have been used in mining. Simple weighting of wet bulb and dry bulb, e.g. the so-called Belgian Effective Scale, W.B. − 0·1 (D.B.-W.B.), or the Wet Bulb Globe Thermometer Index (W.B.G.T.), or its variants (e.g. 0·15 D.B. + 0·15 W.B.) have been used effectively for particular limited purposes, but they are inadequate for use over a wide range of combinations of environmental conditions. The wet bulb value has been used intermittently since the time of Haldane to indicate the "stress" of mining conditions (Caplan, 1943; Bromilow, 1956); where the air is saturated or nearly so, as in many parts of South African gold mines, and air is still, the W.B. approximates to the E.T. Studies based on such conditions are too restricted to be generalized to situations where the D.B. is markedly different from the W.B. and with different air movements and radiant temperatures.

Thermal Conditions in Mines

Environmental

Conditions within mines and in different mines vary, of course, enormously. The following account is intended merely to exemplify these variations.

On the Witwatersrand at 3,050 m below the surface the virgin rock temperature is about 41°C. Because of wet mining the air may be nearly saturated. At 2,300 m along horizontal tunnels from the shaft the wet bulb in summer may reach 32°C while in working stopes wet bulb temperatures as high as 34°C or higher ("hot" stopes) are usual, while air movements may be below 30 m/min (McIntyre, 1937; Weiner, 1950). It is clear that E.T.'s as high as 33°C (at low air speed) need to be taken into account.

In the Kolar Gold Fields of Mysore State, India, where dry mining obtains, for the same rock temperatures the dry bulb is higher and the wet bulb lower than on the Witwatersrand. Because the geothermic gradient is smaller, at depths of about 2,500 m temperatures of 32 to 36°C wet bulb, with 43 to 49°C dry bulb and air movements up to 60 m/min are encountered in stopes and development ends (Caplan, 1943). After air conditioning was installed temperatures were approximately 27–32°C wet bulb, 38–49°C dry bulb and air velocities about 30–60 m/min. These figures correspond to E.T.'s in the range of 29 to 35°C and probably higher because of the elevated surface temperatures.

Ladell (1955) has recorded conditions in gold mines and collieries in West Africa. In the Ashanti gold mind at Obuasi, stope temperatures ranged from 28 to 36°C, wet bulb values from 27·5 to 35·5°C. In about half the stopes the dry bulb was over 33°C with humidities above 90 per cent. Effective temperatures of 32–34°C were not unusual, since air movement was often about 18–21 m/min. In a West African colliery (Ladell, 1948) conditions were not so severe, but hewers and tubmen worked in some places at E.T.'s as high as 33°C.

In the Mount Isa Mine, Australia (Wyndham *et al.*, 1967), very severe conditions obtain. A variety of physical tasks have to be performed at wet bulb temperatures as high as 41°C, dry bulb 49°C, globe temperature of 54·5°C and air movement 9 m/min. Combinations of wet bulb and dry bulb of 32/52 with low air movements corresponding to C.E.T.'s of 37°C and (nominal) P4SR's of about 10 litres for calorie expenditures of about 125 kcal/m²/h are encountered.

Energy Cost of Mining Tasks

Estimates of the cost of many tasks underground have been made in gold mines (Morrison, Wyndham, Mienie and Strydom, 1968) and collieries (Garry, Passmore, Warnock and Durnin, 1955; Humphreys and Lind, 1962; Moss, 1935). The metabolic costs of jobs vary from low levels, e.g. for sitting, driving or standing, 55–65 kilocalories per square metre per hour ($kcals/m^2/h$) to extremely high values, e.g. when crawling uphill or shovelling rock into high cars, 400 $kcal/m^2/h$. Strictly speaking, the external work should be taken into account in estimating the total energy usage, but as the mechanical efficiency for most tasks is probably of the order of 10 per cent and because of great individual variability this correction is generally neglected. An increase of 25 $kcal/m^2/h$ can be taken roughly as increasing the P4SR value by about 0·61 at E.T.'s of 32°C and by 0·31 at E.T. of 28°C (Smith, 1955). During a 6 or 8 hour shift the pattern may in some cases be one of relatively continuous medium, light, or fairly heavy work. Morrison *et al.* (1968) note that labourers usually maintain a steady shovelling rate with frequent short rest pauses of a few seconds. For most of the shift the average labourer will expend about 250 $kcal/m^2/h$ or about 200 $kcal/m^2/h$ allowing for external work. On the other hand, a complete coal getting shift may involve a number of different tasks with a complex pattern of rest pauses, light work and bouts or peaks of heavy activity. Time analyses by Humphreys and Lind (1962) of shifts when the miner cleared his stint showed that 40 per cent of the time was spent sitting or standing but accounted for only 16 per cent of the total expenditure; whereas loading required 30 per cent of shift time and 47 per cent of the total expenditure. The total energy expenditure was on average 2,000 kcal for a shift of just under 8 hours—about 145 $kcal/m^2/h$.

When assessing conditions in terms of thermal stress obviously the whole rhythm of work must be taken into account. The peak tasks must be identified. Even when mechanization displaces manual labour, as in the collieries of the United Kingdom, there will still be men (as Humphreys and Lind point out) using pick and shovel at parts of the face inaccessible to the machine. Ladell (1948) indicated that in a Nigerian colliery, almost entirely unmechanized, the workers avoided heat stress by taking frequent rests and by taking time off in nearby well-ventilated and cooler roads to cool off. In the much more severe conditions of an Ashanti gold mine where "no illnesses directly attributable to heat had been reported" he found again that men avoided heat stress by a slackening of work rates, by frequent rest pauses and by having a lengthy enforced withdrawal during blasting at midshift into cooler well-ventilated areas.

Limits for Work in Mines

Physiological Considerations

Much attention has been given to the problem of prescribing levels of heat stress to enable mining to be carried out efficiently and without risk of heat casualties. Where account has been taken of all the relevant factors, environmental and metabolic, differences in prescribed levels may be attributable very largely to differences in the state of acclimatization.

Another important consideration is the criterion used in establishing tolerance limits. It is feasible to adopt a criterion which will give an "upper or maximum tolerable limit" (Weiner and Lind, 1955). By testing large numbers of men under a variety of hot conditions, a P4SR value of 4·5 litres was arrived at as defining "the situation in which an increasing number of fit acclimatized men found conditions beyond their endurance" (Macpherson, 1960). The value for the upper tolerable limit for unacclimatized men in P4SR terms is 3 litres (Lind, 1963). This level is similar to that of Eichńa, Ashe, Bean and Shelley (1945), who found that above a C.E.T. of 33°C young, fit, well-acclimatized and well-motivated acclimatized subjects found difficulty in completing 4 hours of continuous moderately hard work (about 150 kcal/m²/h). Several other investigations, including those in South African mines (Wyndham, Bouwer, Devine and Patterson, 1953), in the Kolar gold field and in Belgium give similar values. Clearly, a criterion for subjects at the very limit of their tolerance is not relevant to the performance of work at high levels over a long shift day after day, which requires that the subject attain a steady state within the homeostatic limits of his circulatory and heat regulatory system.

To meet this, Wyndham *et al.* (1953) and Lind (1960), used a criterion based on the work of Nielsen (1938) who showed that for a given steady work rate, the rectal temperature is maintained at an equilibrium level over a wide range of external temperatures. This temperature level is thus a function of the metabolic rate and not of climatic stress—but only up to a critical external temperature; above this the original plateau is not maintained. Further increases in environmental temperature result in progressively marked increases in equilibrium levels. Wyndham *et al.* (1953) using highly acclimatized African miners showed that the rectal temperature was maintained at the primary plateau level, up to a C.E.T. of 32°C for light work, up to 30·6°C for moderate work and up to 28·9°C for hard work. Lind's (1963) experiments were specifically concerned with the performance of British coal miners who are not artificially acclimatized or in practice subjected to acclimatizing exposures. For those subjects, not highly acclimatized but well trained for the work, a C.E.T. of 30°C for light work, of 28°C for moderate work and 26·5°C for hard work was obtained (W.H.O., 1969). It is

15

interesting that these E.T. values of 26·5°C for hard work and 32°C for light work were the limits empirically arrived at by Yaglou as long ago as 1937. These values would appear to be the most reliably established so far using this "Nielsen" criterion for highly and poorly acclimatized subjects. The recommendation of C.E.T. 28°C for full coal production is supported for German mines by Brüner (1959).

An alternative approach which also takes account of the homeothermic capacity was proposed by Wyndham, Strydom, Morrison, Williams, Bredell, Maritz and Munro in 1965. The two major channels controlling heat loss at high temperatures—heat conduction through the skin and evaporative loss from the skin—possess a responsiveness showing a characteristic sigmoid relationship to the rectal temperature. Over the range of about 37°C to about 38·5°C the increase in conduction and sweat rate with rise in rectal temperature is large. As temperatures increase still further the rate of increase of conduction and sweat rate falls off, and at rectal temperatures between 39°C and 39·5°C these channels are responding at full capacity. Wyndham *et al.* (1967) proposed "that work in heat can be regarded as 'easy' when the workmen's rectal temperature does not rise above 38·5°C (oral temperature 38°C)" and that "heat stress is 'excessive' when rectal temperature rose above 39°C (oral temperature 38·5°C)." They have applied these criteria in the severe conditions of the Mount Isa Mine, Queensland. Regression analysis indicates that a rectal temperature of 38·5°C corresponds to a heat load in P4SR terms of 3·8 litres. The shift should be reduced to 6 hours when P4SR's reach this level. The 3·8 P4SR conditions correspond to a C.E.T. (basic) of 31–31·5°C. The work rate of 125 kcal/m²/h is midway between light and heavy. By this criterion the corresponding C.E.T. for a work rate of 150 kcal/m²/h would be about 30·5°C. This is quite close to the value of 30°C obtained from the "Nielsen" criterion for a work rate of 150–160 kcal/m²/h both values applying of course to well-acclimatized subjects. This "critical" value equates with a P4SR of 3·5 l/min (Weiner and Lind, 1955).

These interesting and differing approaches employed in studies of the last 20 years would appear to have yielded a substantial measure of agreement as to conditions in which highly or poorly unacclimatized men can be expected to carry out work within physiologically acceptable limits. For moderate work (150 kcal/m²/h) the C.E.T. values can be taken respectively as 30°C and 28°C and these correspond to P4SR values of 3·5 and 2·3 litres for subjects moderately acclimatized.

It will be clear that mining conditions can be monitored in two ways. One is for the ventilation officer to take all the environmental measurements and to make an estimate of the work load. From this either the P4SR is calculated or the C.E.T. The C.E.T. is much the easier to calculate, and given an estimate of the work rate, the above standards could be applied. Simplified graphs for P4SR 3·8 and 5·0 litres have been presented by Wyndham *et al.* (1967). The second method would be for a trained official to take frequent body temperatures, a method used very effectively by Ladell in his studies of West African mines. It is strongly advocated by Wyndham *et al.* (1965) because, in the South African mines, the prescription of a C.E.T. of 30°C as a standard for moderately hard work for well acclimatized miners has not been sufficient to eliminate all cases of heat stroke (Wyndham *et al.*, 1967).

What is not to be encouraged is the use, as an "index", of the wet-bulb temperature alone or in simple combination with the dry-bulb. There is no doubt that the wet-bulb temperature does not closely mirror body temperature levels or other physiological responses.

Performance

A variety of tasks, skilled and semi-skilled, have been studied under hot conditions and the changes in output, in number of errors, or speed and accuracy of performance determined. Only a few such studies have been performed specifically in relation to mining situations.

Laboratory studies, reviewed by Bell and Provins (1962), indicate that in addition to the influence of the environment the efficiency of performance is related to the complexity and duration of the task, the skill, the attitude and motivation of the operator. Moreover, there are large individual variations quite apart from the factors mentioned. Incentive and motivation seem particularly important, since a large variety of different laboratory tests—for dexterity, vigilance, morse code signalling, mental multiplication—do not show statistically appreciable deterioration until an E.T. of about 29–30°C, that is in conditions well above the "comfort zone". (Weiner and Lind, 1955.) Highly skilled performers have shown deterioration in conditions as high as 33°C or even 35°C.

These figures would lead us to expect that the standards set on a physiological basis for mining would not be affected by the psychological component in these tasks. Indeed, under experimental conditions of close supervision, Strydom and his colleagues (1963) showed that the output of well-acclimatized labourers shovelling rock into mine cars continuously over a 5-hour shift only began to fall off when hot conditions reached wet-bulb temperatures over 30°C. At 31°C the fall is only 10 per cent—corresponding to a C.E.T. of 30°C with air movement of 30 m/min. Under less well-supervised conditions or with lesser motivation efficiency may fall off at lower temperatures. Caplan and Lindsay (1946) set labourers to bore holes in granite and considered that efficiency began to fall off between 28 and 29·5°C (wet-bulb).

For British coal mines the evidence is that moderate physical work can be carried out by average fit and poorly acclimatized miners at a C.E.T. of 28°C. Yet observations at the coal face showed that men working in seams at E.T. 27°C had a working efficiency 41 per cent less than that of men working at an E.T. of 19°C (Vernon, Bedford and Warner, 1927). This coincides with the opinion of Cadman (1913).

It is clearly of practical importance to ascertain how far working output and efficiency under actual mining conditions conform to expectations derived from extensive laboratory experiments, but the evidence from everyday working situations remains meagre.

As regards the influence of temperature on accident liability little new information has been forthcoming since Bedford and his colleagues wrote "Men working at temperatures below 70°F (21°C) (D.B.) had the lowest accident rates, and those at temperatures of 80°F (27°C) or over had the highest. . . . In pits at 80°F (27°C) or over there was a sharp increase in accident frequency from the 30 to 39 age group to the 40 to 49 group." (Bedford, 1940).

Tolerance Times

There are situations where the combined stress of the climate, the physical work and the clothing worn is so severe that bodily temperature equilibrium cannot be achieved. In such conditions which occur in mining as well as in the steel industry and the services (Bell and Walters, 1969) it is necessary to specify those limits of tolerance for men both working and resting, over a wide range of conditions. Attention has been given to these problems in the mining industry, particularly in relation to the needs of rescue personnel, and recommendations have been made by Roantree (1951) for the Kolar gold field, and by Lind, Hellon, Jones, Weiner and Fraser (1955).

Rescue teams engaged on underground operations such as fire fighting are exposed to a combination of very severe circumstances— heavy loads have to be carried, sand-bag walls have to be built, the gas-protective respiratory apparatus alone may weigh 15 kg and temperatures as high as 32°C wet bulb and over may be encountered, while ventilation may be virtually absent. This combination of hard work and heat stress is highly conducive to syncopal collapse and great vigilance is required from captains of rescue terms to detect signs of incipient exhaustion, since the failure of one man jeopardizes the whole team. To specify the safe limits for a whole team demands, therefore, that account be taken of the variability of heat tolerance and fitness displayed by a group of men of rather wide age differences, physique, and in everyday occupation. In the recommendations mentioned above a good margin is allowed for to cover the responses of men with the shortest tolerance times. The other major consideration is the criterion of tolerance to be adopted. In the experiments on which the recommendations were based the attainment of a rectal temperature of 38·8°C was chosen as the "end-point", a decision justifiable on physiological grounds, as well as the condition of the men judged by the observer. Recommended tolerance times, both for men not acclimatized to heat and those for acclimatized men are given by Lind (1963). Limits for seated men and for several levels of work are also available. A "code of practice" is presented in the memorandum by Lind *et al.* (1955). For example, in saturated environments of 32°C rescue teams would be allowed 50 minutes' exposure if acclimatized, but 32 if not. At 38°C the corresponding allowances are 29 and 19 minutes respectively.

Heat Disorders in Mining

In the literature concerning the various disorders ascribable to hot environments there is some confusion about their nomenclature and relationships. As Weiner and Horne (1958) and Leithead and Lind (1964) argue in detail one can readily recognize the various disorders as distinct entities based on particular disturbances of physiological functioning. Indeed, it is possible to reproduce these syndromes by deliberate measures to interfere with one or other of the systems concerned with homeostatic adjustment to heat stress (Weiner, 1971).

The successful adjustment of workers to hot mining conditions requires, as we have seen, an efficient functioning of the heat regulatory system and the cardiovascular system. Two disorders of major importance in mining arise from failure in these systems—heat stroke (hyperpyrexia) and heat syncope (circulatory deficiency heat exhaustion). In addition to the adjustments needed for the maintenance of heat balance, long continued exposure requires that the salt and water losses inseparable from high sweat rates should be continuously and fully met. If not, other forms of heat exhaustion may develop—water deficiency heat exhaustion and salt deficiency heat exhaustion (including heat cramps). Another disorder encountered in mines is prickly heat.

The nomenclature used here, though cumbersome, gives recognition to the specific pathogenetic features of each of the disorders. Thus, heatstroke results from failure of the hypothalamic heat centres or the sweat glands (or both); circulatory deficiency heat exhaustion is ascribable to the circulatory pooling that may occur in the distended small vessels and veins immediately after cessation of work and particularly in the standing position with a corresponding reduction of venous return to the heart; water deficiency heat exhaustion results from a reduction in blood volume and total extracellular fluid volume, the dehydration leading to an increase in osmotic pressure in the water compartments of the body; salt deficiency heat exhaustion is brought about by a negative sodium balance when more salt is lost by sweating and the urine than is ingested and here too there is a contraction of blood volume with a lowering in the sodium and chloride level. Prickly heat results from some not clearly understood form of damage to the sweat gland duct associated with maceration of the skin by the continuous presence of unevaporated sweat.

The nomenclature retains the term "heat exhaustion" in respect of three syndromes which as a group stand in contrast to heat stroke. The term "exhaustion" is preserved (though it needs to be clearly qualified) not merely because it continues to be used widely. In fact, much of the symptomatology is due to some form of circulatory insufficiency in all three conditions. The aetiology, pathogenesis, pathology, treatment and prevention of the disorders mentioned here in connection with mining (and several others) are described in detail in the publications already cited and to which reference should be made. The incidence and distribution of these conditions in mining is poorly documented.

Heat stroke, which is the most serious clinically of the heat disorders, has been recognized in its clinical form in the Rand gold mines for a very long time (Dreosti, 1937) and its prevention as well as treatment is taken very seriously. Selection and systematic acclimatization have been in force throughout the industry for a long time (Dreosti, 1937; Wyndham, Strydom, Morrison, Bredell, van Graan, Holdsworth, van Remburg, Munro and Levin, 1966) and fatalities have fallen to very low levels (Wyndham, 1962). Despite the large scale and expensive acclimatization procedures isolated cases have occurred at temperatures below those which on physiological grounds, are acceptable and indeed tolerated by the vast majority of workers (Wyndham, 1962). This finding serves to emphasize the mysteriousness of the predisposition evidently present in a small minority (about 2 per 1,000 at risk per year) who are liable to be struck down. Sporadic cases have occurred in European coal miners. In the light of the careful documentation by the Witwatersrand physiologists and medical officers it is very remarkable that on the Kolar gold field (Caplan, 1943) and in a West African gold mine (Ladell, 1955), both with many situations of extreme heat stress, as described above, heat stroke has apparently never been reported. Fatal and non-fatal cases of heat stroke are notifiable in South Africa by law.

The lay term "heat collapse" has been used to describe heat casualties in the Armed Services, in heat waves, as well as in mining. The cases of heat collapse analysed with great care by Caplan (1943) in his well-known paper on the gold mines, are found in fact to be very largely distinguishable as falling into the separate categories of heat syncope and of salt and water deficiency.

Heat syncope, or simple circulatory deficiency heat exhaustion, is probably the most common form of heat disability, affecting as it does men in a poor state of fitness and acclimatization and particularly when febrile illness coexists. Dreosti (1937) in a 3-year period admitted from a population of about 9,000 at risk some 100 uncomplicated cases. In 2 years at the Kolar gold field Caplan (1943) attended to 170 "mild" heat casualties of whom one-third were probably simple heat syncope, i.e. about 30 per year.

The salt deficiency heat exhaustion syndrome occurs in the South

African mining industry at a frequency of about 2 per 1,000 employees per annum. On the Kolar field a reduced plasma chloride was noted in 70 per cent of all cases of heat "exhaustion" in underground workers. The recent introduction of a slowly released oral sodium chloride preparation (Clarkson, Curtis, Jewkes, Jones, Luck, de Wardener, and Phillips, 1971) may be of value in reducing the incidence of the salt deficiency heat exhaustion syndrome in miners. In hot conditions in industry heat exhaustion due purely to lack of drinking water is probably rarely encountered. Some measure of dehydration is known to occur, the so-called "voluntary" dehydration, when men do not replace all the water lost even though ample fluid is available and it is only during meals that the water deficit is made up. There is evidence that physical performance can be measurably impaired by this voluntary "water debt" (Strydom, van Graan and Holdsworth, 1965). It is likely that dehydration in the mining industry is associated with salt depletion.

Prickly heat (miliaria rubra) according to Loewenthal and Hins (1964) is an important cause of morbidity in the gold mines of South Africa. Its incidence is rising with the extension of deep level mining to the hotter underground conditions in the Orange Free State. The condition is reported also among deep level coal miners in Australia (Johnson, 1962; McGeoch, 1958). On the Rand prickly heat is of clinical importance in the chronic case or when complications occur. The great majority of cases with a single attack do not report sick.

Low Temperatures

Low temperatures are unlikely to be encountered in deep mines even in extreme northern and southern latitudes owing to the geothermic gradient. In shallow or drift mines on the other hand cold conditions can be troublesome not only in cold countries but in winter in temperate zones. They should not, however, give rise to serious ill health (the relationship between cold and the Raynaud's phenomenon in miners is discussed in Chapter 7). Appropriate preventive measures should not be difficult to apply. Effective protective clothing should be supplied and if this fails to solve the problem means to increase the ambient temperature must be provided. In this connection the potentially irritant effects of fumes from braziers, sometimes used to provide local warmth, should be borne in mind.

References

Bedford, T. (1940, reprinted 1966), "Environmental warmth and its measurement." *Medical Research Council War Memorandum No. 17.* H.M.S.O., London.

Bell, C. R. and Provins, K. A. (1962), "The effects of high temperature environmental conditions on human performance." *Journal of Occupational Medicine,* **4,** 202.

Bell, C. R. and Walters, J. D. (1969), "Reactions of men working in hot and humid conditions." *Journal of Applied Physiology,* **27,** 684.

Bromilow, J. G. (1956–7), "Conditioning of the ventilating air in coal mines." *Transactions of the Institute of Mining Engineers*, **116**, 537.

Brüner, H. (1959), "Arbeitsmöglichkeiten unter Tage bei erschwerters klimatischen Bedingungen." *Arbeitsphysiologie*, **18**, 31.

Cadman, J. (1913), "Notes on the effect of temperature in mines in Great Britain." *Transactions of the Institute of Mining Engineers*, **45**, 509.

Caplan, A. (1943), "A critical analysis of collapse in underground workers on the Kolar Gold Field." *Transactions of the Institute of Mining and Metallurgy*, **53**, 95.

Caplan, A. and Lindsay, J. K. (1946), "Effect of high temperatures on efficiency in deep mines." *Bulletin of the Institute of Mining and Metallurgy* (Lond.), No. 480.

Clarkson, E. M., Curtis, J. R., Jewkes, R. J., Jones, B. E., Luck, V. A., de Wardener, H. E. and Phillips, N. (1971), "Slow sodium: An oral slowly released sodium chloride preparation." *British Medical Journal*, **3**, 604.

Dreosti, A. O. (1935), "The results of some investigations into the medical aspect of deep mining on the Witwatersrand." *J. Chem. Metall. Min. Soc. S. Afr.*, **36**, 102.

Dreosti, A. O. (1937), "Pathological reactions produced by work in hot and humid environments in the Witwatersrand Gold Mines." *S. Afr. med. J. Sci.*, **2**, 29.

Eichña, L. W., Ashe, W. F., Bean, W. B. and Shelley, W. B. (1945), "Upper limits of environmental heat and humidity tolerated by acclimatized men working in hot environments." *J. industr. Hyg. & Tox.*, **27**, 59.

Garry, R. C., Passmore, R., Warnock, G. M. and Durnin, J. V. (1955), "Expenditure of energy and the consumption of food by miners and clerks, Fife, Scotland." *Spec. Rep. Ser. Med. Res. Coun. (Lond.)*, No. 289.

Humphreys, P. W. and Lind, A. R. (1962), "The energy expenditure of coal miners at work." *British Journal of Industrial Medicine*, **19**, 264.

Johnson, A. (1962), "Industrial dermatoses." *New Zealand Medical Journal*, **61**, 38.

Ladell, W. S. S. (1948), "Some physiological observations on West African Coal Miners." *British Journal of Industrial Medicine*, **5**, 16.

Ladell, W. S. S. (1955), "Physiological observations on men working in supposedly limiting environments in a West African gold mine." *British Journal of Industrial Medicine*, **12**, 111.

Leithead, C. S. and Lind, A. R. (1964), *Heat Stress and Heat Disorders*. Cassell, London.

Lind, A. R. (1960), "Determination of environmental limits for everyday industrial work." *Industrial Medicine and Surgery*, **29**, 515.

Lind, A. R. (1963), "Tolerable limits for prolonged and intermittent exposures to heat." In *Temperature—its Measurement and Control in Science and Industry*, p. 337. *Vol. 3*, part 3, Chapman and Hall, London.

Lind, A. R., Hellon, R. F., Jones, R. M., Weiner, J. S. and Fraser, D. C. (1955), "Reactions of mines-rescue personnel to work in hot environments." *Med. Res. Memo. No. 1*. London: National Coal Board.

Loewenthal, L. J. A. and Hins, S. C. (1964), "The aetiology of malaria." *South African Medical Journal*, **38**, 613.

Macpherson, R. K. (1960), "Physiological responses to hot environments." *Spec. Rep. Ser. Med. Res. Council*, No. 298. H.M.S.O., London.

McArdle, B., Dunham, W., Holling, H. E., Ladell, W. S. S., Scott, J. W., Thomson, M. L. and Weiner, J. S. (1947), "The prediction of the physiological effects of warm and hot environments: The P4SR index." *Med. Res. Coun. (Lond.) R.N.P. Rep. 47/391.*

McGeogh, A. H. (1958), Concluding paragraph to "Some social aspects of industrial dermatitis," by J. H. T. Davies, p. 181, in Proceedings of a meeting of the Dermatological Association of Australia. *Australian Journal of Dermatology*, **4**, 189.

McIntyre, J. T. (1937), "Deep mine ventilation problems in South Africa." *South African Journal of Science*, **33**, 153.

Morrison, J. F., Wyndham, C. H., Mienie, B. and Strydom, N. B. (1968), *Journal of the South African Institute of Mining and Metallurgy*, 185.

Moss, K. N. (1923), "Some effects of high air temperatures and muscular exertion upon colliers." *Proceedings of the Royal Society*, **B. 95,** 181.

Moss, K. N. (1935), "The energy output of coal miners during work." *Transactions of the Institute of Mining Engineers, London*, **89,** 132.

Nielsen, M. (1938), "Die regulation der Korportemperatur bei muskelarkeit." *Skand. Arch. Physiol.*, **79,** 193.

Roantree, W. B. (1951), "Work in high air temperatures in a fire in Mysore Mine, Kolar Gold Field." *Trans. Inst. Min. & Metall.*, **60,** 513.

Smith, F. E. (1955), "Indices of heat stress." *Med. Res. Council Memo. No. 29.* H.M.S.O., London.

Strydom, N. B., Wyndham, C. H., Cooke, H. M., Maritz, J. S., Bredell, G. A. G., Morrison, J. F., Peter, J. and Williams, C. G. (1963), *Federation Proceedings*, **22,** 893.

Strydom, N. B., van Graan, C. H. and Holdsworth, L. D. (1965), "The water requirements of humans." *Journal of Occupational Medicine*, **7,** 581.

Vernon, H. M. (1923), Special Report Series No. 73, Part V, p. 128, Privy Council, Medical Research Committee. H.M.S.O. London.

Vernon, H. M., Bedford, T. and Warner, C. G. (1927), "The relation of atmospheric conditions to the working capacity and accident rate of miners." *Rep. industr. Fatig. Res. Bd. Lond.*, No. 39.

Weiner, J. S. (1950), "Observations on the working ability of Bantu mine workers with reference to acclimatization to hot humid conditions." *British Journal of Industrial Medicine*, **7,** 17.

Weiner, J. S. (In Press), "Heat Disorders." In *Textbook of Tropical Medicine.* (Ed.) A. Woodruff. London: Churchill.

Weiner, J. S. and Lind, A. R. (1955), "Working capacity in hot and humid conditions." *The Manager (Lond.)*, **23,** 853.

Weiner, J. S. and Horne, G. O. (1958), "A classification of heat illness." *British Medical Journal*, **i,** 1533.

W.H.O. (1969), "Health factors involved in working under conditions of heat stress." *World Health Organization Technical Report Series*, No. 412.

Wyndham, C. H. (1962), "Tolerable limits of air conditions for men at work in hot mines." *Ergonomics*, **5,** 115.

Wyndham, C. H., Allan, A. McD., Bredell, G. A. G. and Andrew, R. (1967), "Assessing the heat stress and establishing the limits for work in a hot mine." *British Journal of Industrial Medicine*, **24,** 255.

Wyndham, C. H., Bouwer, V. O. M., Patterson, H. E. and Devine, M. E. (1953), "Practical aspects of recent physiological studies in Witwatersrand Gold Mines." *J. Chem. Met. Min. (S. Africa)*, **53,** 287.

Wyndham, C. H., Strydom, N. B., Morrison, J. F., du Toit, F. D. and Kraan, J. G. (1954), "A new method of acclimatization to heat." *Arbeitsphysiologie*, **15,** 375.

Wyndham, C. H., Strydom, N. B., Morrison, J. F., Williams, C. G., Bredell, G. A. G., Maritz, J. S. and Munro, A. (1965), "Criteria for physiological limits for work in heat." *Journal of Applied Physiology*, **20,** 37.

Wyndham, C. H., Strydom, N. B., Morrison, J. F., Bredell, G. A. G., van Graan, C. H., Holdsworth, L., van Rensburg, A., Munro, A. and Levin, A. (1966), "A test of the effectiveness of acclimatization procedures in the gold mining industry." *Journal of Applied Physiology*, **21,** 1586.

Yaglou, C. P. (1937), "Abnormal air conditions in industry: their effects on workers and methods of control." *Journal of Industrial Hygiene and Toxicology*, **19,** 12.

Chapter 14

Mine Gases

The gases encountered in mines are met with elsewhere in industry; the particular hazards they present in mining depend on the ventilation of underground workings. As toxic gases are more frequently encountered in coal mining rather than in metalliferous mining much of this chapter will therefore relate to the former. The pollution of mine atmospheres by radioactive gases is dealt with in Chapter 6.

Air is drawn up the 'upcast' shaft of a mine after it has passed through the mine roadways and along coal faces. Fresh air is distributed throughout the mine workings to ensure that faces and headings are adequately ventilated. Disused workings are seldom included in the ventilation system and when they are entered the possibility of asphyxiation should always be borne in mind.

An important aspect of ventilation in coal mines is the dilution of methane to acceptable levels. When gas emission from the strata is high this may require a considerable volume and velocity of air along the coal face.

Sulphuretted hydrogen occasionally occurs naturally in a mine. No other toxic gases are found underground except in the presence of a fire. The principal dangers associated with mine gases are explosive concentrations of methane and oxygen deficiency leading to asphyxia. Warning of these may be given by a flame safety lamp whereas a fire will produce smoke and a characteristic smell. With a flame lamp an official with an intact sense of smell can make an underground inspection by himself with small danger from mine gas.

Methane

Methane, which is odourless and tasteless, is present in virtually all undisturbed coal seams. When the gas is released by mining operations it usually enters the mine atmosphere slowly, the percentage in the return airway increasing if there is a fall in barometric pressure. Certain seams, however, are characterized by sudden large emissions of methane and on occasion by violent outbursts of the gas when large fragments of coal may be thrown considerable distances and dense clouds of coal dust generated.

The principal danger of methane is its ability to form an explosive mixture with air. If ignited the explosion can trigger off a much more violent coal dust explosion. The amount of methane in roadways and on the coal face must thus be kept well below explosive levels. Where the concentrations are not unduly high this can be achieved by adequate ventilation. Where there is a great deal of methane in the coal seam it is, in addition, necessary to bore into the strata above the coal face and to collect the gas in a methane drainage system.

In 'gassy' mines lighting must be of a type not liable to ignite methane, and until the advent of the electric lamp it was provided by the flame safety lamp. This is based on the principle that the flame from exploding methane is so cooled by wire gauze that it does not pass through it. A lamp can, therefore, be constructed in which the flame is surrounded by gauze; any explosion caused by the flame will be contained inside the lamp and the flame will merely blow itself out. Flame safety lamps are still extensively used as an empirical method of detecting methane and oxygen deficiency. The flame, when appropriately adjusted, will show a faint blue cap if methane is present. The size and shape of this gas cap gives the percentage of methane in the mine air; the conventional lamp will show concentrations of 1·25 to 5 per cent. Some safety lamps use the Garforth principle by which samples of the atmosphere are injected into the lamp; by this method up to 20 per cent methane can be detected. Methanometers are used for the more accurate assessment of the concentration of the gas.

Methane is lighter than air; in certain circumstances the speed of ventilation in a roadway will not be sufficient to overcome the buoyancy of the methane which will form a layer and spread along the roadway above the air. Such layering can carry a flame for long distances. An increase in the ventilation or of the turbulence in the roadway will mix the gas with the air; such mixing is not reversible.

Mixtures of methane and fresh air are explosive when the percentage of methane ranges from 5 to 15 per cent. A gas mixture too rich to explode will burn at an interface with fresh air.

When an underground fire breaks out or a 'heating' due to spontaneous combustion occurs the emergency is usually dealt with by isolating the affected area from the general ventilation system. The roadways in the vicinity are sealed by the erection of 'stoppings'. Behind such stoppings the oxygen content of the atmosphere will fall. As the oxygen decreases, the range within which a methane explosion can take place narrows, the upper explosive limit of 15 per cent decreasing and the two explosive limits drawing closer together in consequence. The two will meet when the oxygen decreases to a figure of about 12 per cent; below this no explosion will occur. The explosive limits are shown graphically in the form of Coward's triangle (Fig. 1).

Occasionally the gases behind the stopping contain an appreciable amount of hydrogen in which case the Coward's triangle has a different shape and explosions can occur with a lower percentage of oxygen. The shape of the triangle can also be varied by high concentrations of carbon monoxide.

Methane will only cause asphyxiation underground if the amount is so large that the oxygen is diluted below respirable levels; this is only likely to happen if there is a sudden emission of gas. Such an emission can sweep along a coal face displacing the air. The asphyxiation caused is of the quiet type since there is no build up of carbon dioxide.

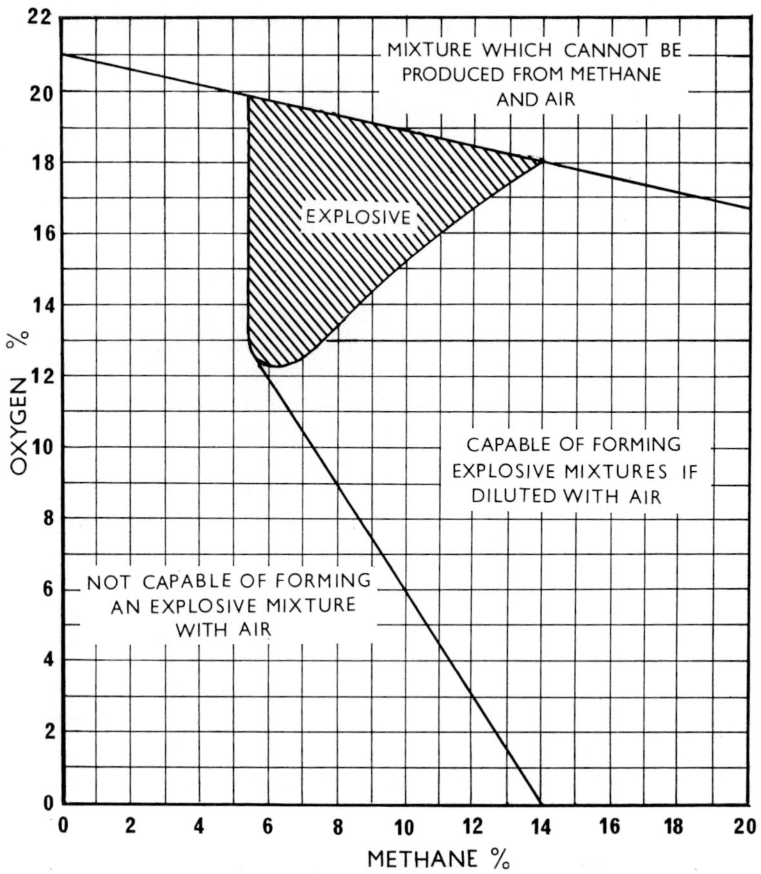

Fig. 1. The explosive limits of methane—Coward's Triangle.

Oxygen Deficiency

When a coal seam is exposed the coal will slowly oxidize. At a working face this will be of little consequence, but in an unused and therefore unventilated district there will be a decrease in the amount of oxygen in the atmosphere and an increase in the carbon dioxide. If a safety lamp is set with a one centimetre yellow flame in fresh air this will shorten as the concentration of oxygen falls and the blue base will increase in height. The lamp is usually extinguished at an oxygen concentration of 17 per cent but this figure will depend upon the lighter fuel used.

In fresh air at sea level the concentration of oxygen in inhaled air is about 21 per cent. The body at rest is not significantly affected until the oxygen concentration falls to 14 per cent. At rest, therefore, it is possible to survive without blurring of consciousness in an atmosphere not quite sufficient to enable a safety lamp to burn. The situation changes materially, however, when the subject exercises; in such an atmosphere the oxygen will not be able to diffuse through the alveolar wall fast enough and there will be a gap or gradient between the alveolar oxygen tension and that in the blood leaving the pulmonary capillaries. At this point desaturation of the arterial blood takes place and anoxia results. An anoxia of this type caused by a combination of exercise and oxygen deficiency in the atmosphere will, once it commences, develop rapidly. A miner walking or working in an oxygen deficient atmosphere is in danger of rapid loss of consciousness.

The relationship between exercise, oxygen saturation of the blood and the oxygen concentration in the atmosphere is shown in Table 1.

Table 1

Percentage Oxygen in Air at 760 mm Hg.

Amount of Exercise	21	20	19	18	17	16	15	14
Resting	x	x	x	x	x	x	x	x
Walking	x	x	x	x	x	x	x	y
Hurrying, Moderate Work	x	x	x	x	x	y	y	y
Heavy Work	x	x	x	x	y	y	y	y

x = oxygen saturation adequate.
y = desaturation likely.

It will be apparent that a miner can perform heavy work until the atmospheric oxygen falls below 18 per cent. Thereafter the rapid onset of unconsciousness is an increasing danger (Muir, 1971).

Carbon Monoxide

Carbon monoxide commonly occurs in mines after explosions of either inflammable gas or coal dust. It will also be present during underground heatings and fires, while small amounts are produced by shotfiring.

When there has been an explosion underground the resulting mixture of gases contains carbon dioxide, carbon monoxide, nitrogen and its oxides, water vapour, unconsumed oxygen, unconsumed methane and traces of gas distilled from coal by the passage of the flame. The undiluted gaseous mixture may contain from 2 to 10 per cent of carbon monoxide, with an oxygen content less than 5 per cent. Underground heatings and fires will produce much the same mixtures of gases, with perhaps a higher percentage of oxygen. Although carbon monoxide itself is without smell it is practically never found in the pure state in mine air. A mixture of gases containing it in various proportions usually has a characteristic odour well known to rescue men and fire fighting teams.

At collieries where the coal is liable to spontaneous combustion small amounts of carbon monoxide may be continuously present in the return air. A valuable measurement in such cases is the carbon monoxide/ oxygen deficiency ratio. This is the ratio between the percentage of carbon monoxide in the air and the percentage of oxygen absorbed from the air during its passage through the mine up to the sampling point (multiplied by 100 to give a convenient number). Each face has its own typical value; the ratio is independent of the quantity of ventilation. The rate of evolution of carbon monoxide increases as the temperature of the coal rises and the CO/O_2 deficiency ratio can thus be used to detect spontaneous heatings at an early stage and to mark their progress. It is also an essential measurement in assessing the progress of underground fires (National Coal Board, 1970).

The particular danger of carbon monoxide underground arises from its lack of dilution. An automobile exhaust contains about 4 per cent carbon monoxide—enough to kill a man after a few breaths, but tests made in still air in heavy traffic seldom show as much as 100 parts per million. A lethal concentration of carbon monoxide produced by an underground fire or explosion undergoes little dilution until the gas reaches the upcast shaft. Any man in the path of the gas cloud may be asphyxiated. Of all deaths due to colliery explosions 80 to 90 per cent are caused by carbon monoxide poisoning.

The affinity of carbon monoxide for haemoglobin is about 250 times that of oxygen. By combining to form carboxyhaemoglobin it temporarily deprives the haemoglobin of its oxygen carrying power. It also interferes with the function of the remaining haemoglobin as the dissociation curve of haemoglobin is shifted to the left. A subject with 40 per cent haemoglobin is severely anaemic, but one with 60 per cent carboxyhaemoglobin may be dead. Although carboxyhaemoglobin is more stable than oxyhaemoglobin dissociation takes place in an atmosphere of oxygen or ordinary air, the dissociation being proportional to the partial pressure of oxygen. The erythrocytes (red blood cells) do not appear to be damaged in any way by saturation with the gas and can readily resume their function as oxygen carriers. Carbon monoxide may, however, interfere with certain enzyme systems.

Concentration of Carbon Monoxide in Blood

Small amounts of carbon monoxide are present in the blood of most people living in urban surroundings. Smokers commonly have about

5 per cent carboxyhaemoglobin in their blood and saturations of nearly 20 per cent have been reported. These small concentrations are not enough to cause symptoms which will not usually occur if the blood saturation is less than 20 per cent. The main symptom with concentrations of 20 to 30 per cent is headache; this is of a characteristic throbbing type. When the concentration reaches about 30 per cent additional symptoms are experienced; these include nausea, vertigo, ringing in the ears, dyspnoea on exertion and muscular weakness and incoordination. The muscular weakness, incoordination and vertigo increase rapidly with saturations of up to 50 per cent and collapse may occur at this stage. Concentrations above 50 per cent may be lethal.

It is however a mistake and possibly a dangerous one, to assume that poisoning will always produce an orderly escalation of symptoms. Drinker (1938) states:

"The subtlety of these mental effects cannot be too much emphasized. The person affected may be brought to the very verge of unconsciousness without appreciating in the least degree that anything is wrong. This is particularly true when relatively high concentrations of carbon monoxide are encountered. We have seen a man, gassed as part of an experiment, scoff at the idea that anything was amiss, only to fall unconscious on attempting to leave the room. One cannot count on headache, dizziness, or nausea to warn of disaster or to wake the victim who is poisoned during sleep."

Considerable reservations are thus necessary concerning the unpredictability of the symptoms, particularly where the concentration of carbon monoxide in the blood is between 30 and 50 per cent.

It is possible to summarize the effects of various blood saturations as:

Below 20 per cent	No symptoms
20 to 30 per cent	Throbbing headache
30 to 50 per cent	Dizziness, nausea, muscular weakness, danger of collapse.
50 per cent and above	Unconsciousness and death.

After death a well-known and striking sign of carbon monoxide poisoning is the pink colour of the skin produced by the hypostatic blood. This sign is not seen in the living patient who is commonly pale (Matthew, 1971).

Effects of Various Concentrations of Carbon Monoxide in Air

The effects of various concentrations of carbon monoxide in air on man have been summarized by Forbes, Sargent and Roughton (1945). See Fig. 2. It will be noted that a subject who starts with no carbon monoxide in his blood absorbs it quickly at first whatever the concentration; the speed of absorption later slows down and eventually the

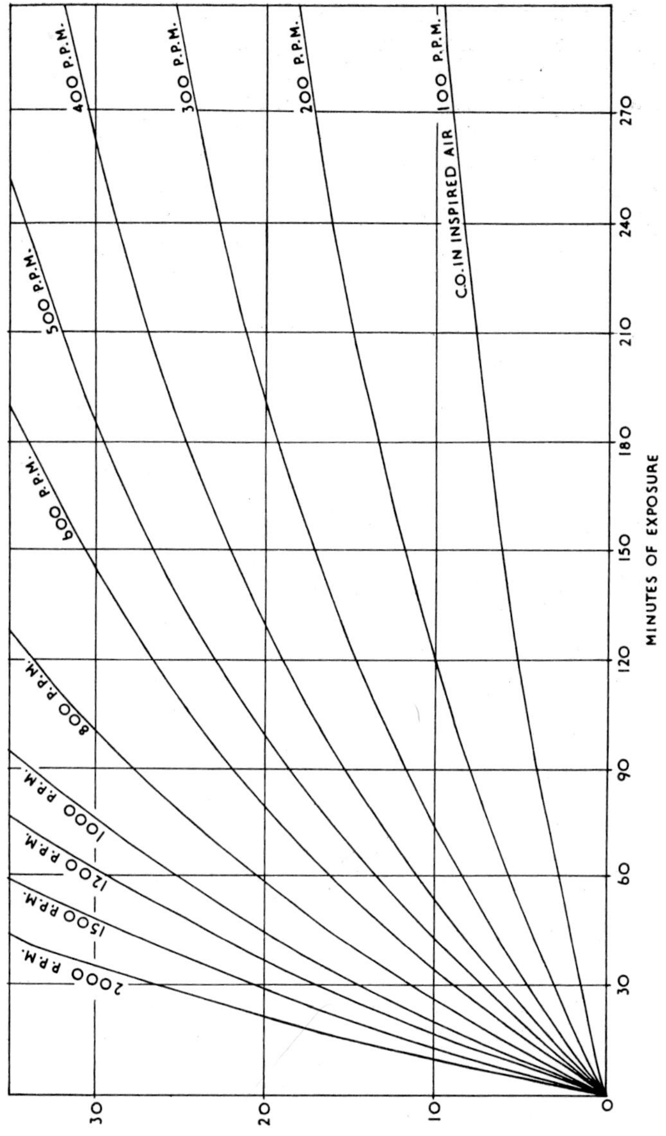

FIG. 2. Uptake of carbon monoxide by man engaging in light activity.

blood reaches equilibrium. If the subject then breathes air or oxygen the concentration will fall exponentially.

For fuller details of the effects of carbon monoxide reference should be made to the proceedings of the Conference on the Biological Effects of Carbon Monoxide, held recently in New York (New York Academy of Sciences, 1970).

In carbon monoxide poisoning the important factors are, the initial concentration in the blood, the concentration in the air, the length of exposure and the amount of exercise taken. Individual variations in response will obviously occur. The very young and the very old are more susceptible; such conditions as anaemia, heart disease, asthma, chronic bronchitis and thyroid disease increase susceptibility.

Acclimatization to the anoxia may occur. However, it is not attained rapidly and it is fairly certain that conditions in the mining industry will rarely be such as to lead to it.

It is sometimes helpful to calculate approximately the danger from small concentrations of carbon monoxide. For this purpose the formula

$$b = \frac{4ate}{100}$$

may be found useful where:

$b =$ blood saturation of carboxyhaemoglobin expressed as a percentage,
$a =$ air concentration of carbon monoxide in parts per million,
$t =$ time of exposure in hours,
$e =$ a factor to allow for the amount of exercise taken during exposure, the factor being $1 =$ rest, $2 =$ walking, $3 =$ working.

Thus:

A length of return airway near the shaft bottom is contaminated with 400 parts per million of carbon monoxide. It takes men a quarter of an hour to walk along this roadway. Is this dangerous?
Then:

$$b = \frac{4ate}{100} = \frac{4 \times 400 \times 0{\cdot}25 \times 2}{100} = 8 \text{ per cent saturated.}$$

It is therefore possible for these men to walk the distance without developing any symptoms.

The formula is inaccurate at high concentrations and for long exposure, but these are not the circumstances where it is likely to be needed and the inaccuracies lie on the side of safety.

Canaries

Canaries are still used in some coal mines for detecting carbon monoxide and are a reliable method of warning of the higher concentrations. On occasion, however, a miner has been working in a fairly

16

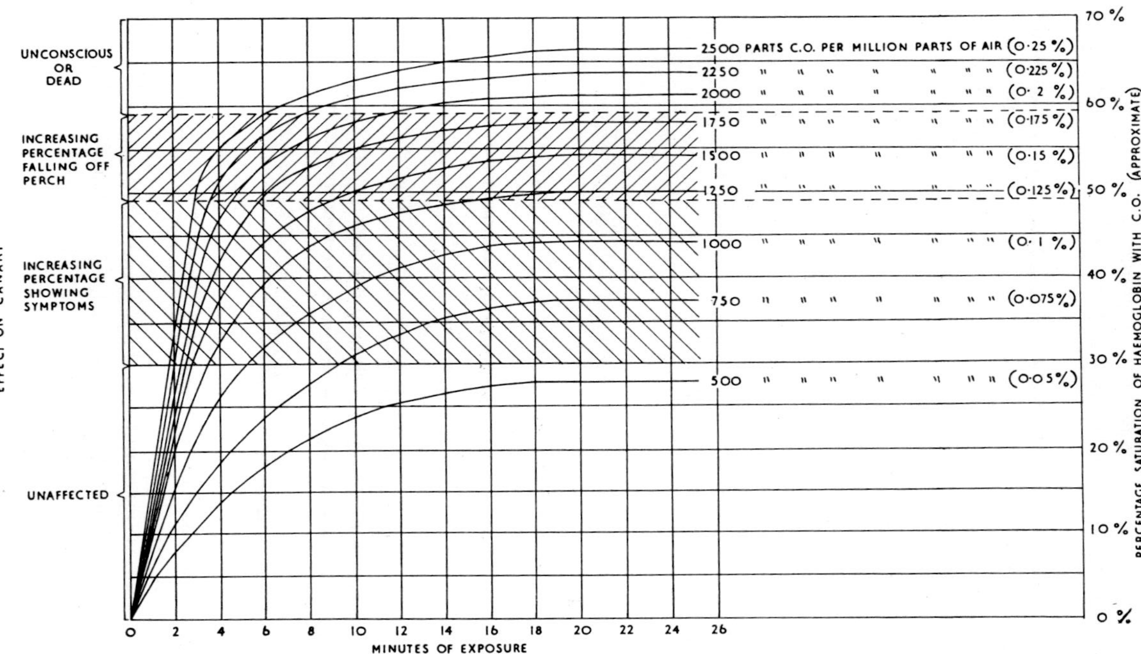

FIG. 3. Effects on canaries of various concentrations of carbon monoxide.

low concentration of carbon monoxide and has developed symptoms while the canary he had with him was apparently unaffected. The effects of various concentrations of carbon monoxide on canaries are shown in Fig. 3.

A canary's blood reaches equilibrium a great deal faster than that of a human being. The blood concentration levels off in about 20 minutes, whereas the corresponding period for a resting man exceeds

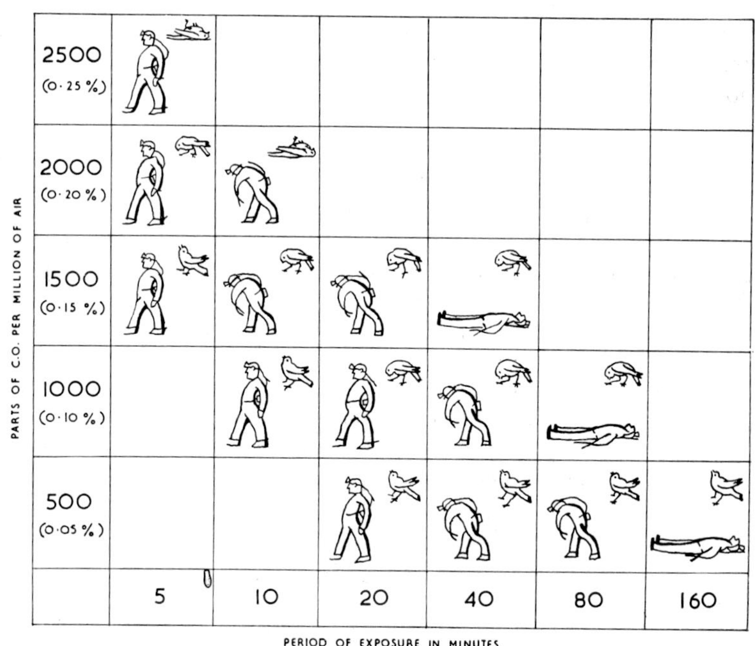

FIG. 4. Exposure to carbon monoxide: effects on man and canary.

6 hours. In an atmospheric concentration of 2500 parts per million a canary will fall off its perch in about 4 minutes; a resting man will probably feel no effects in 20 minutes. In comparatively high concentrations of carbon monoxide therefore the canary will have considerable value as a warning to the man carrying it. If Figs. 2 and 3 are compared, however, it will be seen that it takes approximately two or three times as much carbon monoxide to produce symptoms equivalent to those in human beings. A canary can live in an atmosphere containing 500 parts of carbon monoxide per million, apparently without ill effects; a man will eventually show marked symptoms (Spencer, 1959). See Fig. 4.

Estimation of Carbon Monoxide

(*a*) In the air

The concentration may be estimated quickly, though not very accurately, by means of detector tubes. These consist of granules of silica gel impregnated with a chemical contained in a sealed glass tube. The sealed ends of the detector tube are broken off and a fixed volume of expired air is drawn through it at a specified rate by a simple hand pump. The length (in some cases the colour) of stain produced is measured and gives a fair estimate of the concentration of carbon monoxide. The concentration may be measured more accurately by means of a non-dispersive infra-red analyser which may be used to monitor and record continuously the ambient concentrations.

(*b*) In the blood

The percentage of carbon monoxide in the blood can be measured by taking a blood sample; this however takes time whereas it is usually important to have an estimate immediately. The amount of carbon monoxide in the expired air correlates well with the blood concentration and measurement of this concentration in expired air samples gives a good idea of the blood level.

When a patient suffering from carbon monoxide is brought into fresh air the dissociation of the carboxyhaemoglobin will follow an exponential curve, the percentage falling to half its previous level about every 4 hours at rest. The dissociation is faster in young men and slower in those over fifty and will obviously depend on the pulmonary ventilation and on the partial pressure of oxygen.

Treatment

The giving of pure oxygen instead of air will increase the rate at which carboxyhaemoglobin is dissociated. Breathing is not likely to be depressed in carbon monoxide poisoning unless the patient is moribund. The use of carbogen (7 per cent carbon dioxide, 93 per cent oxygen) serves no useful purpose and could well be harmful. The treatment of choice, oxygen at two atmospheres pressure, can only be applied when the patient has been brought out of the mine and taken to a special centre.

Oxides of Nitrogen

These occur in the exhausts from diesel engines and also in the fumes from shotfiring and other explosions. The term 'oxides of nitrogen' is generally used for the toxic oxides (i.e. excluding nitrous oxide, N_2O). The principal oxides are nitric oxide and the more poisonous nitrogen dioxide. Samples of air taken at loading points and in the driver's cab on diesel engines give average concentrations of nitrogen dioxide of about one part per million. This figure and those obtained similarly for nitric oxide are well below the recommended limits. Fumes from shot-firing contain oxides of nitrogen and mining operations should be so arranged that men are not exposed to harmful concentrations. Sometimes during shotfiring explosive cartridges are incompletely detonated and merely burn slowly giving off unusually large amounts of oxides of nitrogen.

A particular danger of nitrogen dioxide inhalation is the delayed onset of pulmonary oedema which may be fatal.

Sulphuretted Hydrogen

Sulphuretted hydrogen may be present during an underground fire. It can also arise from the reaction of acidic mine waters with naturally occurring pyrites. It is a poisonous gas in concentrations as low as 100 parts per million and has on occasion caused the deaths of miners. Compared with the other noxious gases it is rarely encountered and is more of a nuisance than a hazard.

Sulphur Dioxide

Where a mine shaft is naturally wet sub-zero temperatures may be dangerous as ice may form and drop down the shaft causing serious damage. It is therefore necessary to keep the length of the shaft above freezing point. Adequate heating systems to warm the downcast air are usually installed in mines where several months of sub-zero temperatures are experienced every year; where the problem occurs on odd days, however, makeshift measures may be employed. One of these is the lighting of coke fires around the top of the shaft, the heat (and the smoke) being drawn down it. This somewhat inefficient method of preventing ice formation will disseminate a considerable amount of sulphur dioxide in the mine workings. In these circumstances the gas may well exacerbate chest symptoms among some miners.

Unusual Gases Produced by Fires

When materials such as poly-vinyl-chloride belting and electric cable sheathing are decomposed by heat a number of other toxic gases such as hydrochloric acid in vapour form, hydrogen cyanide, phosgene and chlorine may be evolved. These gases may be dangerous as they are not diluted as they would be on the surface.

References

Drinker, C. K. (1938), *Carbon Monoxide Asphyxia*, p. 64. Oxford University Press, London.

Forbes, W. H., Sargent, F., Roughton, F. J. W. (1945), "The rate of carbon monoxide uptake by normal men." *American Journal of Physiology*, **143**, 594.

Matthew, H. (1971), "Acute poisoning; some myths and misconceptions." *British Medical Journal*, **1**, 519.

Muir, D. C. F. (1971), Personal communication.

National Coal Board (1970), "Noxious gases underground." National Coal Board, London.

New York Academy of Sciences (1970), Proceedings of the Conference on the Biological Effects of Carbon Monoxide. Ed. R. F. Cockburn. *Annals of the New York Academy of Sciences*, **174**, pp. 1–430.

Spencer, T. D. (1959), "Effects of carbon monoxide on man and on canaries." *Transaction of the Institute of Mining Engineers*, **118**, 518.

Chapter 15

Noise

Measurement of Noise

The human ear has a protective system by which sounds are damped down as they get louder and which can perhaps be described as analogous to the contraction of the pupil when exposed to bright light. This means that the ear behaves rather as a logarithmic device when it assesses loudness of a sound and any instrument used to measure sound levels must follow this logarithmic pattern. The instrument used for the routine measurement of noise is the sound level meter. The system of measurement utilises steps or ratios of tenfold intensity known as Bels; for practical purposes a unit of one-tenth of a Bel (the deciBel, usually contracted to dB) is used. Thus noise which registers on a sound level meter as, say, 70 dB has ten times the intensity of a sound of 60 dB but does not of course sound ten times as loud to the human ear (American Industrial Hygiene Association, 1966).

Ears are not equally responsive to all frequencies so that two sounds of the same intensity but different frequencies will not necessarily sound equally loud. In an attempt to allow for this, various "weighting" scales have been incorporated into sound level meters so that an overall figure for the intensity of the noise can be given which approximates to the impression on the human ear. Of the three weighting scales commonly used (A, B and C), scale A has increasingly found favour and it is now usual to express intensity of noise as dBA, the decibel value on the A scale. When a worker is exposed to noise for eight hours a day it is considered that this will not cause any disability if the intensity is 85 dBA or less; however, susceptibility varies widely

For research purposes a sound level meter will be used which gives an octave band analysis of the noise being studied. For routine use, however, an instrument which provides a dBA reading will be sufficient. In mines where an explosion risk exists the sound level meter must be intrinsically safe and pass the tests of the appropriate inspectorate.

Measurement of Hearing

The examination of hearing can only be carried out satisfactorily in very quiet surroundings. If the hearing of men at a number of mines is to be tested it will probably be found necessary to use a mobile audiometric van.

Ambient noise at even a moderately quiet part of the surface is likely to reach 70 or 80 dBA on occasion whereas for the examination of hearing a figure of 40 dB must not be exceeded. The necessary attenuation can be obtained with the van alone at the higher frequencies but particularly at frequencies below 250 Hz such a reduction will only be obtained by the use of a sound-proof van incorporating inside it an audiometric booth. Such an audiometric van will be heavy but can be towed from one mine to the next.

Apart from the need for mobility of the examination room, audiometry in the mining industry has no special problems which do not apply to industry in general. Special mention should, however, be made of the question of temporary deafness. It is well known that exposure to noise is liable to cause a transient loss of hearing called temporary threshold shift; the time taken for recovery will vary, depending chiefly on the intensity of the noise exposure and it is prudent to allow a period of from 24 to 48 hours before audiometric examination is carried out. This requirement will cause difficulties in any industry but for underground workers these become acute. It will seldom be possible (as it often is in surface industry) to arrange for the miner to have a quiet job for the first hour or two on a Monday morning until he has attended for examination. Audiometry must be completed before the normal time for the commencement of the shift. The carrying out of any large scale research survey under these conditions will create considerable problems.

Regular visits by the audiometric van to a miners' hospital or rehabilitation unit can facilitate audiometric examination of many miners in a short time under very suitable conditions and ready co-operation should be forthcoming. This solution does not of course, enable a study to be made of the results of exposure of a group of men to one particular machine. Reasons will be given later why this objection is not as great as it may appear at first sight.

Estimation of Noise Hazards

Effects of Noise

Noise can cause interference with performance and efficiency, annoyance, fatigue and hearing loss. Although the importance of the mental and psychological effects of noise are not questioned they are very difficult to evaluate; many of them are of a highly individual and personal nature.

The effects of noise on hearing are well known and will only be briefly described here. The results of exposure to prolonged noise will depend on a number of factors which include its overall intensity, the duration of exposure in months and years, and the susceptibility of the individual to noise induced hearing loss.

The first sign is a small depression in the audiogram between 3000 and 6000 Hz, commonly at 4000 Hz. If exposure to noise continues the dip at 4000Hz deepens but remains predominantly in the same frequency range. 4000 Hz is a shorter frequency than that of the highest note on a piano and hearing loss at this level will be quite unnoticed; it is however detectable by audiometry.

With further exposure the deterioration of hearing at 4000 Hz will slow down but there will be a gradual extension to higher and lower frequencies. As the hearing at 3000 Hz and below is invaded the subject will begin to suffer from the all-important effect of noise induced hearing loss, interference with speech communication. Serious handicap occurs when there is significant hearing loss at 2000 Hz and below. Typical audiograms for three degrees of noise induced hearing loss are shown in Fig. 1. The effect on speech communication of hearing loss at these frequencies is illustrated in Table 1 (Burns, 1968).

Table 1

*Classes of hearing ability based on average value of hearing levels at 500, 1000, and 2000 Hz.**

Class	Degree of handicap	Average hearing level dB	Ability to understand ordinary speech
A	Not signficant	Less than 25	No significant difficulty with faint speech.
B	Slight	25 to less than 40	Difficulty only with faint speech
C	Mild	40 to less than 55	Frequent difficulty with normal speech.
D	Marked	55 to less than 70	Frequent difficulty with loud speech.
E	Severe	70 to less than 90	Shouted or amplified speech only understood.
F	Extreme	90	Usually even amplified speech not understood.

* These hearing levels, in dB, apply to the better ear; if the average for the poorer ear is 25 dB or more than that for the better ear, add 5 dB to the average for the latter.

Assessment of Noise Hazard by Audiometric Surveys: Selection of a Suitable Group

If the effect of noise on a given population is to be ascertained it is first necessary to exclude from the survey those whose deafness is or may be due to other causes.

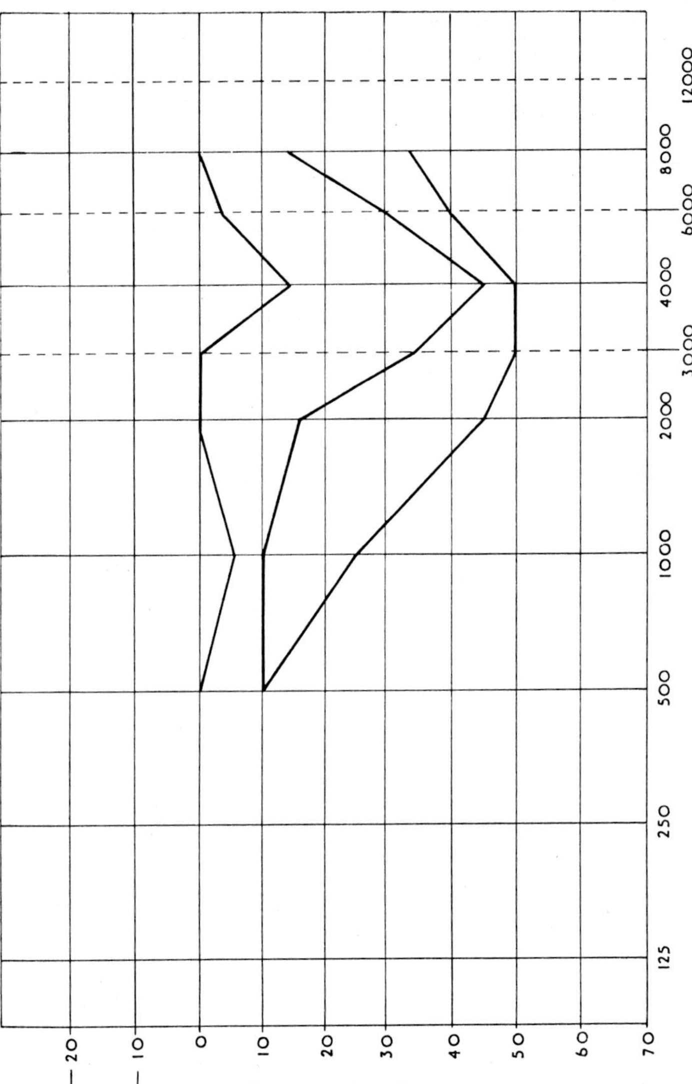

FIG. 1. Audiograms showing various degrees of noise induced hearing loss. A hearing level of 0 dB indicates normality.

The first of these can conveniently be grouped under the term 'pathology', here used to mean causes such as otitis media, otosclerosis, Menière's disease and a large number of less common conditions (Sataloff, 1957). This does not include temporary causes such as wax in the ears or a cold in the head.

The next large group which must be excluded consists of men who have suffered acoustic trauma. This is the condition of sudden aural damage resulting from short term intense exposure. Where miners are exposed to noise from loud explosions it would be impossible to differentiate the effect on their hearing from that caused by continuous exposure to noise. Shot-firing must be considered as a possible cause of acoustic trauma; fortunately the need to limit the size of the explosion for other reasons will often ensure that the intensity of the noise is not high. Many underground workers, however, have served in the armed forces or shoot as a hobby, and an arbitrary basis must be adopted on which it is decided whether or not they can be used in the survey. In addition there are those who have received treatment with a drug which can permanently effect hearing such as streptomycin and also those who have suffered from concussion and may in consequence show an audiogram similar to that caused by noise induced hearing loss.

The selection of the group will, therefore, require the completion of a questionnaire of the type shown in Appendix 1, a clinical examination and removal of wax where necessary. If the exclusion procedure has been successful the two remaining causes of deafness will be noise induced hearing loss and deterioration of hearing due to age.

Presbycusis

Presbycusis is the normal or physiological loss of hearing with advancing age. It appears to be due to various degrees of deterioration in the middle ear, the organ of Corti, the eighth nerve and to ageing processes in the brain. The effect is directly related to frequency—the higher the frequency the greater the deterioration. The speed at which hearing loss progresses varies widely among individuals; there is no hard and fast rule as to the time of onset or rate of progress.

Hinchcliffe (1959) examined the hearing of a random sample of people from a rural population in Scotland who had no ear disease or exposure to excessive noise. By this method he produced smoothed curves showing the expected loss due to age at the various frequencies, the graphs differing somewhat according to sex. The effect of age on hearing is shown in the audiograms in Fig. 2.

A study of noise induced hearing loss in a group of workmen would be very difficult if all those who might be subject to presbycusis were excluded. It is usual, therefore, to assess the effects of noise by subtracting the expected loss due to age from the actual hearing loss found at each frequency, thereby giving figures for age-corrected hearing loss.

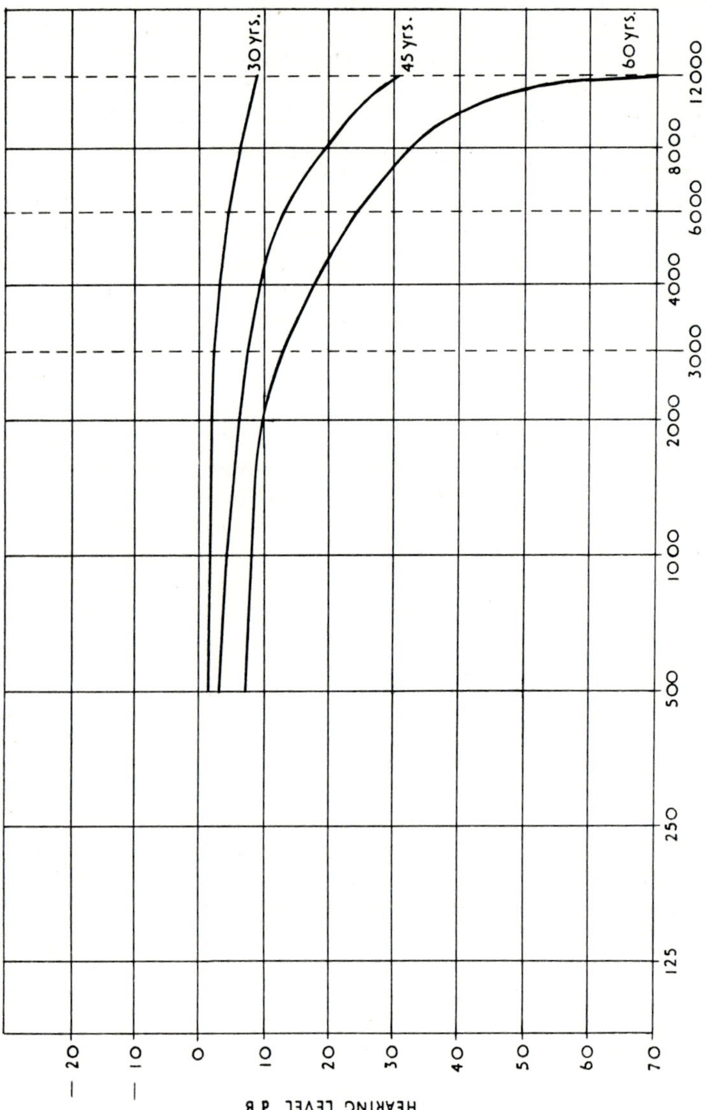

Fig. 2. Audiograms showing the average presbycusis at 30, 45, and 60 years of age.

Although such a procedure is obviously liable to give erroneous results for individuals, in the case of average figures for groups its has been widely used and has given valuable information on the relationship between hearing loss and noise exposure (Burns, 1968).

Noise Induced Hearing Loss

By excluding pathological conditions, acoustic trauma, drug induced hearing loss and also allowing for presbycusis with, in addition, further adjustments for the length of individual exposure it is possible to observe in some detail the effect on a group of workmen of an exposure to a constant level of noise for 8 hours a day, 5 days a week.

It is at this point that study of the noise exposure of underground workers encounters serious difficulty. The noise exposure of the miner is seldom the same for years or even months at a time. The machines he uses will change and those used for the same purpose may produce very different noise levels. New methods of working will entail the use of different types of machine; most underground noise is of an intermittent variety and much of it lasts only for an average of two or three hours a shift with wide daily variations. Finally, a miner's exposure to any noise is discontinuous in that he may at any time change to a different underground job with little or no noise exposure. This situation is in complete contrast, say, to that of an operative in a cotton mill exposed eight hours a day to a constant noise for years on end.

In consequence it is very difficult to assess the danger of hearing loss among miners. Audiograms tend to show less damage than might be expected, due presumably to the intermittent nature of the noise and the miner's discontinuous exposure to it.

Possibility of using Temporary Threshold Shift in Audiometric Surveys

These difficulties make it tempting to consider the possibility of obtaining information from the degree of temporary deafness experienced by a miner when exposed to a particular noise. However, the following difficulties make this impracticable. First, the relationship between permanent threshold shift (P.T.S.) and temporary threshold shift (T.T.S.) remains uncertain (Burns and Robinson, 1970). There is the further difficulty that the T.T.S. should be measured very soon after the cessation of exposure to noise. It is usually considered that consistent figures will be obtained by measuring the threshold shift two minutes after exposure to noise has ceased (Kryter, Ward, Miller and Eldredge, 1966). This period can be extended by a few minutes with the aid of suitable correcting factors but study of T.T.S., say 20 minutes after the miner has finished work, is not considered of any value. By the very nature of mining, therefore, the study of T.T.S. would entail formidable obstacles.

It appears clear that the measurement of temporary threshold shift does not at present show any signs of being of value in assessing the danger of permanent damage to hearing in underground workers.

Preventive Measures

Underground noise is a special problem and only a few of the preventive measures used in surface industry are of value. Much of the noise underground arises from equipment such as booster fans and mining machines. Miners are only exposed to the noise from the fans as they walk past them and in the latter case only the machine men are exposed for much of their working shift. Conditions underground do not give rise to the problem of reverberation which is common in surface installations. It is these ameliorating circumstances together with the intermittency of exposure already discussed that have prevented noise in mining from becoming a greater hazard.

Certainly the noise produced by many of the machines would be enough to produce marked noise induced hearing loss if the miner were exposed for a regular 8 hour day—see Appendix 2. The worst offenders are pneumatic machines; in the coal mining industry the coal face may have too high an output of methane for electricity to be considered safe and pneumatic machines will be used in consequence, particularly at the return end of the face in long wall mining; in mining generally the pneumatic drill tends to be more powerful than the electric drill and to be used as a preliminary to shot-firing when hard rock is encountered.

There is little hope that much can be done to suppress the noise from those machines already in use. It is seldom possible to construct a noisy machine and then, as an afterthought, to suppress the noise it produces. The occasional success only underlines the large majority of failures. If noise is to be decreased this must be part of the thinking of the designer at the earliest stages of planning.

Manufacturers are being urged to produce less noisy machinery and it is important that manufacturers of mining machinery should not be excepted. The approach to noise attenuation of mining machines should be in three stages. The first is that of recording noise levels, on a standard basis, for machines at present in use and also for new machines under development. The noise hazard of a new machine can in this way be considered at an early stage and it will sometimes be found possible to substitute a quieter machine for one likely to produce harmful noise.

The second stage is to ask the manufacturers to indicate the noise levels produced by a new machine. This approach helps to make the manufacturers noise-conscious which in turn will be likely to lead to an attempt by them to take some action to decrease the noise produced by the machines they are selling.

The third stage is the inclusion in the specification for new machines of a noise level which should not be exceeded by the machine when in use.

The chances of success by such an approach are better than they would appear at first sight. Many industries using engineering equipment will be following a broadly similar policy and the mining industry will be only one of those exerting pressure on manufacturers.

Certainly such pressure is overdue. Machines used in all types of mining are becoming larger and more powerful; both an increase of load and an increase of speed will lead to a considerable increase of gear noise; the constant striving for higher machine utilisation will mean that noise levels are high over a larger proportion of the shift. It is very likely indeed that the hazard of noise underground will increase unless considerable efforts are made by manufacturers to prevent it.

The main difficulty in following this policy is that manufacturers may well find it cheaper to produce a noisy machine than a quiet one and mining companies may be reluctant to pay the extra cost. The willingness to pay more for a less noisy machine will probably be a major factor in deciding whether underground noise is to become more or less of a hazard.

If the use of very noisy machinery underground is unavoidable recourse to hearing protection becomes necessary. Where the noise levels are very high but the miner is exposed for only a small part of his shift, it is practicable to introduce a system of ear muffs.

The muffs must be of a type that can be worn in conjunction with a safety helmet while maintaining sufficient pressure against the ears. The muffs may be attached to the helmet in such a way that they can be folded up on to it when not in use; this gives satisfactory protection initially but there is some doubt whether the muffs continue to be held tightly enough against the ears after a few months use. Another type consists of the usual spring headpiece joining the two muffs which, instead of fitting over the top of the head, passes round the back of the neck. An additional supporting band passes over the head to hold the ear muffs in place—this can be made of a material which fits easily under the helmet.

In underground conditions, particularly in hot mines, ear muffs will quickly become dirty; they will also be liable to receive rough treatment. It is essential, therefore, that an ear muff maintenance system is installed with a separate pair for each man. It must be possible to dismantle the muffs easily both to facilitate daily cleaning and so that worn or damaged components can be replaced.

Ear muffs feel comfortable when first worn but most men find them difficult to wear for any length of time. Sweating inside the muffs is uncomfortable and the sensation of isolation from the environment is difficult to tolerate. They are therefore suitable only where protection is needed for short intervals.

Ear plugs must fit tightly if they are to be efficient; but it is possible to obtain plugs which fit efficiently yet are comfortable (Bell, 1966). Fibreglass wool plugs have the advantage that they can be thrown away at the end of the shift; the user must learn how to prepare and insert them. The conditions of work underground, particularly if hot and dusty, and the intermittent nature of the noise encountered usually make it impracticable to institute the regular use of ear plugs by miners exposed to noise. If a miner is exposed to noise severe enough to cause tinnitus or temporary threshold shift, and therefore enough to be of concern to him, it is likely to be caused by machinery producing high noise levels for short periods of time. In this situation the only effective protection will be by ear muffs.

Appendix 1

QUESTIONNAIRE ON HEARING

Survey Site... Date.................................

Name... Date of Birth.................................

Address ....

Interviewer ....

Occupational History

Section A
 (1) Present Occupation?
 (2) Number of years in the job?
 (3) Is this job noisy?
 (4) If so, do you at any time have to shout to be heard?
 (5) Do you wear ear protection?
 (6) If yes, what type?
 (7) Previous occupation, if any?
 (8) Number of years?
 (9) Was this job noisy?
(10) If noisy, did you wear ear protection?
Remarks:

Acoustic Trauma

Section B
 (1) Have you ever used a rifle, or other gun, or served in a gun crew?
 (2) If yes, state what type and whether a few or a great number of rounds fired.
 (3) Have you ever used any type of firearm in sporting activities?
 (4) If yes, state what type and number of rounds fired?
 (5) In either of these instances did you use ear protection?
 (6) If yes, state what type of ear plug.

Otological History

Section C
 (1) Do you have, or have you had, pains in the ears? If yes, state which ear and when.
 (2) Do you have, or have you had, running ears, discharge, or abscesses in the ears?
      If yes, state which ear and when.

(3) Have you ever had an injury to the ear? If yes, state what injury, which ear and when this occurred.
(4) Has your eardrum ever been punctured? If yes, state which ear and when.
(5) Have you ever had an operation on your ear or mastoid? If yes, state which ear and when.
(6) Have you ever been unconscious due to an injury to the head? If yes, state when and how long you were unconscious.
(7) Do you have noises (ringing, hissing or buzzing) in ears or head? If yes, complete section C.1.
(8) Do you suffer, or have you suffered from attacks of dizziness or giddiness? If yes, complete section C.2.
(9) Have you ever had injections of Streptomycin? If yes, complete section C.3.
(10) Have you ever had to take Quinine for any illness? If yes, complete section C.3.
(11) Have you ever had any of the following illnesses? Mumps.............................
     Meningitis............................. Malaria.............................
(12) Is there any family history of deafness?
(13) Can you recall any incident that may have affected your hearing at any item (e.g. an explosion, a blow on the ear)? If yes complete section C.3.

Section C.1.
Do you have noises (ringing, hissing or buzzing) in the ears or head?
  (i) When did these noises first start?
  (ii) Which ear is affected?
  (iii) Do the noises bother you?
  (iv) Are they present all the time or on and off?
  (v) If the noises are continual, do they vary in loudness?
  (vi) If only on and off, how often do they appear?

Section C.2.
Do you suffer, or have you suffered, from attacks of dizziness or giddiness?
  (i) Do they give you a sensation of the room or yourself going round?
  (ii) When did these attacks first start?
  (iii) How long do they last?
  (iv) Are they brought on by moving the head, rising or stooping?
  (v) Do you feel sick or actually vomit during these attacks?
  (vi) Do you lose consciousness when they start?
  (vii) Do these attacks produce pressure or noises in the ear?

Section C.3.
Have you ever had injections of streptomycin?
  (i) When and for what?
  (ii) For how long a period?
  (iii) Following these injections, did you have any after effects? (e.g. difficulty in focussing with the eyes or unsteadiness in walking)?
Have you ever had to take quinine for any illness?
  (i) When and for what?
  (ii) For how long a period?
  (iii) Did it produce noises in the ears?
Can you recall any incident that may have affected your hearing at any time, (e.g. an explosion, a blow on the ear, etc.)?

Present State of Hearing

Section D
(1) Do you at all times hear normally (except when you have a cold)? If no, complete section D.1.

Section D.1.
   (i) Is the hearing:
       (a) Sometimes normal?
       (b) Never normal, but better sometimes than others?
       (c) Getting worse?
       (d) Neither better nor worse?
  (ii) Do you have difficulty when a group of people are talking?
 (iii) Do you have difficulty in person to person conversation?
  (iv) Is there any distortion of sound?
   (v) Can you hear better or worse in noisy surroundings?
  (vi) Can you have the radio too loud?
 (vii) Do you have difficulty in deciding which direction sounds come from?
(viii) Do you wear a hearing aid? If yes (a) Is this satisfactory or not?
                                          (b) What type of aid?

Section E
   (1) Have you ever had your hearing tested with a machine before? If yes,
    (i) When?
   (ii) Where?
  (iii) Why?

Nose

Section F
   (1) Do you have a cold at the moment?
   (2) Do you suffer from hay fever?
   (3) Do you suffer from a thick yellow discharge from the nose? (If yes, state for
       how long).

Clinical Examination

Section G
Normal—
Abnormal—See Section G.1.
Section G.1.

Hearing Survey: Clinical Findings

Name.. Serial No...
                                                                Right   *Left*

Nose: (Anterior Rhinoscopy)
     Mucopus:
     Polyp:
     Other abnormality:
Mouth:
     Edentulous:
Ears:
(a) External Appearances
       Congenital abnormality of pinna:
       Post-auricular scar:
       Endauricular scar:
(b) Meatus
       Completely occluded by wax:
       Stenosis/Atresia:
       Radical/modified radical mastoid cavily:
       Otitis Externa: Acute
                       Chronic: Active
                                Inactive

(c) Drums
       Abnormal landmarks:
       Inflammatory appearances:
       Immobile:
       Hairline and/or bubbles:
       Chalk patch:
       Generalized opacity:
       Scarred:
       Perforated: Dry
                  Moist
(d) Tuning Fork tests
       Weber: Forehead
             Vertex
       Rinné

Appendix 2

Examples of Noise Levels Found in New South Wales Coal Mines

Sound pressure level in decibels (reference ·0002 microbar)

Noise source	Range dBA	dBA	Frequencies (Hz)								
			31	63	125	250	500	1000	2000	4000	8000
Coal preparation plant	95–102	96	90	86	92	93	93	92	90	83	72
Workshop—boiler maker	70– 99	88	75	87	93	89	81	76	70	64	57
Workshop—general	70– 76	72	74	70	69	72	70	70	74	60	57
Continuous miner	92–102	96	94	88	94	94	94	90	86	85	80
Shuttle car	80– 92	86	74	84	80	80	76	77	74	70	68
Mobile Loader—at face	94– 98	97	84	86	98	96	95	92	86	77	70
Mobile Loader—behind continuous miner	94– 96	94	84	93	94	93	91	90	87	80	71
Coal cutter	88– 98	96	85	85	88	90	90	88	82	78	76
Front end loader—heavy	92–106	104	90	106	110	100	100	96	94	85	76
Transporter—light	86– 96	90	96	96	92	92	90	90	86	80	72
Roofbolter—compressed air percussion	100–128	114	93	108	112	111	114	115	114	114	115
Roofbolter hydraulic rotary	84– 90	86	83	85	90	82	81	70	76	76	76
Shaftsinking—compressed air equipment	102–120	115	90	114	116	118	114	110	108	108	104
Mobile coal drill	80– 86	85	70	70	70	80	84	81	83	74	70
Transfer point	88– 96	94	66	70	74	90	92	90	88	76	68
Man transport—battery	84– 94	94	98	105	96	90	85	80	74	68	58
Man transport—Diesel personnel car	83– 94	94	98	110	94	98	92	82	72	66	61

References

American Industrial Hygiene Association (1966), *Industrial Noise Manual.* 2nd edition. American Industrial Hygiene Association, Detroit.

Bell, A. (1966), *Noise.* World Health Organisation, Geneva.

Burns, W. (1968), *Noise and Man.* John Murray, London.

Burns, W. and Robinson, D. W. (1970), *Hearing and Noise in Industry.* Her Majesty's Stationery Office, London.

Hinchcliffe, R. (1959), "The threshold of hearing as a function of age." *Acustica,* **9,** 304.

Kryter, D. K., Ward, W. D., Miller, J. D. and Eldredge, D. H. (1966), "Hazardous exposure to intermittent and steady-state noise." *Journal of the Acoustic Society of America,* **39,** 451.

Sataloff, J. (1957), *Industrial Deafness,* p. 28–44. McGraw-Hill, New York.

Chapter 16

Accidents

Introduction

Systematic research into the safety of underground mining operations can identify not only the extent of accidents causing injury but also the patterns in which different categories of accidents occur. In this way a factual basis can be provided on which to plan and implement safety programmes. This chapter reviews several such approaches to underground safety. Although a good deal of the information is based on the extensive body of research carried out in gold mines in South Africa, the methods and findings are likely to be relevant to other mining situations. In the first part a distinction is made between accidents and injuries and the liability of different parts of the body to injury is indicated. Then the various factors which contribute towards accidents and injuries are grouped into three categories, as suggested by Gordon (1949), for analysis and discussion:

(i) The *host*—factors associated with the injured worker himself;
(ii) the *agent*—objects instrumental in causing injury; and
(iii) the *environment*—circumstances surrounding the injury.

Though these factors are considered consecutively their complex inter-relationship must be borne in mind. The final part of the chapter deals briefly with accident prevention.

Accidents, Injuries and the Extent of the Problem

Accident and Injury Rates

Two important aspects of accidental events have been mentioned above, namely the risk or probability that an accident will occur and, if it does, the probability that a worker will be injured.

If a total of n workers are employed for a given period of time, they may be divided into three categories as follows:

(*a*) The number of workers who *are not involved* in accidents.
(*b*) The number of workers who are involved in accidents but who *are not injured.*
(*c*) The number of workers who are involved in accidents and who *are injured.*

Then $n = (a + b + c)$ and the total risk or probability of injury is c/n. For example, if 4,000 workers are employed and 6 injuries occur during a given period of time (let us say one month), then the probability of an individual worker being injured is 6/4,000 or 0·0015 per month. The injury risk for an individual is usually small and it is often more convenient to express the risk as the injury rate for a group of workers. Without changing the implications of the figures the injury rate in this example could be stated as 0·15 injuries per 100 workers per month, or as 1·5 injuries per 1,000 workers per month. The base period should be long enough to make c large enough to provide a reliable index.

The probability that a worker will be involved in an "accident" in the given time is $(b + c)/n$, and the probability that a worker who is involved in an accident will in fact be injured is $c/(b + c)$.

But
$$\frac{c}{n} = \frac{b + c}{n} \times \frac{c}{b + c}$$

Thus,

the probability that a worker
will be injured $\qquad$ = the probability of an accident
$\times$ the probability of an injury
in the event of an accident.

It is clear, therefore, that there are two possible ways in which the total injury risk can be reduced. One is to reduce the likelihood of an accident and the other is to reduce the risk of injury when an accident does occur.

Several difficulties occur when compiling statistics about accidents as means for devising safer working conditions. An important problem is that it is usually impractical to collect information about b. Many unplanned and accidental events occur but because they do not result in injury they are not recognized as "accidents". In fact, in the more hazardous occupations such as mining, "accident" and "injury" tend to be regarded as synonymous. With b undetermined it is, of course, impossible to calculate $(b + c)/n$, that is the probability of workers being involved in accidents with or without injury, and consequently to examine trends in this regard. Consequently, accident statistics usually concentrate on the number of injuries c and the injury rate c/n.

Another problem is the definition of what will be and what will not be included as an "injury" when analysing accident statistics. Most concern is caused by fatalities and injuries which require hospital admission, and less concern about the more numerous minor injuries such as small cuts, scratches, sprains and strains, which do not interfere unduly with the victims' well being, or with work performance. Indeed statistics published for the mining industries as a whole seldom include minor injuries. In this chapter, injuries are grouped in increasing order of severity as follows:

(i) Minor injuries: First aid treatments involving lost working time of less than one shift.

(ii) Admissions to hospital: Injuries involving hospital admission for at least one working shift.

(iii) Fatalities.

Jensen (1970) found that fatality and injury rates bore little relationship to one another, possibly because of the comparatively small number of fatalities and the consequent wide fluctuations in the fatality rate between mines and from one year to another. Although fatality rates are often used to gauge the safety records of mines, Jensen concluded that hospital admissions, while themselves not ideal for the purpose, constituted a more reliable index provided that record keepers did not manipulate injury records to give favourable impressions of safety on their mines. Fatality records are, of course, immune to such manipulation.

At first sight there may appear to be no disadvantage in emphasizing serious injuries in accident statistics. However, the more serious the injury the lower the probability of its occurrence and improved safety measures further reduce this risk. Consequently the number of cases at a mine which fall into categories (ii) and (iii) above may become too few in a reasonable period of time to permit worthwhile analysis, particularly if they are further subdivided, for example, in terms of different job categories or different managers' sections within the mine.

Thus, Bettencourt and Jensen (1970) have argued that the more numerous minor or "dressing station" injuries which occur at a mine should permit a quicker and a more reliable analysis of the accidents causing them and consequently better designed measures for accident prevention. There is certainly no evidence to suggest that accidents resulting in minor injuries are unimportant when investigating accident causation.

Parts of Body Injured

The vulnerability of different parts of the body to injury is of particular relevance to efforts to reduce the risk of injury in the event of an accident, for example, by protective clothing. Bettencourt, Bold and Jensen (1967), Bettencourt and Jensen (1967) and Van Graan and Morrison (1967) have shown differences between hospital admissions and minor injuries, relating to the parts of the body which were injured. Whereas the majority of minor injuries involved hands, most admissions to hospital were due to leg injuries. These findings are illustrated in Figure 1. The percentages shown in the figure may also be regarded as conditional probabilities for the occurrence of the different injuries. Thus, given that a minor injury had occurred the probability that it was a hand injury was about 0·53, while given that a hospital admission had occurred, the probability that it was for a hand injury was only about 0·28, but the probability that it was for a leg injury was about 0·33.

To permit them to claim that the incidence of more serious injuries could be predicted from the incidence of minor injuries, Bettencourt and Jensen (1970) found it necessary to reconcile the distributions of minor injuries and admissions to hospital. They suggested that the higher proportion of leg injuries among hospital cases may have been

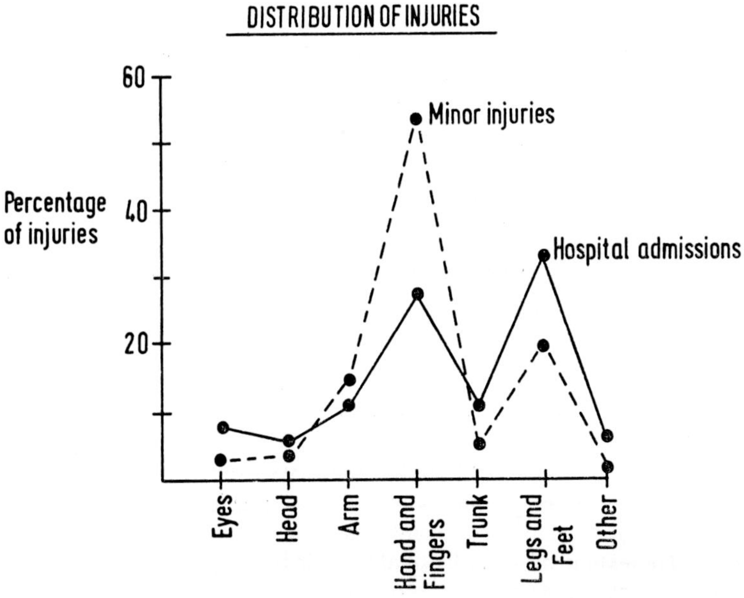

DISTRIBUTION OF INJURIES

Fig. 1.

an artefact which occurred because admission to hospital did not adequately reflect the seriousness of an injury. These writers pointed out that a worker with a hand injury may be placed on convalescent light duty and not classed as an admission to hospital, whereas a worker with a leg injury of "equal severity" may have had to remain in bed.

This argument clearly depends upon the definition of "severity". For example, is a fracture of the hand as "severe" as a fractured leg? The only practical basis on which to assess the severity of an injury appears to be the extent to which it interferes with work attendance and Bettencourt *et al.* (1967) have presented evidence confirming that leg injuries result in the loss of more shifts per casualty than do other injuries, particularly hand injuries (Table 1).

By reconciling the distributions of minor injuries and hospital admissions, Bettencourt and Jensen (1970) came to the conclusion that minor injuries can provide a reliable basis for designing programmes for accident prevention. In so doing they appear to have come to the right conclusion but for the wrong reason. With interest focused on the study of "accidental events" which resulted in injuries rather than on injuries themselves, an understanding of accidental events should be attainable through a study of *either* the minor injuries *or* hospital admissions, *or* both, regardless of the similarity or lack of similarity between probability distributions such as those illustrated in Figure 1.

Table 1

Average Shifts Lost per Casualty as Result of Injury to Different Parts of Body

Part of Body Injured	Average Shifts Lost per Casualty
Lower leg	51·8
Pelvis	50·8
Thigh	47·1
Upper arm	36·7
Back	30·2
Ankle	26·0
Wrist	19·1
Fingers	18·0

Host Factors in Injury Accidents

A worker may behave in such a way that he precipitates an accidental event and consequently contributes to his own injury or to that of others. The extent of an individual's contribution to an accident may be obscured by the circumstances of the incident itself. When examining the relevant circumstances the fact that his behaviour at the time may have been beyond his control, in the sense that it was characteristic of his particular personality, may be overlooked. In other words, it is sometimes forgotten that some workers, because of their personal attributes, may be more susceptible or vulnerable to accidents than others.

The literature on accidents abounds with discussions of the concept of "accident proneness" as an explanation for the fact that some people are involved in more accidents than others and that the majority of accidents usually occur among a comparatively small proportion of the population at risk. Haddon, Suchman and Klein (1964) have identified and discussed different aspects of accident proneness but have pointed out that, as a psychological concept, accident proneness must be viewed as only one possible explanation for individual variations in accident rates, in addition to such considerations as exposure to hazards, capacity for correctly judging hazards, and response to stress.

Several research studies in the gold mining industry have examined the contribution of individual differences to the incidence of mining injury accidents and the findings of a number of these may be summarized as follows:

Age and Experience

Relationships between injury accident rates and the age or the experience of the victims have been established for several different types of accident unrelated to mining (Haddon *et al.*, 1964); it would seem reasonable to expect that in mining work also, experienced men would be less likely to be involved in accidents than inexperienced men. Further, if men are employed for any length of time in mining then there must clearly be a positive correlation between their age and their mining experience, and it would therefore also seem reasonable to expect that there would be a higher probability of accident and injury among younger miners.

However, Bettencourt (1967a) has analysed the minor injuries occurring among drilling crews and stope team labourers on a gold mine and although he noted a tendency for injury rates to fall as men reached the age of 34 to 37 and then to rise, this relationship was not statistically significant.

In a subsequent re-analysis of the available research data, Bettencourt and Jensen (1970) have shown the necessity for distinguishing between mining experience (total experience in mining) and job experience (experience in a particular mining job). These investigators found a correlation coefficient of $+0.61$ between age and mining experience but an insignificant correlation coefficient of $+0.10$ between age and job experience. However, job experience was found to be strongly associated with the occurrence of injuries among drilling crews and stope team labourers, as shown in Figure 2. Regardless of the men's total mining experience, higher injury rates occurred during the first four months of job experience.

These findings have shown that although the risk of injury is generally less for older men (with more mining experience), the influence of changes of job and unfamiliarity with new jobs (involving less job experience) should not be overlooked when considering the likelihood of accidents among mineworkers. Supervisors should thus pay special attention to workers who are placed on jobs with which they are unfamiliar.

Aggressiveness

Numerous investigators have examined the relationships between personality and involvement in accidents, and much of the research has been concerned with individual "aggressiveness" and the part it plays in accident causation. For example, Krall (1953) found that among children "accident repeaters" displayed more aggressive behaviour and fewer inhibitions and Porterfield (1960) has suggested "that aggressive hazardous driving is likely to be characteristic of persons similar to those who have suicidal or homicidal or both tendencies". Findings such as these imply that at least certain types of accident may be avoided by careful selection of workers by means of personality tests: that this is feasible has been confirmed in the case of motor bus drivers (Shaw, 1959; de Ridder, 1961; Sichel, 1965).

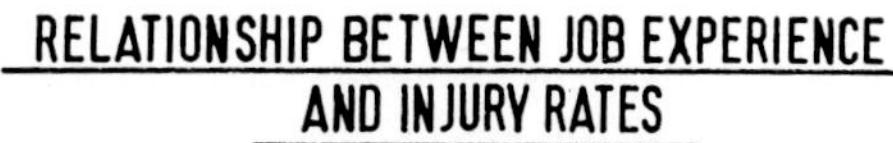

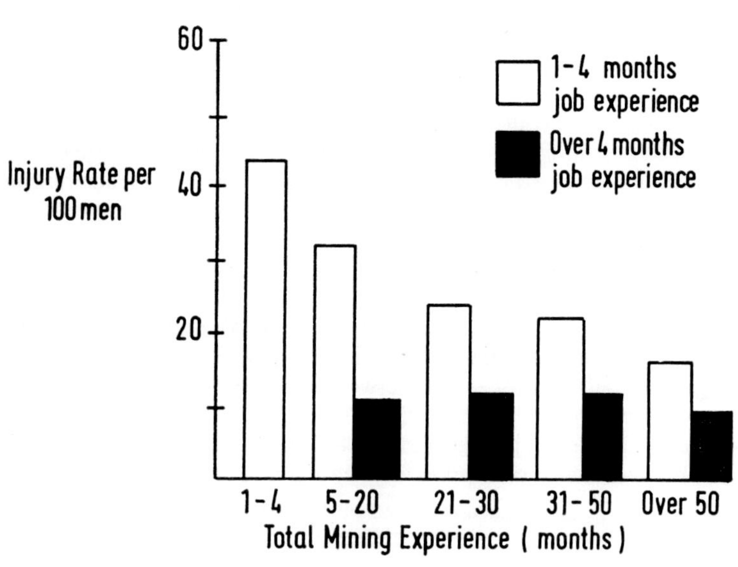

Fig. 2.

In the gold mining industry the use of personality tests, particularly projective tests of the thematic apperception type (T.A.T.) has excited considerable interest as a possible means for identifying workers with an accident potential when selecting underground locomotive drivers. Various attempts to this end have been reviewed by Wortley and Nativel (1969) but they found that the tests had not been successful in reducing accident rates, and concluded that:

(i) some accidents are probably caused or contributed to by personality factors;

(ii) it is possible in certain circumstances to predict these personality factors from a test like the T.A.T.; but

(iii) these accidents are totally obscured by the greater number of accidents arising from other causes.

These conclusions about the limited importance of the relationship between scores on projective personality tests and locomotive accidents may well apply also to other types of mining accident particularly if, as Wortley and Nativel suggest, poor or inconsistent supervisory practices are a major consideration among the other causes which obscure personality factors in accident causation.

Type of Work

In view of the numerous different job categories involved in mining and the fact that each man is often trained specifically for only one of them, it is appropriate to regard his "job category" as a personal feature of the individual worker and to consider this among the host factors which contribute towards accidents.

As would be expected from the nature of mining work, the large majority of accidents causing injury occur among underground rather than surface job categories of men. Several investigators have reported on the liabilities of different underground mineworkers to accidental injury in terms of their job categories (Bettencourt and Jensen, 1967; Bettencourt *et al.*, 1967; and Jensen, 1970), and although meaningful comparisons between the findings are sometimes hampered as the result of the different ways in which jobs have been grouped, the injury rates for different jobs were found, in general, to be of the order shown in Table 2. Although in this table the figures for minor injuries are of the

Table 2

Injury Rates for Different Underground Job Categories

Job Category	Minor Injuries Rate per 100 per month	Hospital Admissions Rate per 100 per year
Drilling Crews	16	18
Scraper winch operators	12	11
Other stope labour	7	9
Stope labour supervisors	11	16
Locomotive crews	6	14
All other labour	Not given	4
Mine average	8	9

same magnitude as the corresponding figures for hospital admissions, it must be noted that the minor injuries are per 100 workers per month while the hospital admissions are per 100 workers per year.

The injury rate has thus been shown to be highest among stope workers and particularly among those working at the rock face.

Jensen (1970) has observed that almost two-thirds of all the injuries recorded in one study occurred in stopes and his figures suggest that more than a third of these were sustained during drilling, cleaning and barring operations.

Although jobs differ widely in the risk of injury which they entail, the distributions of injuries over the body are much the same for different types of work. For example, Table 3 shows the anatomical distributions for minor injuries and more serious injuries requiring

Table 3

Distribution of Injuries per Cent for Different Job Categories

Part of Body Injured	Drill Operators		Scraper Winch Operators		Pipes and Tracks Workers		Locomotive Drivers		Locomotive Guards	
	M	H	M	H	M	H	M	H	M	H
Eyes	2·6	9·1	3·5	9·0	1·1	3·9	—	3·6	3·2	4·1
Head	4·9	4·3	4·8	2·7	5·0	4·9	23·1	9·8	9·7	11·0
Shoulder	3·7	2·5	1·0	2·6	2·2	2·4	1·9	1·0	1·6	1·4
Arm	21·1	18·5	20·2	12·1	13·8	10·7	7·7	9·3	8·0	4·2
Hand	10·7	3·6	12·5	5·6	8·3	2·4	7·7	3·1	9·7	2·8
Fingers	39·9	22·5	50·5	25·0	56·4	32·4	48·1	34·1	41·9	32·4
Trunk	3·2	9·3	1·3	10·4	2·2	10·2	—	9·7	8·1	16·5
Leg	7·1	19·9	3·5	22·0	5·0	21·1	3·8	13·5	9·7	15·9
Foot	4·2	9·2	0·6	9·8	5·0	11·5	7·7	14·9	4·8	11·7
Other	2·6	1·1	2·2	0·8	1·1	0·5	—	1·0	3·2	—
Total	100	100	100	100	100	100	100	100	100	100

Key: M = Minor injuries.
        H = Injuries requiring hospital admissions.

hospital admission for five job categories which entailed very different activities. It will be observed that although the distributions for minor injuries were not the same for those requiring admission to hospital, there were only relatively few differences within these classifications between jobs.

Despite differences in the work involved in drill operating, scraper winch operating, and pipes and tracks labouring, injury patterns were much alike. Greater differences occurred between the injury distributions for these jobs and those for locomotive drivers and guards, but even these differences were not large (Fig. 3).

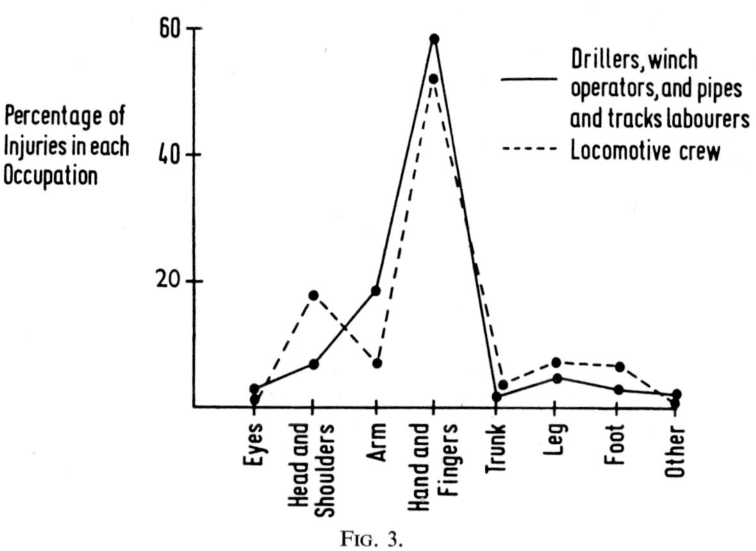

Fig. 3.

Work Activity at Time of Accident

Many different activities are involved in each work category and it is convenient, therefore, to consider these also as host factors. As was shown in Table 2 injury rates are higher in stope jobs than in other work categories, and in two studies minor injuries were examined in terms of the actual activities in which stope workers were engaged at the time when they were injured (Bettencourt *et al.*, 1967; and Bettencourt, 1967a). The majority of minor injuries in stopes occurred during the handling of material, then came those occurring during drilling activities. The "handling material" injuries occurred predominantly while rock was being handled and while material was being transported in stopes. These findings are not surprising in view of the fact that broken rock is sharp and rough to handle, that material has to be transported over its irregular surface and that most minor injuries were inflicted on hands and arms (Fig. 1).

The activities of drilling crews and "stope team" labourers were then singled out for separate study. It was found that the drilling crew were at maximum hazard while they were operating the drill itself, usually as the result of falls of rock, and that their other activities contributed comparatively little to their injury rates. Stope team labourers were injured most frequently while lashing (shovelling rock) and while installing supports.

Other Host Factors

The relationships between injuries and several other host variables have been examined by different investigators but without any findings of great significance emerging.

Nelson (1964) studied the relationship between accidents and a large number of neuropsychological and sociological factors among 251 underground locomotive drivers and guards, but did not find any major correlations. Individual differences, related to brain function and experience, accounted for only 6 per cent of the variance among injuries resulting from locomotive accidents. Similarly, individual differences in behaviour patterns and reaction times comprised only 6 per cent of the variance of data from records of disciplinary action against locomotive crew.

During this investigation, the attitudes of locomotive crew towards the mine, their jobs and their supervisors were compared with the incidence of accidents (Hall, 1965). The analysis did not identify any factors related to attitudes which could be considered as predisposing workers towards accidents or injury.

Agents Causing Injury

The instrument or agent which causes injury in a work accident depends upon the worker's job category and the particular work activity in which he is engaged at the time. When considered together with the vulnerability of different parts of the body to injury, information about the agent of injury is useful in designing effective measures to safeguard against injury in the event of an accident.

The agents causing the more serious injuries underground have been analysed in a study of seven gold mines (Bettencourt *et al.*, 1967). The results of this study are summarized in Table 4 which shows that "rock" was the main agent causing serious injury, accounting for nearly 44 per cent of admissions to hospital, while a further 27 per cent of the injuries were inflicted by mechanical devices. The majority of the "rock" injuries occurred as the result of unexpected falls of rock.

Information about the agents causing minor injuries is less extensive. However, the analysis of minor injuries among drilling crews and stope team labourers (Bettencourt, 1967a), has shown that "rock" may

Table 4

Agents Causing Hospital Admissions

Agent	Injuries (%)	
Rock:		43·3
Falls from hanging	23·3	
Other falls	16·9	
Other (rolling, handling, flying chips)	3·1	
Transport Devices:		20·5
Locomotives, trucks, cocopans and		
hoppers	8·5	
Scotch cars and loaders	12·0	
Materials:		12·9
Timbers, packs, props	4·1	
Rails, pipes and cables	3·6	
Other	5·2	
Scraping Machinery:		6·9
Winches, pulleys, snatch blocks	3·5	
Scoops and ropes	3·4	
Chemical agents including explosives		6·8
Other		9·6
Total		100

account for as much as 80 per cent of minor injuries in these job categories. In this case, less than half (about 40 per cent) of the injuries occurred as the result of falls of rock and the majority occurred when parts of the body, especially hands, were struck against the rock while working.

Environmental Factors Contributing to Injuries

The influences of the physical environment are implicit in the foregoing discussion of injuries and injury rates, but in addition to the more obvious physical hazards there are several other factors which may be considered to be part of the worker's "environment". These include, for example, the locality in which the worker is required to work, the time of day, the day of the week, and the attitudes of his superiors towards the work in general and safety in particular.

Locality of Work

The place where the accident causing injury involves a worker is obviously linked to a considerable extent to his particular job category

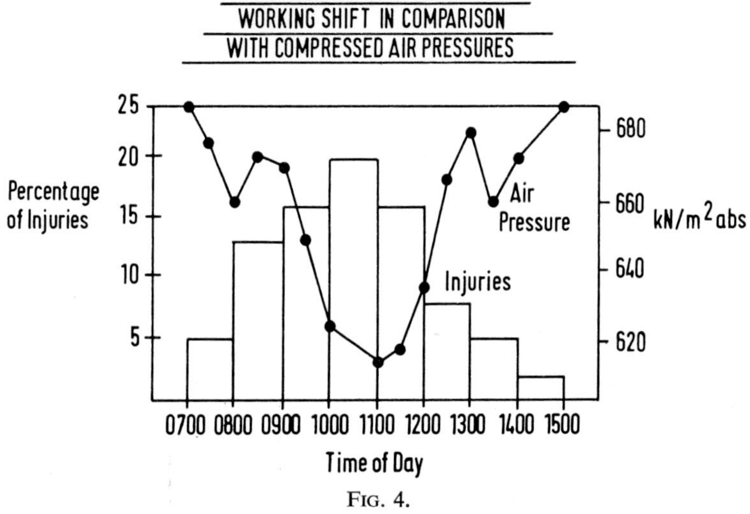

Fig. 4.

and in Table 2 it has already been shown that the stope is the locality where most injuries are suffered.

Wortley and Strohbach (1969) have reported on the sites where underground locomotives in one gold mine were involved in accidents (with or without injuries) and events which could have resulted in accidents. As shown in Table 5, more than one half of these accidents occurred on haulages and in cross cuts.

Findings such as these are valuable in indicating where improved precautionary measures are needed to reduce the risk of accidents and the injuries arising from them.

Time of Day

An examination of the distribution of injuries during the workng shift (Bettencourt and Jensen, 1967, 1970) has shown that more thian half of the accidents at one mine occurred during the last three-hour period (09.00 to 12.00) of the first half of the day shift (Fig. 4). The distribution of injuries was proportional to pneumatic drilling activities as shown by compressed air pressures at shafts, and this suggested that the risk of injury rose as pressure increased for production output. Bettencourt and Jensen (1970) have pointed out, however, that other factors may

Table 5

*Localities of Accidents and Potential Accidents involving
Underground Locomotives*

Locality	Accidents and Potential Accidents
	(%)
Along straight haulage (not at a switch)	36·6
In cross cut	23·1
At a switch	15·4
At a ventilation door	6·4
At tips	4·5
At bend in haulage	3·2
In developing end	3·2
In tramming loop	3·2
At a stop point in haulage	1·9
In fitting shop repair bay	1·3
At station cross cut	0·6
At working place	0·6
Total	100·0

have accounted for this relationship. For example, during the early part
of the shift, while the working place was being made safe, workers were
subject to closer supervision and may have taken greater care to work
safely.

In their study of locomotive accidents, Wortley and Strohbach (1969)
found a fairly constant number of incidents (accidents and potential
accidents) during the day shift but a very much larger number during
the night shift despite the fact that the locomotives were in almost
continual use during both the day and night shifts. Only 28 per cent of
the accidents occurred during the 10 hours of the day shift compared
with 72 per cent during the 12 hours of the night shift. These investigators attributed the increase in accidents during the night shift to the
decrease in supervision at that time.

Day of the Week

Wortley and Strohbach (1969) have also reported on the distribution
of underground locomotive accidents over the six working days of the
week. The majority of these occurred on Monday and Friday (44 per
cent) and far fewer in mid-week on Wednesday and Thursday (26 per
cent).

The accident rate appears to have moved in parallel with the production rate, Saturday being least productive and having the lowest accident
rate as the result of its unpopularity as a working day. Although the
total number of accidents was too few to permit firm conclusions to be

drawn the results also suggest that attitudes towards production and safety may change during the course of a week and that accident patterns may change accordingly. If this is so, it has important implications for training and for supervisory practices which are aimed at accident prevention.

Physical Environment

Mining takes place in a hostile physical environment. If ore reefs are narrow, stoping widths may be just sufficient to permit men to work effectively, and may be as little as one metre. In some mines the reef dips up to 90 degrees, and at deep levels temperatures and humidities are extremely high. Working conditions, particularly in stopes, may tend to be uncomfortable and tiring. In addition, the danger of rock bursts and rock falls is always present.

Van Graan and Morrison (1967) have examined the relationship between the number of hospital admissions and the declination (dip) and width of stopes on 44 mines. Stoping width appeared to be unrelated to frequency of accidents but a positive correlation was observed between stope declination and hospital admissions. Jensen (1970) has stated the correlation coefficient for this relationship as +0·5. Steeply dipping stopes can be expected to present a greater risk of injury due to rolling rock and to men slipping and falling.

Underground mining operations result in stresses in the rock which may culminate in rockbursts and other rock failures as work proceeds, unless operations are designed so as to prevent energy from being released destructively in this way. Bettencourt (1969) has found significant positive correlations with coefficients of the order of 0·68 to 0·93 between the occurrence of injuries and the energy release rates on one mine over a period of four and a half years, thus confirming the view that adequate consideration of energy release constitutes a major factor in preventing injuries resulting from rock falls.

Attitudes of Managers and Supervisors Towards Safety

Mineworkers are subject not only to a particular physical environment and climate underground, but also to a "supervisory climate" in the attitudes of managers and supervisors towards working practices, accidents, injuries and accident prevention. This supervisory climate is likely to have an important effect on the adequacy of safety measures in the work situation and in the adherence of mineworkers to working practices which are known to be safe.

There is, however, a continuing dilemma inherent in the mining situation which faces managers and supervisors. On the one hand they are reluctant to expose their workers to known dangers which may result in injury, while on the other hand their business objectives are measured in terms of production and this necessitates exposure to these hazards.

Jensen (1970) has reported on two studies involving interviews with 109 subjects drawn from all levels of management and production personnel. Management was found to attach considerable importance to the establishment and observance of "standard" practices and procedures for all aspects of underground work as a means of attaining both high production and low accident rates. However, it was conceded that maintenance of production levels tended to receive first consideration and that pressures in this direction tended to create attitudes which had an adverse effect on safety. Concern for safety and concern for production are not easily reconciled and a number of accident research projects have suggested that the conflict between them is one of the fundamental considerations in accident causation (Nelson, 1964; Krenzer, 1965; Wortley and Strohbach, 1969; Jensen, 1970). Jensen, Strochbach and Bold (1967) found that supervisors themselves confirmed this contention. When questioned about the causes of accidents 34 per cent of the responses indicated "production pressures" and 37 per cent suggested "negligence or carelessness" (Table 6).

Table 6

*Principal Causes of Underground Accidents Reported by
166 Supervisory Staff*

Cause	*Number of Responses*
	(%)
Negligence or carelessness	37
Production pressures	34
Lack of knowledge about unsafe conditions	13
Inadequate supervision and discipline	9
Psychological and physiological states (e.g. fatigue, tension)	7
Total	100

Preoccupation with productivity may result in a lack of attention to such matters as accident patterns, injury rates and the risks inherent in different job categories. Lack of knowledge of such aspects of the accident problem is also likely to reduce safety for men working underground. The extent to which 104 rockbreakers (supervisors), shift bosses and mine overseers were familiar with accident patterns on their own mine was examined by Bettencourt (1967b). He found that, in general, knowledge about injury rates among production personnel was poor and that there was a tendency to underestimate them in important job categories such as drilling and stope team work. Mine overseers and shift bosses were found to be only slightly superior to rockbreakers in this respect. Bettencourt concluded that lack of knowledge about accidents among controlling personnel may have had a significant bearing on the limited success which preventive and supervisory programmes aimed at accident prevention had achieved.

Prevention of Accidents and Injuries

During the preceding discussion of the sources, nature and extent of accidents and injuries, possible ways in which they may be prevented have been mentioned explicitly or implied. Basically, two approaches to "accident" prevention may be used, independently or jointly. One aims at the inculcation of an awareness at all levels of personnel of the importance of the accident problem, and the imparting of knowledge which is properly understood and applied to reduce the risk of "accidents". The means available for this approach centre largely around initial and subsequent training, safety incentives, safety competitions and the like. The other approach aims at preventing injuries in the event of an accident. One of the main means for accomplishing this is the provision of suitable clothing to protect the exposed parts of a worker's body from injury.

Safety Training and Propaganda

A large proportion (50 per cent) of the responses illustrated in Table 6 attributes accidents to causes which can be remedied only by training and propaganda, namely negligence or carelessness and lack of knowledge. This was confirmed to some extent by responses in the same study to a question about the most important procedures for accident prevention.

Thus one of the principal functions of the training organization at a mine is to emphasize continually the importance of safe working habits while training workers in job skills. To this end extensive use may be made of recognized training techniques, including the use of lectures, slides, posters and films. However, the success of training procedures which are aimed at the development of attitudes favourable to accident prevention, or at a change to more favourable attitudes, is evaluated less easily than training which is concerned with the teaching of skills. It is possible, therefore, for safety training to deteriorate into programmes which are administered routinely but with doubtful effectiveness. The same remarks apply to propaganda aimed at accident prevention and which makes use of the same techniques as formal training programmes.

For example, Jensen (1966) discovered several inadequacies in the techniques used for safety training and propaganda, and has emphasized, in particular, the need for the formulation of specific measurable objectives for safety training and the systematic checking of trainees' comprehension of safety training material.

Commenting on the imperviousness of "negligence" to propaganda, incentives, coercion or any other authority-backed methods, Jensen *et al.* (1967) have recommended an approach which avoids vague concepts of safety and accident prevention, and makes hazards and the consequence of negligence as concrete as possible through real-life case-studies and factual material drawn from the situation in which the men are employed.

Safety Bonuses

It is fairly common practice to award a periodic bonus to the supervisor of a particular mine section if his safety record is satisfactory. The basis on which the latter is judged is not always clear and may include the maintenance of safe conditions underground as judged by his superior, and the injury rate in his section. The bonus may be associated with different aspects of accident prevention each month to focus attention on these different aspects.

In two studies which investigated attitudes towards bonus incentives for safety, at a total of ten mines (Jensen, 1966; Jensen *et al.*, 1967), it was found that whereas, in theory, safety bonuses should have been a worthwhile means of encouraging interest in safety, there were problems in administering the schemes in such a way as to attain the desired ends. In most cases, the subjects interviewed were critical of the bonus system and indicated that it did not receive their whole-hearted support.

Jensen (1966, 1970) has attributed this lack of support to two factors. Firstly, he has stated that the criteria on which "safety" will be judged are seldom clearly stated in operational terms. He has suggested, for example, that the objective for a particular supervisor could be to change the statistical distribution of accident rates in a specified manner for a specified group over a given period of time. Set in these terms objectives should become both logical and fair.

Secondly, Jensen has emphasized that an incentive scheme must have the whole-hearted support of managers, supervisors, and workers, and has pointed out the need for extensive and continuing consultation between management and those to whom the incentive will apply to ensure this mutual support.

Safety Campaigns and Competitions

Where they have been introduced, inter-mine competitions appear to have contributed in no small measure to improvements in accident rates through the years.

Many mines also conduct internal safety competitions on an inter-sectional basis. Jensen *et al.* (1967) found that although the usefulness of these competitions was generally accepted the most frequent criticism referred to the fact that not all workers in the winning section shared in the prizes. For example, a prize may have been awarded only to the supervisor of the winning section.

Although the concepts of probability and chance distributions are unlikely to be fully understood by workers, they are quick to appreciate the inequity of a judgment which is determined by an "Act of God", for example, if a fall of rock injures three men but if the fall had occurred six feet further away it would have injured no one. The views expressed by Jensen about the need for safety incentives to be based on statistical parameters, apply equally to safety competitions.

Safety Departments

Different mines follow different policies in so far as safety departments are concerned. Some have well-developed departments headed by people with considerable expertise in the field of accident prevention and who emphasize activities which are forward looking in the sense that they aim at accident "prevention". Other mines have safety officers who are less progressive, being primarily concerned with the maintenance of injury records and statistics and in investigating accidents which have already resulted in serious injuries. Yet other mines do not have safety departments as such but prefer to foster the concept that each manager and supervisor is his own safety officer and that he cannot relieve himself of responsibility for safety in his section by calling on the services of a safety department. The particular outlook of managers and supervisors at these mines may, of course, be either progressive or retrospective.

Jensen *et al.* (1967) in a study of gold mines (presumably all with safety departments) found that the safety officers and safety departments were not always held in high regard. The functions of safety departments were thought to be too restricted and safety officers were said often to be inadequate for their jobs and lacking in authority to enforce safety practices and regulations. These investigators have commented as follows in this connection.

"The apparent weakness of safety departments reflects management's attitudes towards the functions of such departments but is also due to the shortage of qualified and trained safety personnel in the mining industry. Often it is not realized that safety is a highly specialized field requiring technical knowledge in statistics, psychology, and ergonomics. Certain personality attributes and a high degree of familiarity with the industrial situation in which the safety engineer works are also necessary. Most mine safety officers have only the last qualification."

The remedy here appears to be the use, as safety officers, of competent mining engineers with authority to enforce safe working practices, and the reorganization of safety departments along more effective lines.

Thus Briggs (1953) found that accident rates on a mine were reduced from 298/1000 labourers/year to 82/1000 labourers/year over a period of three years following a reorganization of the safety department, and then further to 43/1000 labourers/year over the next seven years.

Protective Clothing

The effectiveness of protective clothing in reducing the risk of injury in the event of an accident has been examined by van Graan and Morrison (1967). At mines at which leg guards were not issued, injuries necessitating admission to hospital were 92 per cent higher and minor injuries were 200 per cent higher than at mines at which leg guards were issued to the whole labour force. Similarly, the proportion of hospital cases at mines issuing gloves was not much lower than that at mines not using gloves, but the proportion of minor injuries was very much higher at the latter. Information about the effectiveness of goggles and arm guards was less conclusive.

On the basis of these findings the investigators decided that serious injuries could not be prevented by the use of protective clothing but that the severity of the injury could be reduced and many minor injuries such as scratches, cuts and bruises could be prevented. However, the effectiveness of such clothing depends upon the willingness of the workers to wear it in the intended way, and it was found that certain clothing caused discomfort and was tiring to wear, for example, leg guards, and that critical dimensions of the clothing were not always appropriate to the anthropometric measurements of the workers concerned. It is important, therefore, that protective clothing should not only be effective in preventing injuries but must also be well-designed and acceptable to the workers, otherwise it is unlikely to be worn correctly, if at all.

References

Bettencourt, J. J. (1967a), "An analysis of injuries to drilling crews and stope team labourers on a mine." Unpublished report, Chamber of Mines of South Africa, Johannesburg.

Bettencourt, J. J. (1967b), "A questionnaire on underground accidents administered to personnel on a mine." Unpublished report, Chamber of Mines of South Africa, Johannesburg.

Bettencourt, J. J. (1969), "The relationship between the number of injuries arising from falls of ground and the amounts of energy released per unit area mined." Unpublished report, Chamber of Mines of South Africa, Johannesburg.

Bettencourt, J. J., Bold, A. and Jensen, A. (1967), "An analysis of underground accidents on seven gold mines." Unpublished report, Chamber of Mines of South Africa, Johannesburg.

Bettencourt, J. J. and Jensen, A. (1967), "An analysis of underground accidents in a gold mine." Unpublished report, Chamber of Mines of South Africa, Johannesburg.

Bettencourt, J. J. and Jensen, A. (1970), "A statistical analysis of accidents to Bantu personnel in the gold mining industry." *Journal of South African Institute of Mining and Metallurgy*, **71**, 105.

Briggs, R. C. (1953), "Safety organization in a mine." *Chemical Metallurgical and Mining Society of South Africa Journal*, **54**, 157.

De Ridder, J. C. (1961), *The Personality of the Urban African in South Africa*. Routledge and Kegan Paul, London.

Gordon, J. E. (1949), "The epidemiology of accidents." *American Journal of Public Health*, **39**, 504.

Haddon, W., Suchman, E. A. and Klein, D. (1964), *Accident Research: Methods and Approaches*. Harper and Row, New York.

Hall, S. K. P. (1965), "African loco drivers: A study of their backgrounds and attitudes related to incidence of accidents." Contract Report C/Pers 107, National Institute for Personnel Research (South Africa), Johannesburg.

Jensen, A. (1966), "Attitudes and practices in regard to certain aspects of safety on a gold mine." Unpublished report, Chamber of Mines of South Africa, Johannesburg.

Jensen, A. (1970), "A review of personnel research in the gold mining industry," Ph.D. thesis, University of Witwatersrand, Johannesburg.

Jensen, A., Strohbach, H. J. B. R. and Bold, A. (1967), "Attitudes towards accident prevention among gold mine personnel." Unpublished report, Chamber of Mines of South Africa, Johannesburg.

Krall, V. (1953), "Personality characteristics of accident repeating children." *Journal of Abnormal and Social Psychology*, **48**, 99.

Krenzer, O. (1965), "Underground locomotive accidents in gold mines." Contract Report C/Pers 121, National Institute for Personnel Research (South Africa), Johannesburg.

Nelson, G. K. (1964), "A pilot study of underground locomotive accidents in a gold mine." Contract Report C/Pers 84, National Institute for Personnel Research (South Africa), Johannesburg.

Porterfield, A. L. (1960), "Traffic fatalities, suicide and homicide." *American Sociological Review*, **25**, 897.

Shaw, L. (1959), "Special selection procedures developed for African bus drivers with a view to accident prevention." *South African Mechanical Engineer*, **9**, 29.

Sichel, H. S. (1965), "The statistical estimation of individual accident liability." *Traffic Safety Research Review*, **9**, 8.

Van Graan, C. H. and Morrison, J. F. (1967), "The relationship between the use of protective clothing, the safety organization and accident rates in the gold mines." Unpublished report, Chamber of Mines of South Africa, Johannesburg.

Wortley, R. H. and Nativel, P. (1969), "The thematic apperception test as a predictor of locomotive accidents." Unpublished report, Chamber of Mines of South Africa, Johannesburg.

Wortley, R. H. and Strohbach, H. J. B. R. (1969), "A case study of locomotive accidents in a gold mine." Unpublished report, Chamber of Mines of South Africa, Johannesburg.

Chapter 17

Emergency Surgery

Introduction

The doctor who is called to a mine to treat a seriously injured patient must be prepared to meet situations of unusual difficulty.

In considering the various surgical emergencies the management of the most difficult of all—the desperate case in which the victim has been trapped by an extremity and can only be released by immediate amputation—is one to which special consideration must be given.

In all serious cases, and particularly in the example quoted, the problem of traumatic shock will be a source of anxiety, since it carries a continuous threat to the life of the patient.

It is also important to emphasize that the dangers of traumatic shock are almost certain to be made worse by the often unavoidable delay, even in less serious cases, in evacuating casualties from distant and difficult underground workings to mine shaft, surface and hospital. Some discussion of shock is therefore necessary.

Traumatic Shock

Definition

Traumatic shock has been defined as a condition arising from diminished vascular volume due to internal and/or external loss of blood and fluids. This leads to decreased tissue perfusion and cellular hypoxia with anaerobic metabolism and metabolic acidosis. Progressive cellular malfunction and destruction may lead to organ failure beginning with the kidney and affecting other organs (Blakemore and Fitts, 1969a).

Sequence of Events

The mechanisms operating in shock may be described thus: the fall in blood volume causes first a fall in central venous pressure and then a low cardiac output; the blood pressure falls when vasoconstriction is inadequate to compensate for the fall in cardiac output. At each stage compensatory activity in the sympathetic nervous system gives rise to signs of the classical shock syndrome, sweating, venous constriction, pallor and tachycardia (Walters, 1969).

Clinical Picture

The clinical picture will vary with circumstances, and is largely dependent on the volume of blood and fluids lost. It is difficult to quantify this loss except by the patient's response to replacement. It is now accepted that significant and even serious blood loss may follow closed fractures. Examples of blood loss cited by Blakemore and Fitts (1969b) follow: with a simple major fracture of the femur, blood loss into the thigh may be 500 to 1,500 ml, or 10 to 30 per cent of the total blood volume of an adult; with larger wounds, and particularly fractures of the pelvis, this may increase to two or three litres, or half the total blood volume. With extensive fractures of the pelvis and retroperitoneal haemorrhage greater losses have been recorded. The presence of tachycardia and an arterial blood pressure that remains below 80 mm Hg. systolic generally indicate blood loss of greater than 1,000 ml and often as much as 1,500 to 2,000 ml.

The doctor facing this sort of emergency will have to estimate the degree of shock by such means as he has to hand, namely, the probable extent of the injuries, the appearance of the casualty, his pulse rate and pressure, and his arterial blood pressure. In this situation we must regard the pulse pressure as the most reliable index of the circulatory state (McGowan and Walters, 1966). Weil and Shubin (1967a) have published the following useful table showing the correlation of clinical findings and the magnitude of volume deficit.

Severity of shock	Clinical findings	Reduction in blood volume
Mild	Minimal tachycardia. Slight decrease in blood pressure. Mild evidence of peripheral vasoconstriction with cool hands and feet.	15–25% (750–1,250 ml)
Moderate	Tachycardia 100–120. Decreased pulse pressure. Systolic B.P. 90–100 mm Hg. Restlessness. Increased sweating. Pallor. Oliguria.	25–35% (1,250–1,750 ml)
Severe	Tachycardia over 120. B.P. below 60 mm Hg. systolic, and frequently unobtainable by cuff. Mental stupor. Extreme pallor. Cold extremities. Anuria.	Up to 50% (2,500 ml) (Based on a blood volume of 7% in a 70 kg male of medium build.)

Therapy

In haemorrhage and most forms of trauma the need is to make good the loss, namely, whole blood. During the interval in which blood is being prepared and properly cross-matched, isotonic saline solution or clinical dextran solution will often adequately support the circulation, and a reasonably satisfactory blood pressure may be obtained by the rapid intravenous infusion of a litre or more of one of these solutions.

Dextran is a polymer of glucose. Preparations of this substance with a high molecular weight are comparable to plasma in providing colloid osmotic pressure but are more rapidly lost in the urine. About 50 per cent remains in the circulation after eight to twenty-four hours (Blakemore and Fitts, 1969c). The important thing is to inject a suitable solution in sufficient quantity to maintain the filling of the heart. Gruber (1969) has emphasized the significance of volume in the aphorism, "with great simplification one might say that it is not so important *what* one gives, if one just gives *enough* and *in time*". As care is required to avoid overloading the vascular space in elderly patients, this is best allowed for by recommending an average intravenous amount of fluid (see below).

In the circumstances which we are considering, such exactitudes as estimation of central venous pressure and urinary output have no place, although they will play a very important part in subsequent maintenance in hospital. The same considerations apply to the giving of whole blood which will not be immediately available during the emergency.

Emergency Infusion

In the absence of whole blood the most suitable and readily available solution for intravenous infusion is Macrodex* 6 per cent solution of dextran. Until recently reconstituted dried human plasma was also acceptable, but while plasma is still valuable for specific conditions, e.g. extensive burns, its use as a general corrective for hypovolaemic shock carries disadvantages—its shelf life is comparatively short, reconstitution before use is less simple than starting with a fully prepared alternative, and its use is not devoid of the risk of transmitting infection. Gruber (1969) states that since the incidence of hepatitis after the administration of fresh plasma, stored pooled plasma or dried human plasma is about the same as after blood transfusions, these preparations should not be used for the treatment of shock.

Macrodex is widely used as a plasma volume expander throughout the world. In hypovolaemic shock it is greatly superior to electrolyte solutions and is comparable in its effects to blood or plasma. This preparation, also known as clinical dextran, dextran 70, or Swedish-American dextran, has an average molecular weight of 70,000 corresponding to that of albumen, and the makers state that it is narrowly and carefully fractionated in order to avoid the side effects of the large dextran molecules (Pharmacia A.B., 1968). Macrodex has a shelf life of five years, and has the advantages that it cannot convey infective hepatitis and does not interfere with subsequent blood typing or cross-matching. It is supplied for intravenous use in bottles of 500 ml. In the absence of blood, dextrans are not usually given in quantities exceeding 1,500 ml in the adult (Crocker, 1968).

* A proprietary preparation.

Adjuvants

Whilst there is a place for the infusion of sodium bicarbonate as a readily available and useful buffering agent for the correction of the acidosis resulting from reduced flow of blood or shock, especially if severe, this is properly within the purview of hospital treatment where the pH of arterial blood can be monitored.

Vasopressors should not be used. There is ample evidence that the prolonged use of vasoconstrictor agents in haemorrhagic shock is detrimental. Studies of metabolic effects of vasoconstrictors in hypovolaemia indicate that they do not improve tissue metabolism despite their ability to raise blood pressure to normotensive levels; indeed, the data suggest that after prolonged hypotension they intensify the defect in aerobic metabolism produced by hypovolaemia alone. In contrast, volume replacement with either blood or colloid solutions improves oxidative metabolism (Mills and Moyer, 1965). Weil and Shubin (1967b) state, "Sympathetico-mimetic vasoconstrictor drugs have little or no place in the management of shock due to haemorrhage."

Special Cases

The Crush Syndrome

Bywaters and Beall, who in 1941 described sixteen victims of this syndrome resulting from the aerial bombardment of London, called it 'the crush syndrome', although Bywaters later expressed a preference for the title 'ischaemic muscle necrosis'. Bywaters and McMichael (1953) found the necrosis of muscle was the common aetiological factor in all the cases described, with the development of acute cortical renal ischaemia and tubular blockage by myohaemoglobin.

Crush injury should always be suspected in a patient who has been crushed or trapped by a great weight for a considerable time, and certainly if for as long as one hour. This particularly applies if the part crushed is very muscular, for example the thigh or buttock. The outward signs of crush syndrome will appear on release, and include erythema, blisters, loss of sensation, paralysis or gross swelling of a part which may otherwise be uninjured. The damaged tissues will become swollen, tense and hard, and the distal pulses may disappear. Oligeamic shock will be present (A Field Surgery Pocket Book, 1962).

Bentley and Jeffries (1968a) describe three patients buried in a coal mine by a fall of rock. One of these cases died despite repeated dialysis and full supportive treatment. The other two cases recovered, one o whom also required dialysis. The authors state that this syndrome is likely to be seen in coal mining areas more often than elsewhere because of the peculiar hazards of this occupation, and cite five other cases recorded in coal miners. There is a correlation between the duration of crushing and the extent of renal damage.

In all cases in which crush syndrome is a possibility the hospital should be informed. Morphine should be given. Oral fluids unless contraindicated by vomiting or suspected abdominal injury may be given. Tourniquets or early amputation should not be employed as prophylactic measures against renal failure. Amputation cannot be justified except as the only means of freeing a trapped man (Bentley and Jeffries, 1968b). The crushed limb should be treated by elevation and cooling. On the question of giving oral sodium bicarbonate or intravenous infusion of sodium lactate whilst the patient with crush syndrome is still trapped, the same authors, Bentley and Jeffries (1968b), express the opinion that it is not justifiable to delay release of a trapped man in order to carry out possibly hazardous treatment of doubtful value.

The Patient on Steroids

There is no good indication for physiological doses of steroids in traumatic shock except in those who have Addison's disease or have recently received a prolonged course of steroid therapy (Blakemore and Fitts, 1969d). Occasionally, however, there will be cases where miners are employed whilst on continuous steroid therapy. Within the writer's recent experience there were ten such cases, seven working underground, in a small labour force of four thousand men.

The patient on steroids who becomes a casualty, and especially if subjected to the stress of being trapped with the probability of immediate amputation, is in added danger from suppression of the normal pituitary-adrenal response to stress. The suppressive effect of prolonged corticosteroid therapy on the hypothalamo-pituitary-adrenal axis has been well documented, and as pointed out by Mason (1969) a daily dose of 5 mg prednisone is not free from the danger of adrenal suppression; nor can it be assumed that smaller doses do not have the same effect. The duration of treatment, individual variation, and past dosage are all important, and, of course, suppression may occur long after the steroids have been withdrawn. Adrenals which are adequate ordinarily may be grossly inadequate in conditions of stress when the need for corticosteroids is sharply increased. There is also evidence that in patients with chronic asthma intermittent corticosteroid therapy is no more effective than continuous (daily) treatment in preserving the response of the hypothalamo-pituitary-adrenal axis to stress (Malone, Grant and Percy-Robb, 1970).

The symptoms of acute adrenal insufficiency are often sudden with rapid progression. They closely resemble those of severe shock, and may include nausea, vomiting, and abdominal pain, eventually terminating in coma and death. When faced with this suspected reaction in a patient known to be, or to have been, on maintenance steroid therapy an intramuscular injection of cortisone cover should be given without delay. In a discussion of surgical operation on those vulnerable to adrenal suppression Bayliss (1966) advocates intramuscular injection of 100–200 mg cortisone acetate on completion of the operation. The writer carries in his emergency equipment hydrocortisone sodium succinate (soluble) 100 mg with 2 ml of pyrogen-free sterile water for intramuscular injection.

Amputation

Immediate Amputation by Machinery

Contact with unguarded moving machinery is the commonest cause of immediate amputation or avulsion of a limb. Whilst such accidents are rare they do occur sometimes. The writer has seen the late result in a man who caught his hand in a conveyor belt and suffered a complete forequarter amputation, losing at once his whole right upper extremity including scapula and clavicle. In this type of emergency efficient and speedy management may be life saving. The principles of treatment will be control of haemorrhage, if necessary by packing, application of large wound dressings, and immediate evacuation from the mine, keeping the area of injury under continuous observation, and seeing that advance information reaches hospital.

The Trapped Man

The case for immediate surgical amputation will arise when the casualty is found to be in such a critical situation that he is held fast by a grossly damaged limb and his liberation, and almost certainly survival, are dependent upon his being cut free without delay. Examples are:

  (i) A man pinned by an extremity caught by an extensive fall of roof, or by moving machinery, or equipment.

  (ii) Upper or lower extremity partially amputated and firmly held in cutting machinery, haulage gear, or a wire rope.

It is just conceivable that in exceptionally favourable circumstances, as when the accident has occurred at a mine close to a large hospital, the problem of freeing a trapped man could be left to a mobile surgical team. It is, however, essential to remember that the alerting of a hospital team which includes anaesthetist and surgeon, with all equipment, must necessarily take time, requiring detachment from immediate duties, mobilization, and travel.

It is therefore assumed that the situation is demonstrably so urgent that the burdens of decision and action have to be borne by a single medical officer—the man on the spot—whether the emergency has occurred on the surface or underground.

Ethics of Amputation

Gordon-Taylor (1942) in his ten commandments for amputation puts the need for a second opinion as the first commandment. In referring to amputation in bone and joint injuries Watson-Jones (1941) says, "The decision to adopt this unusual and drastic measure should always be supported by a second opinion."

In the mine a second medical opinion will not be available, nor will it be necessary to obtain it, since the decision to amputate will not be based so much on pathology as on the extreme urgency and physical difficulties of a particular situation. Here the choice is between cutting the casualty free or seeing him die, still trapped, while awaiting help. The doctor would be well-advised to have the opinion of a mining engineer or of an experienced miner, that the magnitude of the mechanical problem is such that amputation is imperative. In practice no difficulty on this score is to be expected; there will have been time before the doctor's arrival to study the situation and to attempt to release the patient with all the engineering resources available.

Aims

The aims of the doctor are twofold, and must not be lost sight of at any time. They are:

(i) Free the patient with the utmost speed compatible with the control of pain.

(ii) Get the patient to hospital at the earliest moment possible.

Any procedure that is given priority over the above objectives, and especially anything deliberate that delays them, will have to be weighed against the paramount claim of speed in amputation and evacuation.

Control of Pain: the Conscious Patient

Anaesthesia in the underground workings of a mine is beset with certain problems. Explosive anaesthetic agents may be ruled out, and in the situation we visualize—a trapped patient in severe shock—nitrous oxide or intravenous anaesthesia are contraindicated.

It is assumed that the casualty will have received already a pain-killing drug such as morphine 16 mg, or omnopon* 30 mg. The method of controlling pain here recommended is based on a combination of trilene inhalation analgesia together with skin and deep tissue infiltration with 0·25 per cent lignocaine (lindocaine*: xylocaine*) with adrenaline 1 in 500,000. The maximum dose of lignocaine in the strength advised is 200 ml.

The use of analgesic trilene* (trichloroethylene) 0·3 to 0·5 per cent air mixtures from draw-over apparatus to supplement local anaesthesia is of great value (Boulton, 1966; Boulton, 1967a).

The acutely injured patient bordering on shock, or who has been in and out of shock, will require less anaesthesia, no matter what agent is

* A proprietary preparation.

19

used. Shock itself decreases cerebral function and lowers the pain threshold. Experimental work has shown that the symptomatology of shock is closely related to the adequacy of cerebral blood flow. When this flow is critically reduced, the symptoms of shock appear, and thus the presence of shock indicates cerebral anoxia and depression (Blakemore and Fitts, 1969e).

Every situation will have to be judged on its merits, speed always claiming priority. If it is feasible, the proposed line of section (as close to the source of trauma as possible) should be cleaned up with cetrimide; the operator should then infiltrate the skin with lignocaine using the 20 gauge 25 mm (1 in.) long or similar needle, completing the encirclement of the limb as far as conditions will allow. Next proceed to infiltration of deeper tissue using a 76 mm (3 in.) long 20 gauge needle; the object is to infiltrate as much deep tissue as possible including compressed tissue distal to the bone to be sectioned. The advice of Boulton (1967b) should be remembered, "Provided the needle point is kept moving intravascular injection of any quantity of solution is unlikely."

When the deep-tissue infiltration has been completed the operator must fill the trilene apparatus and start the administration of trilene; depending on the type of apparatus in use the two strengths offered are either 'weak' and 'strong' or 'minimum' and 'maximum'. Start with the stronger. The trapped man may be expected to welcome the analgesic inhalation as an escape from pain. The doctor must appoint a reliable assistant, preferably with a knowledge of first aid, ready to take his place as trilene administrator, while he himself proceeds to the amputation. The assistant should be instructed how to place the head and jaw so as to maintain an open airway while he continues trilene analgesia, keeping a careful watch on respiration throughout.

Equipment

Emergency amputation equipment should include a fairly elaborate collection of instruments and other surgical requirements held in a state of readiness at one or more central points, or of a more modest outfit carried by an individual medical officer, or both. In practice it will be found that requirements will be met by equipment for trilene analgesia and lignocaine infiltration, together with sterilized amputation knife, saw, osteotome and mallet, bone-cutting forceps, surgical scissors, artery forceps, ligatures and dressings.

Practical Difficulties

Much time may have elapsed between the accident and the doctor's arrival. This will be reflected in the patient's condition. Bear in mind the possibility of crush injury as a complication. Haste is all-important, and there will be neither time nor place for the niceties of surgical technique.

Washing-up and skin preparation are neither desirable nor possible. The field of operation will be extensively contaminated. Under the circumstances the best efforts might reduce this by a negligible margin and valuable time would be lost in a futile exercise. It may be necessary to remove clothing, and the skin will have to be cleaned sufficiently to enable the extent of the injuries and the point of section to be seen. For this a small bottle of 1 per cent cetrimide is suitable.

Space for manoeuvre is likely to vary from the difficult to the almost impossible. In view of the time factor alluded to above, it is to be expected that in some cases at least space for action will have been cleared by the time the doctor has arrived.

Technique of Amputation
  (i) If the casualty is conscious obtain his consent to operation.
 (ii) Use a tourniquet. It is realized that in severe shock there will be little or no bleeding, but a tourniquet is a necessity.
(iii) Be quick.
 (iv) Use the long knife.
  (v) The amputation must be as low as possible. The sole aim is to complete a traumatic amputation; therefore keep as close to the source of trauma as possible.
 (vi) If the bone has already been severely damaged or partially broken close to the site of the original trauma, time will be saved by completing the section at that point. If sectioned bone is not available it will be necessary to saw, or use the osteotome or bone-cutting forceps. The latter would be suitable for forearm, hand, or fingers, tarsus and metatarsus, and the osteotome could be useful for larger bones, particularly where there is insufficient room to use the saw. In many cases the division of tendons and skin remnants will be all that is required.
(vii) Secure vessels by artery forceps, which may be left *in situ*. Sutures are provided in all emergency outfits. Unless transport out of the mine is delayed they will not be required. Only if time permits should vessels be tied off and artery forceps be removed.
(viii) Make no attempt to suture the skin. Cover the wound with sterile dressings and towels, and ample cotton wool padding and bandages.
 (ix) When the patient has been freed, the next procedure will depend on the time it will take to get him to hospital. If this will be within twenty minutes leave the exposed and visible tourniquet on and unloosened. In the more likely event of an expected long journey to the mineshaft loosen the tourniquet and check the stump for haemorrhage. If dry, leave the thoroughly loosened tourniquet

in position. The operator must ensure that his assistant is made responsible for *continuous* observation of the stump, making certain throughout that haemorrhage is arrested.

(x) Before leaving the site of operation make arrangements for later recovery and safe-keeping of the amputated part. (The grounds for amputation are most unlikely to be challenged, but the production of a non-viable limb would be conclusive.)

(xi) Accompany the patient to hospital: pay special regard to the overall protection and observation of the field of operation and to intravenous medication if in use.

After-treatment

After the wound has been dressed and the operation zone has been placed in the charge of the assistant the doctor must see to the patient as a whole. The casualty has had a severe operation without preparation, and if conscious, will have had no premedication except an intramuscular injection of omnopon (or morphine). Make sure the airway is unobstructed and that breathing is satisfactory. It has been established that the Trendelenburg, or head-down, position is deleterious to a patient in shock. Vital capacity is reduced by fifteen to twenty per cent. The flow of blood to the brain is not improved, and the carotid sinuses may misinterpret the position as an increase in pressure and may reduce the degree of vasoconstriction. Elevating the legs alone will empty the lower extremities of blood pooled in the veins and will be equivalent to a small transfusion. This may be helpful (Blakemore and Fitts, 1969d).

See that the patient is sufficiently covered with dry blankets, leaving the dressings covering the stump (and the loosened tourniquet) exposed to full view, and under observation.

Resuscitation

At this stage the main problem in a deeply shocked, and seriously exsanguinated patient, is to maintain his circulation, and thus to combat hypovolaemic shock. While massive quantities of blood are likely to be required, this is properly a task for hospital staff under suitable conditions.

Unless conditions are altogether exceptional a rapid start must now be made with an intravenous infusion to combat hypovolaemic shock, using Macrodex.

For expanding plasma volume Macrodex 6 per cent in normal saline is advised. The intravenous infusion rate is determined by the patient's general condition. In severe shock it should at first be allowed to run in freely, being reduced subsequently as the pulse rate falls and the blood pressure rises. Under the conditions postulated the dose of Macrodex could be between 500 to 1,500 ml.

If attempts to enter a vein with a sharp intravenous needle or cannula are unsuccessful it will be necessary to cut down over a suitable vein (the basic requirements, in addition to those for local anaesthesia, being a scalpel, a 12·5 cm (5 in.) artery forceps, a toothed dissecting forceps, an aneurysm needle, catgut, sharp-pointed scissors and a blunt-ended cannula). In dire emergency the vein which can be entered is the best vein. If entry into antecubital veins is not successful, dorsal veins of the hand, the great saphenous anterior to the internal malleolus, or larger veins may be used, not excluding the possibility of using a large vein in the stump. (In the latter case the tourniquet will, of course, be fully released, and left loosely round the limb in case of stump haemorrhage, in which event the infusion must be stopped and the tourniquet retightened immediately.)

In the evacuation of the patient medical supervision should include particular attention to an unimpeded airway, control of haemorrhage and meticulous supervision of the intravenous infusion bottle and tubing: care will be necessary in controlling the rate of flow, especially with the first and fast-running bottle, when it will be vital to make sure that the tube is clipped in good time before the change of bottles.

Speed in execution and speed in transport must always take priority, and those in charge must never lose sight of the fact that the sooner the patient is in specialist hands in hospital the better his chances of survival will be.

References

A Field Surgery Pocket Book (1962), pp. F1 and F2. H.M.S.O., London.

Bayliss, R. I. S. (1966), In *Price's Textbook of the Practice of Medicine* (10th edition): *The adrenal glands*, p. 439. The Oxford University Press, London, New York, Bombay.

Bentley, G. and Jeffries, T. E. (1968a), "The crush syndrome in coal miners." *Journal of Bone and Joint Surgery*, Vol. 50-B, 588.

Bentley, G. and Jeffries, T. E. (1968b), "The crush syndrome in coal miners." *Journal of Bone and Joint Surgery*, Vol. 50-B, 592.

Blakemore, W. S. and Fitts, W. T. Jnr. (1969a), *Management of the Injured Patient*, p. 314. Harper and Row, New York, Evanston and London.

Blakemore, W. S. and Fitts, W. T. Jnr. (1969b), *Management of the Injured Patient*, p. 305. Harper and Row, New York, Evanston and London.

Blakemore, W. S. and Fitts, W. T. Jnr. (1969c), *Management of the Injured Patient*, p. 307. Harper and Row, New York, Evanston and London.

Blakemore, W. S. and Fitts, W. T. Jnr. (1969d), *Management of the Injured Patient*, p. 313. Harper and Row, New York, Evanston and London.

Blakemore, W. S. and Fitts, W. T. Jnr. (1969e), *Management of the Injured Patient*, p. 326. Harper and Row, New York, Evanston and London.

Boulton, T. B. (1966), "Anaesthesia in difficult situations." *Anaesthesia*, **21,** 513.

Boulton, T. B. (1967a), "Anaesthesia in difficult situations: The use of local analgesia." *Anaesthesia*, **22,** 104.

Boulton, T. B. (1967b), *Anaesthesia*, **22,** 115.

Bywaters, E. G. C. and McMichael, J. (1953), *Crush Syndrome in the History of the Second World War: Surgery*, p. 73. H.M.S.O., London.

Crocker, M. C. (1968), "Fluids for emergency conditions: (A review with special reference to disaster situations)." *Anaesthesia*, **23**, 421.

Gordon-Taylor, G. (1942), "On amputation: ten commandments." *Lancet*, **1**, 669.

Gruber, U. F. (1969), "Volume expansion and flow promotion in shock." *Postgraduate Medical Journal*, **45**, No. 526, 534.

Malone, D. N. S., Grant, I. W. B., Percy-Robb, I. W. (1970), "Hypothalamo-pituitary-adrenal function in asthmatic patients receiving long-term corticosteroid therapy." *Lancet*, **2**, 733.

Mason, R. M. (1969), "Chronic rheumatic diseases." *The Medical Annual*, p. 439. John Wright and Sons, Bristol.

McGowan, G. K. and Walters, G. (1966), "A clinical study of surgical shock." *Lancet*, **I**, 611.

Mills, L. C. and Moyer, J. H. (1965), *Shock and Hypotension, Pathogenesis and Treatment: The Use of Vasopressors in Haemorrhagic Shock*, p. 403. Grune and Stratton, New York and London.

Pharmacia AB, Uppsala, Sweden (1968), *Blood Flow Improvement*, pp. X and XI.

Walters, G. (1969), "Factors in the assessment of clinical shock." *Postgraduate Medical Journal*, **45**, 497.

Watson-Jones, R. (1941), *Fractures and other Bone and Joint Injuries* (2nd edition), p. 160. E. & S. Livingstone, Edinburgh.

Weil, M. H. and Shubin, H. (1967a), *The Diagnosis and Treatment of Shock*, p. 118. The Williams and Wilkins Company, Baltimore.

Weil, M. H. and Shubin, H. (1967b), *The Diagnosis and Treatment of Shock*, p. 125. The Williams and Wilkins Company, Baltimore.

Chapter 18

Medical Aspects of Mines Rescue

Whenever there is an explosion, a fire, or a heating at a mine an atmosphere may be produced containing poisonous gases or lacking sufficient oxygen to sustain life. An emergency service is, therefore, necessary which will provide men trained in the use of self-contained breathing apparatus. Such an organization is usually referred to as a mines rescue service.

The title can perhaps be misleading, conjuring up a picture of rescue workers saving trapped or asphyxiated miners. Although their work will occasionally include such dramatic events, most of their time will be spent in controlling underground fires. A rescue service has many similarities to a fire brigade; most of the differences are due to the special ways of dealing with fires underground.

Rescue Apparatus

The first practical self-contained breathing apparatus was produced by Henry A. Fleuss in 1878. It was used successfully at the Seaham Colliery fire in England in 1880–1881. There was little interest in the subject for the next 20 years. The Draeger apparatus was introduced in Germany in 1903. The Pneumatogen apparatus which supplied oxygen by chemical means was developed in 1904 in Austria. In 1906 the first liquid air apparatus, the Aerolith, was also produced in Austria. French scientists designed the Tissot apparatus in 1907 (McAdam and Davidson, 1947).

A closed-circuit self-contained breathing apparatus (see Chapter 19) works on a few simple principles. Sufficient oxygen is carried by the wearer to enable him to do hard work for about two hours. Any oxygen not used by the wearer is re-circulated in the apparatus and re-breathed; the carbon dioxide breathed out is absorbed by passing the exhaled air through caustic soda or soda lime granules (Davis, 1947). The re-circulation is essential; the actual use of oxygen by the body when working hard rises to about two litres per minute. Over 300 litres, enough to last for well over two hours, can be provided in a cylinder weighing 4·5 kg (10 lb). If the inhaled oxygen were not re-circulated but was discharged to atmosphere 10 or 20 times as much would be needed.

Most apparatus in present use depends on either compressed oxygen or liquid oxygen. Liquid oxygen has the advantage that the inhaled air from the apparatus is cool for a longer period; its disadvantage is that once the apparatus is charged the oxygen will boil off continuously and it cannot, therefore, be used for intermittent spells of work; the compressed oxygen apparatus can be turned on and off as required. A rescue apparatus is heavy; a modern liquid oxygen apparatus fully charged and ready for use weighs about 14 kg (31 lb) and a compressed oxygen apparatus 17 kg (37 lb). In addition, working in rescue apparatus is much more strenuous than merely working with this weight around the shoulders; a compressed oxygen apparatus is much easier to work in when uncoupled than when coupled up.

Under certain conditions pure oxygen can be harmful. Breathed for more than six hours continuously it can give rise to retro-sternal discomfort and may damage the pulmonary epithelium—the so-called Lorrain-Smith effect. This hazard is unimportant when healthy men are using oxygen for a maximum of two hours (Standing Medical Advisory Committee, 1969). In very rare cases a potential danger will arise if rescue men wear self-contained apparatus to reach trapped miners through a flooded roadway which requires them to travel under water at any depth. Oxygen poisoning due to increase in pressure will certainly occur at depths of water greater than 10 m (33 ft) unless appropriate dilution of the oxygen with nitrogen or helium has been carried out. The use of oxygen carries with it a much increased risk of fire.

Work of the Rescue Man

Underground fires at mines are not common enough to justify the retention of large numbers of full-time rescue workers. On the other hand when an incident does occur teams are likely to be required continuously and 500 individual attendances by rescue men would not be an unusual figure for a fire lasting three days; a large proportion of the actual work will, therefore, be carried out by part-time men.

The general pattern of organization usually consists of central rescue stations situated within half an hour's travelling time of the mines they serve. Where the demand justifies it these stations will have enough permanent staff to provide a first team to go underground at any time. Where mines are sparse the rescue station will have only enough permanent men to carry out instruction and conduct rescue practices. Isolated mines will not be covered for first call by any rescue station and should possess a special rescue room with apparatus of their own. In all cases the main burden of rescue work will fall on mineworkers who are also part-time rescue men. This has represented a considerable advantage from the medical point of view; the work of the miner has been so arduous that it has acted as an automatic check that the man doing it is fit and in training. The amount of heavy, physical work is generally tending to decrease; where this change is occurring there is an increasing need for a form of medical examination which ensures that the miner is fit to undergo severe physical stress.

It takes time to become habituated to rescue apparatus and after training regular realistic practices are necessary. These consist of work at the rescue station in life-like conditions of heat and smoke, underground practices at mines working in apparatus and sessions in a special chamber in hot and humid conditions.

The most common cause of mine fires is spontaneous combustion. In the coal mining industry some seams readily absorb oxygen and then heat up to the point of self-ignition; when these seams are worked constant vigilance is required to detect heatings or fires in their early stages. Electrical equipment underground is now the second greatest fire risk. Until recent times belt conveyors were made of inflammable material and were common sources of fires, usually due to friction. Other dangers are naked lights, friction fires in haulage systems, air compressors and shotfiring. Whatever the cause of the fire the result will be that the roadways will be contaminated with the toxic products of combustion, particularly carbon monoxide. These will not be significantly diluted until they find their way to the upcast shaft. It is, of course, this lack of dilution of its gaseous products which produces the peculiar hazard of an underground fire.

The restriction of ventilation presents the main danger of underground fires; it also indicates the way in which they can be extinguished. Although fire extinguishers and water are used whenever practicable, the commonest defence is the building of "stoppings" to seal off all possible supplies of the air required to support combustion. Temporary stoppings can be erected where there is no danger from gas explosions and where the function of the stopping is solely to prevent the inflow of oxygen to the fire. Often, however, methane will be present; once stoppings are complete this will build up behind them in the fire zone with the chance that it may reach explosive levels. Explosive-proof stoppings must therefore be constructed if inflammable gas is present and there is any possibility of a methane explosion. Such stoppings require a considerable amount of material; a single stopping constructed of sand bags will commonly contain from 50 to 100 tons.

A rescue man will usually be working in heavy and cumbersome apparatus, often in smoke and heat. His tasks would be heavy, even in good conditions and without apparatus. If he becomes exhausted there is a danger that he will fail to breathe entirely through his mouthpiece and will in consequence inhale carbon monoxide. Should he then become a casualty the other team members will have the added task of getting him back to the fresh air base. It is thus essential that he should be not only in good health but in a state of fitness in which he can withstand severe physical stress.

Annual Medical Examination

The initial and annual medical examinations of rescue men require the use of equipment that is not easily portable; ready access is also necessary to the man's previous medical records. They can usually be conveniently combined with one of the practices at the rescue station.

The age limits for rescue men should be 20 to 45 years. A retirement age based on annual assessment of physical fitness causes many difficulties and a fixed age is preferable.

Very small men are not usually suitable for rescue work. The weight to be carried, the speed of travel and the work to be done cannot be varied to any extent and leave the small man at a disadvantage. Any man whose stripped weight is less than 64 kg (140 lb) should not be passed at medical examination or, if this is considered too drastic, such a man should be watched carefully during his initial training to ensure that he is fully able to keep up with his fellows. Very large men are also unfitted for the work; they have difficulty in working in confined surroundings, and in crawling through access tubes. It is uncommon for a man whose stripped weight is 96 kg (210 lb) or more to be suitable for training as a rescue man.

Obviously a new entrant should not be suffering from any material disability. His height/weight/age ratio should be within normal limits, with a chest expansion proportionate to build. There should be good muscular power and development, with good abdominal tone in relaxation. All bones and joints should be normal, with full and thorough range of movement. He should be able to undergo rough travelling and have sufficient reserve left to engage in heavy work at the end of it; able to run, climb up steep hills or ladders, crouch low, crawl, squat comfortably and rise quickly; able to handle tools and do heavy work such as digging, pulling, dragging, heavy lifting and climbing. He requires good average intelligence and it is most important that he should possess a stable personality. The rescue service is no place for a man who is joining to prove his virility.

Pulmonary Function Test

An important part of the annual examination is the regular use of a pulmonary function test; the test requires to be quick and simple, and to give a record which can be compared with results from previous years. The most useful apparatus for this purpose has been found to be the self-recording dry spirometer. A routine trace calls for a minimum of instruction to the patient and gives a permanent record of pulmonary function. From this the Forced Vital Capacity (F.V.C.) and the Forced Expiratory Volume after one second (F.E.V.$_{1.0}$) are immediately available; other measurements such as the F.E.V. for shorter periods than one second, the Maximum Voluntary Ventilation and the percentage forced expiratory volume (see Chapter 5) are all easily made if considered necessary. Particular interest will attach to any change in the F.E.V.$_{1.0}$ and in the forced vital capacity from one annual examination to the next. The ability to examine a series of annual spirometer recordings provides valuable and perhaps essential checks on the findings elicited by history taking and clinical examination.

Exercise Tolerance Test

When a rescue worker receives his annual medical examination it is not sufficient for the doctor merely to look for and note an absence of any pathological condition. None of the ordinary tests carried out by the doctor at a routine medical examination will show how fit a man is to undergo severe exertion.

The commonly used methods for estimating physical fitness in a person who is already known to be free from disease are the static cycle (ergometer), the tread mill, and one of the step tests. There are other more accurate measurements but these are expensive and require specialist knowledge to apply. There appears no reason to think that either the static cycle or the tread mill have any particular advantages over the step tests. The best known step tests are the Harvard Pack Test and the Harvard Step Test. The results of the two tests correlate reasonably well, but the Harvard Step Test relies to a very large extent on the quadriceps, whereas the Pack Test requires the use of most of the large body muscles. In this test a man carries one third of his own weight on his back and, with the aid of handrails, steps up and down from a step 40 cm (16 in) high 30 times a minute for 5 minutes. The pulse is recorded at intervals 3 times in the 5 minutes after the exercise has been completed. The pulse rate during this time follows an exponential curve; the 3 pulse rates provide 3 points on the curve and are sufficient to indicate its shape. This can be expressed as a fitness index. The index reflects fairly accurately the degree of physical fitness of the subject; when a man obtains particularly high figures it is often found that he is in training for some sport such as cycle racing or Rugby football.

Once an exercise tolerance test of this type has been instituted it gives the rescue man and the rescue station superintendent, as well as the doctor, confidence in the fitness of the man to work in the exacting conditions which will sometimes occur. Full-time rescue men are not usually doing as much heavy physical work as they were when working in the mine and are likely to get slightly out of condition. The Harvard Pack Test acts as a check to ensure that they get the exercise they need. Part-time men who have changed during the year to a less arduous job and have then put on weight are sometimes in a similar position. A full description of the Harvard Pack Test is given as an appendix to this chapter.

Electrocardiography

The question arises whether the comprehensive examination proposed above should include an electrocardiogram. It has been suggested that this would be helpful in weeding out those men liable to suffer from angina pectoris or coronary thrombosis. The difficulties of introducing electrocardiography as a routine would be considerable, but the main objection is that the test would not serve the purpose for which it had been introduced. The electrocardiogram might appear quite normal and yet the subject could have a severe coronary thrombosis a week later. On the other hand, a number of electrocardiograms would be equivocal in character and the doctor would probably wish to play safe and exclude the men with these tracings from rescue duties. No man who has what he regards as a special diagnostic test and is thereafter rejected for rescue work is going to be unconcerned or to believe that the result was merely doubtful; a number will develop a cardiac neurosis. It seems fairly certain that this approach would do more harm than good. The best solution at present is for the doctor to be on the look out for a history or symptoms of anginal pain, particularly in the over 40's.

Practices in Hot and Humid Conditions

When a man is working in self-contained rescue equipment he is particularly vulnerable to the effects of hot and humid conditions. A man without an apparatus breathes out saturated air at body temperature and breathes in what is usually cooler, dryer air. The situation is quite different in apparatus; the circulating air is being heated by the chemical action which takes place as the carbon dioxide is absorbed by the soda lime. The air being breathed in is, therefore, hotter than that being breathed out; it is also fully saturated; instead of breathing being one of the ways of dispersing heat it generates heat. Compressed air apparatus has a small cooler which modifies the situation a little—the liquid oxygen apparatus has the advantage that the incoming oxygen is cooler. In both cases, however, the fact remains that the apparatus itself increases the heat which the body must dissipate by sweating.

A miner in hot conditions will work stripped to the waist and cool himself by sweating. Rescue apparatus will often envelop its wearer to such an extent that he has difficulty in losing heat in this way. He is probably doing fairly hard work in addition to carrying his apparatus; the result will be that even in moderate temperatures he is liable to sweat profusely. If in addition he is now asked to work in hot and humid conditions with little or no ventilation heat exhaustion becomes a real danger.

It is clear that as the heat and humidity of the working conditions increase the stage will be reached when the rescue man can no longer be expected to work for the 120 minutes that his apparatus will last. Lind (1955) and Lind, Hellon, Weiner and Jones (1955) therefore carried out research to establish how long men could continue rescue operations in given environmental conditions before reaching a stage when they were in danger of heat exhaustion. Previous experiments showed that when the rectal temperature reached 38·8°C (101·8°F) this was close to the end of a man's endurance. Rescue men, therefore worked under observation in a controlled hot chamber until they felt compelled to give up or until their rectal temperature reached this figure.

Results were obtained for saturated environments for both compressed oxygen and liquid oxygen rescue apparatus. These were expanded so that they applied in addition to non-saturated environments. Details are given in Fig. 4, Chapter 19.

There is considerable individual variation in the response to heat. Improved physical fitness in any one individual will increase that individual's ability to work in hot environments but fitness by itself does not confer heat tolerance. Lind was, therefore, forced to add a more or less arbitrary safety factor to his findings so that the figures shown could be considered as applying to virtually all rescue men.

Men who are to work in hot and humid conditions need to experience them during training. It is common, therefore, for rescue stations to be equipped with a hot chamber where the temperature and humidity can be controlled within narrow limits. Regular practices are carried out by rescue men in the chamber; such practices will habituate men to the effects of heat, they will learn the warning signs that they are pushing themselves too hard and accustom themselves to working at a more suitable rate. This should not be confused with acclimatization which would only take place after many hours of practice under hot conditions and would quickly wear off.

Practices such as these in a chamber under supervision in controlled conditions and with only a door separating the man from cool air are very different from the circumstances envisaged by Lind when setting his limits. Somewhat higher figures for heat and humidity can thus be allowed for practice than would be acceptable in actual underground work.

Medical Supervision at an Incident

Before starting the medical examination of rescue workers at an incident the doctor should find out the conditions in which they are likely to have to work. These will naturally vary considerably. In some cases the work may be easy with very little danger from carbon monoxide poisoning; in others the work may involve severe stress, considerable heat, and exposure to smoke.

Although the majority of men examined will be considered either as fit or unfit, there will be the occasional marginal case with, for example, a slight sore throat, a cold in the head or slight irritation of the eyes, where it may be considered reasonable for the man to carry out his spell of duty if conditions are good, whereas he will be found unfit if he is likely to have to undergo severe stress. Where the carbon monoxide is in concentrations which are potentially lethal, precautions should be stricter and the man declared temporarily unfit if there is the slightest doubt concerning his condition.

It should be possible to find out from the official in charge of the emergency:—

(1) The distance from the shaft bottom to the fresh air base and the extent to which rescue men will have to carry their own apparatus.
(2) The distance from the fresh air base to the actual place of work.
(3) The degree of difficulty of travel between the place of work and the fresh air base.
(4) The type of work the rescue men are likely to have to perform, particularly whether this is light or heavy.
(5) The likely dry bulb and wet bulb temperatures at the place of work.
(6) The degree to which hazard from smoke is likely.
(7) The carbon monoxide content of the air.

It is useful if details of the annual medical examinations and of the fitness index reached in the exercise tolerance test are available.

Each member of the rescue team should be seen individually and out of earshot of his fellow members. The captain should be seen first; he should be asked whether he has doubts about the fitness of any of his team. Where it appears that the information obtained about underground conditions would be helpful to the captain, it should be given to him. This is particularly likely to apply to the carbon monoxide concentration. It will be appreciated that under the stress of hard work the rescue man may inadvertently leak air around his mouth-piece, and if the carbon monoxide concentration is high the captain should impress upon his team the need to take even more than their usual care to avoid this.

At this first examination a history should be taken of any illness or accident since the last annual examination. The rescue man should be asked if he has been off work for any reason at all during the last month, and if so the cause should be ascertained. It should be discovered by direct questioning whether he is suffering from any acute condition of his respiratory tract, any bowel disorder, or any boils or minor complaints. If his apparatus has a mouthpiece rather than an ori-nasal mask he must have an efficient 'bite' to hold his mouth-piece in place and this may be temporarily inadequate if he has recently had teeth extracted.

Miners summoned to rescue work will come from various shifts and a rescue man may be lacking in sleep. This should be treated seriously. Lack of sleep will cause a loss of alertness which could endanger the man's life. He should be asked how many hours of sleep he has had during the last twenty-four and it should be noted whether he is suffering from any undue signs of anxiety or fatigue.

The importance of the actual clinical examination at the time of the incident should not be over-estimated. A full history, particularly of any event since the last annual examination, and a careful check to exclude any recent illness or injury are more important at this stage than the search for symptomless pathology.

Subsequent Examinations at the Incident

After the man's first underground visit he will be much more ready to tell the doctor about any minor illness or anxiety. It occasionally happens that rescue teams are wanted in quick succession, and do not have enough rest between spells of duty. In all cases, therefore, it is necessary to establish the number of hours since completion of the last underground visit and the total length of time spent underground on the last visit.

When teams return to the surface they should again be seen but it is unnecessary to interview each man separately. Meeting the teams will give the doctor a relatively up-to-date picture of the severity of the work, the heat, humidity, the degree of smoke and other material factors.

Roster of Doctors

When a disaster occurs at a mine all available help is required immediately. This may also apply in rescue work where large numbers of men are endangered by an incident or an explosion has led to a number of casualties; usually, however, it takes several days to deal with fires or heatings and arrangements for medical cover must be made accordingly.

There should be a doctor in attendance whenever men are working in rescue apparatus. This means a roster of doctors attending round the clock. Where the available doctors are plentiful a convenient roster is—

08.00 hrs to 14.00 hrs
14.00 hrs to 22.00 hrs
22.00 hrs to 08.00 hrs

This can mean that a doctor need lose only about half a day from his other work where this is pressing. With, say, 10 doctors such a roster can be continued for the length of nearly any fire without too much strain on medical resources. Where doctors are few, 12 hour shifts may have to be undertaken; the strain and the dislocation of other work is, however, out of all proportion to the extra hours worked.

Rarely an attempt to evacuate men from the vicinity of a fire will have been unsuccessful and some may be thought to be still alive; a doctor will then be required at the fresh air base. In such a case a fresh doctor should arrive at the mine every 4 hours. Each doctor can then spend half a shift examining rescue men on the surface and the second half on duty underground.

It would be wrong to give the impression that the doctor's work at an incident is confined to the examination of rescue men. Casualties may require treatment and close touch should be maintained with those in operational control so that he remains fully informed about the underground situation. Visits to the rescue room will reveal the problems that are being met by the rescue teams. In addition it should be remembered that teams waiting to go underground need proper facilities for food, rest and quiet recreation; any deficiency in these should be promptly drawn to the attention of the controller of the incident by the doctor.

Appendix

Harvard Pack Test

The principles of the Harvard Pack Test were laid down in a paper by Johnson, Brouha and Darling (1942) working at Harvard University. The object was to find a rapid simple test of fitness for strenuous exertion. Briefly, the principles on which the test was based were as follows:—

(1) The amount of work involved in the test should give a good "spread" of results, differentiating clearly between those in a good and poor state of physical fitness. It was found that a comparatively easy task will not carry out such a differentiation. A standard exercise that exhausts most, but not all subjects, within 5 minutes gives a much wider spread of measurements.

(2) The pulse rate during recovery from severe exercise follows an exponential curve. It is not, however, necessary to draw this curve as its shape can be gauged accurately enough for practical purposes from three pulse readings, which in turn can easily be translated into a Fitness Index by calculation from a formula or with the aid of a simple table (*vide infra*). The shape of the curve (as shown by the Fitness Index) is a reasonably sensitive measurement of the degree to which a clinically fit person is "in training". This, therefore, avoids the difficulties of having to take a resting pulse before commencing the test with all the errors inherent in such a reading.

(3) Johnson *et al.* did not settle on an exact task but the conditions of exercise laid down by them were:—

(*a*) It must put the cardiovascular system under considerable stress by involving large muscle groups.

(*b*) It must be of such intensity that about a third of all subjects stop from exhaustion within five minutes.

(*c*) It must not demand any unusual type of skill for its successful performance.

(4) Most of their experiments at this time were performed by the subject pulling a "stone boat" loaded so that the subject pulled horizontally a third of his body weight over a flat smooth course at a speed of 1 yard per second for 5 minutes or until he was exhausted.

The accepted Harvard Pack Test developed from these principles and details are as follows.

Equipment

Weighing machine

Stopwatch

A belt made with shoulder straps and containing pockets in which weights can be placed.

Strong box, 40 cm high for stepping, placed with stepping edge 35 cm in front of balancing handles 50 cm long and 50 cm apart, fixed to the wall with their middle about 150 cm above the ground.

Small bags of sand or lead slabs, weighing 2 kg, to add to the load.

Metronome.

Procedure

1. Weigh the subject. Estimate his weight stripped. Explain the nature of the test to the man and tell him that failure to complete it will not necessarily mean that he will cease to be able to be a rescue man.

2. Load up the belt with shoulder straps so that the total added weight is a third of the body weight, correct to 2 kg. The subject then grasps the balancing handles at shoulder height.

3. On the word 'Go' start the stopwatch and the exercise. The subject places one foot on the box, brings up the other foot, *straightens up*, replaces the first foot on the floor, then the other, a natural walking movement. The whole movement must take two seconds only, i.e. he mounts the box 30 times per minute. The time should be taken from the metronome. Continue the exercise for 5 minutes. He should lead off with the same foot each time and not try to alternate. However, one or two changes of leading foot in the course of the test are immaterial.

4. If this is the subject's first attempt at the Pack Test he should be given a very short practice. During this practice he can learn to change

the foot with which he leads without breaking the rhythm of his exercise. It can, at the same time, be explained that he must only do this occasionally.

5. It is in order to let the candidate know at intervals how long he has been exercising so far. Stop the exercise after 5 minutes. At once undo the weighted belt and seat the subject in a comfortable chair.

6. Count the pulse beats, in each of the three intervals—1–1·5, 2–2·5, 4–4·5 minutes after stopping the exercise, i.e. at 6, 7 and 9 minutes on the watch, start the half minute counts.

7. Calculate the 'Fitness Index' according to the formula—

$$\text{F.I.} = \frac{\text{Duration of exercise in seconds}}{2 \times \text{sum of the three counts}} \times 100$$

The calculations given above are simple but somewhat laborious and they can be avoided by using the fitness index table given below.

8. The rescue man should obtain a minimum figure of 75 as his fitness index in this test at his annual examination. If his figure is below this he should exercise to increase his physical fitness so that he can make a further attempt at a later date. In a clinically fit man more physical exercise and a reduction in smoking will improve the fitness index in a comparatively short time.

Notes

The test should be performed *after* the clinical examination when the doctor is convinced of the absence of clinical abnormality and, there-fore, of the man's fitness to attempt it. The doctor should be available during the test although his presence in the same room is not necessary. Very occasionally a man will faint at the end of the test, or even during it.

The height of the box should be constant at 40 cm. In theory this handicaps the short man but in practice this is not found to be im-portant. Varying the height of the box complicates the test and intro-duces an unnecessary source of error.

It is important that the man must raise himself the full 40 cm every time and that the knees and back must be straightened when the man is on the box. It is worth while emphasizing this in the short practice for men who are new to the test.

The Harvard Pack Test is simply a test of physical fitness. The rescue worker will simulate rescue work during all the rest of his training. There is no necessity to modify the test so that it, too, will simulate the work he is to do, e.g. by wearing apparatus during it.

The temperature of surroundings when the test is being carried out should be within reasonable limits, say 13°C–21°C. If the test is carried out in a hot environment lower figures are obtained.

Fitness Index Table

Sum of three counts	Fitness index	Sum of three counts	Fitness index
250	60	150	100
246	61	149	101
242	62	147	102
238	63	146	103
234	64	144	104
231	65	143	105
227	66	142	106
224	67	140	107
221	68	139	108
217	69	138	109
214	70	137	110
211	71	135	111
208	72	134	112
205	73	133	113
203	74	132	114
200	75	130	115
197	76	129	116
195	77	128	117
192	78	127	118
190	79	126	119
188	80	125	120
185	81	124	121
183	82	123	122
181	83	122	123
179	84	121	124
176	85	120	125
174	86	119	126
172	87	118	127
170	88	117	128
169	89	116	129
167	90		
165	91		
163	92		
161	93		
160	94		
158	95		
156	96		
155	97		
153	98		
152	99		

For a fit man the first half of this test feels very easy. Usually, however, the finishing of the test requires considerable determination. Some rescue station superintendents consider this aspect of the test a useful contribution to the assessment of a recruit to the rescue service.

References

1. Davis, R. H. (1947), *Breathing in Irrespirable Atmospheres*, p. 165–230. St. Catherine Press Ltd., London.
2. Johnson, R. E., Brouha, L. and Darling, R. C. (1942), "A test of physical fitness for strenuous exercise." *Revue canadienne de biologie*, **1**, 491.
3. Lind, A. R. (1955), "The influence of inspired air temperature on tolerance to work in the heat." *British Journal of Industrial Medicine*, **12**, 126.
4. Lind, A. R., Hellon, R. S., Weiner, J. S. and Jones, R. M. (1955), "Tolerance of men to work in hot saturated environments with reference to mines rescue operations." *British Journal of Industrial Medicine*, **12**, 296.
5. McAdam, R. and Davidson, D. (1947), *Mine Rescue Work*. Oliver and Boyd, London.
6. Standing Medical Advisory Committee; Report of a Sub-Committee (1969), *Uses and Dangers of Oxygen Therapy*, p. 3. Her Majesty's Stationery Office, Edinburgh.

Chapter 19

Mine Rescue Breathing Apparatus

Introduction

When a man enters an atmosphere containing dangerously high concentrations of noxious gases or dusts, he must be protected against their effects. The choice of protective apparatus is usually determined by the nature and concentration of the contaminant, and by the oxygen concentration in the contaminated atmosphere (which may be too low to support life). Four principal types of equipment may be distinguished: filter respirators, e.g. dust masks; chemical respirators, e.g. self-rescue apparatus; self-contained breathing apparatus and air-line breathing apparatus (Fig. 1).

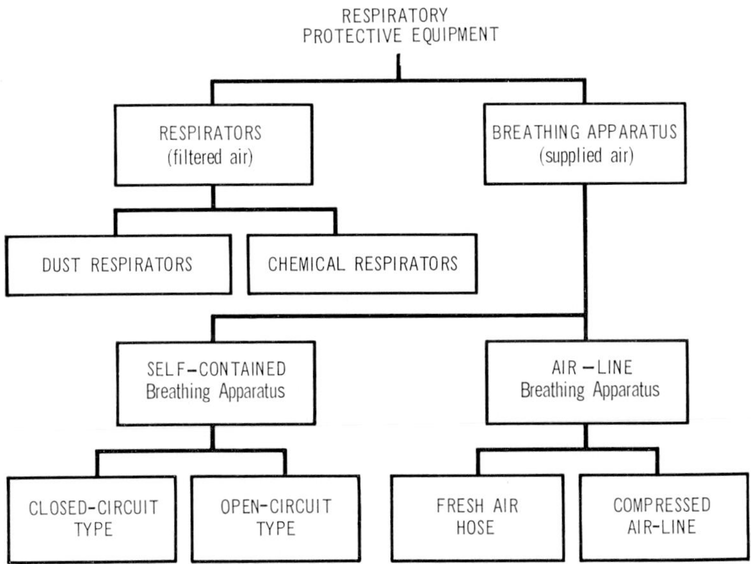

FIG. 1. Types of respiratory protective equipment.

Respirators have no oxygen supply and usually provide only limited protection. Breathing apparatus supplies the user with uncontaminated air or oxygen, and thus provides respiratory protection, irrespective of the nature and concentration of the gases in the surrounding atmosphere.

Breathing apparatus (with supplied air) is needed in mines because of the irrespirable atmospheres that may be present in abandoned, unventilated workings or that may result from fires or explosions. The earliest form of breathing apparatus probably consisted of a length of tubing, or reed, which allowed the user to exist in a foul atmosphere, or under water, while breathing from a fresh air source by the use of his respiratory muscles. Apparatus utilizing this principle are still available; an improved version consisting of a large bore hose together with a hand or motor operated blower (fresh air hose apparatus) is occasionally used in mining. When the air is supplied from a compressed air source (compressed airline apparatus) a longer hose of smaller bore is normally used.

Self-contained breathing apparatus of the open-circuit type use compressed air carried in a cylinder on the back. The wearer breathes from the cylinder through a demand valve, which is lung controlled, and his expired air is released to the atmosphere (vented). This type of apparatus is usually simple in design but has the disadvantage that all the air needed by the wearer must be carried. Its duration is therefore limited to about 30 minutes by the weight and bulk of the apparatus. However, the comparatively recent acceptance of lightweight cylinders, made of a special strength nickel chromium molybdenum steel, has led to the development of apparatus lasting up to about 50 minutes. Open-circuit apparatus of this type are not in general use at present in mines, though the fact that they are easy to use and maintain makes them suitable for such duties as gas-sampling and inspection.

Breathing apparatus to protect men who must enter irrespirable atmospheres in mines is almost always of the self-contained, closed-circuit type, in which the expired air is purified by the chemical absorption of carbon dioxide and is then enriched with oxygen from a supply within the apparatus before being rebreathed. The respiratory circuit must include a flexible breathing bag or counter-lung to hold the expired gases and a relief valve to prevent the build-up of high positive pressures in the apparatus. It is also usual to include two non-return valves to ensure adequate circulation of the expired air through the purifier before rebreathing. The oxygen supply of the apparatus may be obtained from a cylinder containing compressed oxygen or less commonly from the vapourization of liquid air or oxygen. This type of breathing apparatus allows a man to work in foul air for longer periods than are generally possible with the open-circuit type and with greater freedom of movement than is allowed by the fresh air hose type of apparatus. It is mainly for these reasons that the breathing apparatus used in rescue and recovery work in mines is almost entirely of this self-contained closed-circuit type and henceforth in this chapter this only will be considered.

Physiological Requirements

Men trained for mine rescue are often called upon to work in irrespirable atmospheres. Severe physical exertion may be entailed and the breathing apparatus must therefore satisfy very high standards of performance to make the combination of wearer and apparatus a safe and efficient working unit. The more important physiological considerations are, (1) the composition of the inhaled air, (2) the temperature and humidity of the inhaled air and (3) the extra respiratory work imposed by the resistance of the apparatus.

The Composition of the Air Breathed

The air inspired from a closed-circuit breathing apparatus consists of oxygen, carbon dioxide and nitrogen.

When closed-circuit apparatus are used correctly the oxygen concentration will usually be greater than 70 per cent. Such a high concentration is beneficial in reducing the ventilation rate and therefore the respiratory work rate, and also in delaying the onset of fatigue during work. There is some evidence, however, that these beneficial effects are slightly reduced with concentrations as high as 100 per cent (Bannister and Cunningham, 1954).

The carbon dioxide content should ideally be nil. The inhalation of appreciable quantities of carbon dioxide is both undesirable and potentially dangerous, leading to greater ventilatory requirements (Craig, 1955), greater respiratory effort, fatigue and sensations of shortness of breath and suffocation which may be enhanced by the severe psychological stress inherent in underground rescue work and fire fighting. In practice there is a certain unavoidable deadspace in the respiratory circuit, the non-return valves may be imperfect, and the purifier may lose efficiency in the course of a heavy work period. However, with a good apparatus in normal use, the percentage of carbon dioxide inspired at any time will usually be very small. Figure 2 shows the concentration of carbon dioxide likely to be inspired from three frequently used apparatus. The results were obtained using a breathing simulator operating at a tidal volume of 2 litres and 20 cycles per minute, thus giving a minute volume of 40 litres; for the purpose of these tests it was assumed that the expired air contains 5 per cent carbon dioxide.

The nitrogen is present in the respiratory circuit before use and is also derived from the wearer's lungs, and from impurities in the source of oxygen. In most apparatus obtaining their oxygen from high pressure cylinders active efforts must be made to flush the circuit and the lungs several times with oxygen before use. One commonly used method is for the wearer to breathe in oxygen repeatedly from his apparatus and then breathe out to atmosphere. If this is not done a consumption of oxygen at a rate greater than the supply to the circuit can result in a dangerous deficiency. For example, if the apparatus before use has a gas capacity of about 8 litres and if the system is filled with 50 per cent oxygen and 50 per cent nitrogen, then the volume of oxygen in the

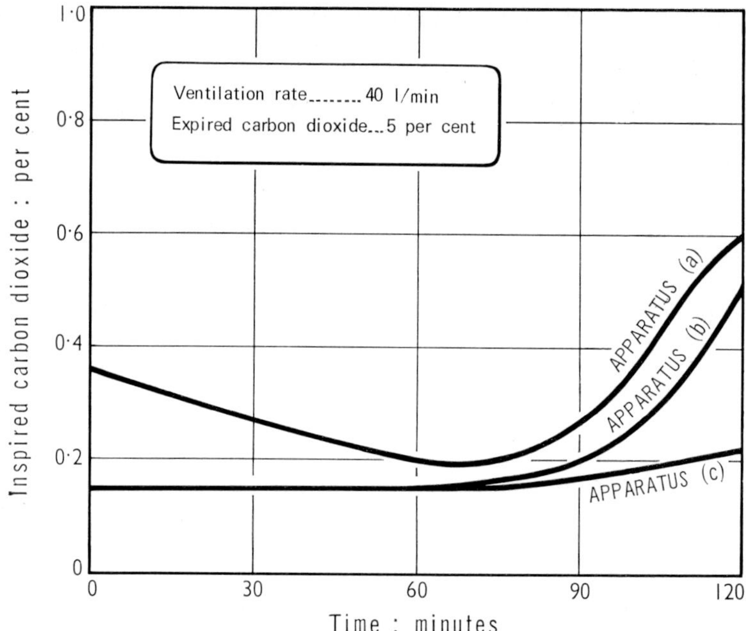

FIG. 2. Inspired carbon dioxide concentration.

apparatus at the outset is 4·0 litres. If the wearer works sufficiently hard to extract from the system 3·5 litres of oxygen more than is supplied, then there will remain in the apparatus only 0·5 litres of oxygen in a total volume of 4·5 litres, i.e. only 11 per cent oxygen. Thus, when the oxygen supply rate is 2 litres per minute and the oxygen consumption rate is 2·5 litres per minute, under these conditions there will be a serious oxygen deficiency within about seven minutes. Some breathing apparatus have a small venting device to ensure that air from the respiratory circuit is frequently vented to the atmosphere; such a system ensures an adequate oxygen concentration throughout the wearing period. If, however, the source of oxygen is the evaporation of liquid oxygen, there is always such a generous supply that this hazard does not arise.

The Temperature and Humidity of the Air Breathed

Work in breathing apparatus is often performed in hot and humid conditions with little or no ventilation. In these circumstances the heat losses from the surface of the body are much reduced. Indeed in certain adverse conditions the body may even be accepting heat from its surroundings. It is therefore desirable that a breathing apparatus should add as little as possible to a man's thermal load and should even provide some cooling. Figure 3 shows the likely rate of heating or cooling of the wearer when wearing breathing apparatus of the compressed oxygen type without a cooler apparatus (a), or with a cooler apparatus (b), or of the liquid oxygen type apparatus (c). The results were obtained

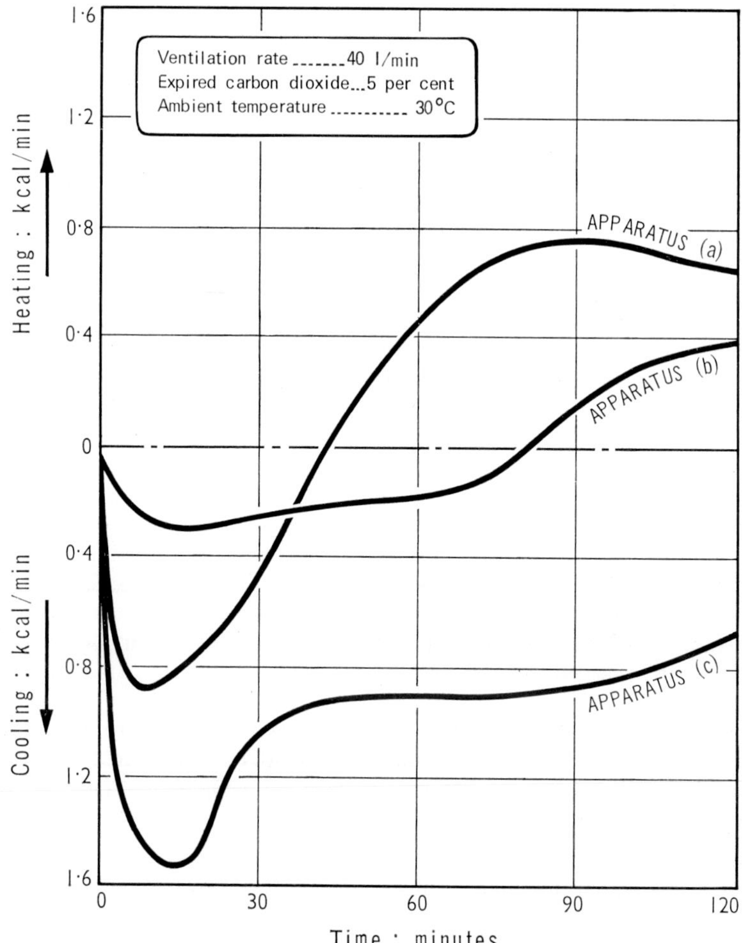

Fig. 3. Respiratory heat exchange.

using a breathing simulator operating at a rate equivalent to reasonably hard work.

When the expired air is passed through the purifier of a breathing apparatus the carbon dioxide is absorbed by the chemical action of caustic alkali, for example, sodium hydroxide or soda lime; these reactions produce heat and water vapour. In both cases the temperature of the air leaving the purifier rises rapidly; it will be saturated and exceed body temperature after about 30 minutes breathing. The cooling or heating effect of the inspired air on the wearer is closely related to its water content, and this is very important in practice. The air leaving the lungs is saturated at body temperature. If the air inhaled has a lower water content, water is evaporated in the respiratory tract. The body supplies the latent heat of evaporation of this water and is thereby cooled. Conversely, if the inspired air contains more water vapour than does air saturated at body temperature, water will be condensed in the respiratory tract and the latent heat of condensation will provide heat to the body. The heat needed to change the temperature of dry air is very much less than that involved in evaporating or condensing out water which is in the saturated air. A large part of the enthalpy (i.e. total heat) of a saturated gas lies in the water vapour. Thus whilst dry air can be inhaled at a temperature well above that of the body and still have a substantial cooling effect, the rate at which air, saturated above body temperature, heats the man increases very rapidly with the temperature of the inhaled air. Theoretically, absolutely dry air at 120°C may still cool the body, yet air saturated at 50°C will have a heating effect on the body of the order of 1·5 kilocalories per minute at a ventilatory rate of 40 litres/minute. This is equivalent to almost a quarter of the total heat production of a man exercising at a level corresponding to a ventilation rate of 40 litres/minute. Much work has been done, notably by Lind and his co-workers (Lind, Hellon, Weiner and Jones, 1955) in defining the period during which it is safe for men to work under various adverse climatic conditions when wearing certain breathing apparatus. In practice, charts are often used which advise on these safe limits; an example from the British Mines Rescue Service is shown in Fig. 4. Some idea of the importance of breathing apparatus providing cool air to breathe may be derived from the fact that the allowable time under particularly adverse climatic conditions may be extended by as much as a quarter by using a thermally 'good' apparatus rather than a 'bad' one.

The Extra Respiratory Work Imposed by the Resistance of the Apparatus
There are two main mechanisms whereby physiological ill effects may arise from external resistance to respiration;

(a) The extra resistance may be so great as to lead to reduced ventilation of the lungs; alternatively efforts to maintain ventilation may cause added fatigue; and

(b) If the resistances to inspiration and expiration are not reasonably well matched, a serious change in the mean intra-thoracic pressure may result. Thus an excessive resistance to expiration will require greater expiratory efforts and higher positive pressure

Wet bulb temperature		A compressed-oxygen apparatus SAFE PERIOD IN MINUTES Dry-bulb temperature									A liquid-oxygen apparatus SAFE PERIOD IN MINUTES Dry-bulb temperature									
°C	°F	26·7	29·4	32·2	35	37·8	40·6	43·3	46·1	48·9	26·7	29·4	32·2	35	37·8	40·6	43·3	46·1	48·9	°C
		80	85	90	95	100	105	110	115	120	80	85	90	95	100	105	110	115	120	°F
22·5	72·5	—	—	—	—	—	—	—	—	59	—	—	—	—	—	—	—	—	—	
23·9	75	—	—	—	—	—	60	59	57	54	—	—	—	—	—	—	—	—	—	
25·3	77·5	—	—	—	60	56	54	53	52	48	—	—	—	—	—	—	—	—	120	
26·7	80	60	60	56	53	50	48	46	44	41	—	—	—	—	—	—	—	120	94	
28·1	82·5	—	50	49	46	44	42	40	38	36	—	—	—	—	120	97	78	65	56	
29·4	85	—	44	42	39	38	36	34	33	32	—	120	101	81	67	58	50	45	40	
30·9	87·5	—	—	37	35	34	32	30	29	28	—	—	59	51	46	41	37	34	31	
32·2	90	—	—	32	31	30	28	27	26	25	—	—	42	38	34	32	29	27	25	
33·6	92·5	—	—	—	27	26	25	24	24	22	—	—	—	30	27	26	24	23	21	
35·0	95	—	—	—	24	23	22	22	21	20	—	—	—	24	23	22	20	19	19	
36·4	97·5	—	—	—	—	22	20	19	19	—	—	—	—	—	20	19	18	17	16	
37·8	100	—	—	—	—	19	—	—	—	—	—	—	—	—	17	16	16	15	15	

FIG. 4. Recommended working times for mines-rescue personnel, wearing self-contained breathing apparatus in hot environmental conditions.

in the chest, which will directly interfere with circulatory efficiency by retarding the return of blood to the heart. When endeavouring to define allowable standards of resistance for a breathing apparatus it is therefore important to consider both the total rate of extra work which the apparatus imposes on the respiratory muscles and also the distribution of this burden between inspiration and expiration.

In research on respiratory protective apparatus most of the studies on the effects of breathing against external resistance have been carried out by Silverman, Lee, Yancey, Amory, Barney and Lee (1945) using equipment in which the pressure necessary to pass a flow of gas was directly proportional to that flow. However, a large part of the resistance to respiration in closed-circuit breathing apparatus arises from tubes and valves in which this simple law does not apply. In these, the necessary pressure rises very much more rapidly than the rate of flow. Furthermore, the closed-circuit apparatus includes an elastic rebreathing bag or counter-lung which imposes a resistance to expiration. But this resistance is not present in inspiration, indeed the elastic tension in the counter-lung tends to re-inflate the patient when he next begins an inspiratory effort. These factors are considered by Cooper (1960) and Senneck (1962) and in greater detail by Cooper (1961).

It is common practice to express allowable resistance in terms of the pressure necessary to drive air through the respiratory circuit at certain stated rates of flow. There is as yet no commonly accepted "ideal" resistance but opinions based on deductions and extrapolations from the work of Silverman *et al.* (1945) are in reasonable agreement as to what comprises a safe external load. Even stricter standards have been suggested for the "comfort" of wearers, and there is good evidence (Bentley, Griffin, Love, Muir and Sweetland, 1972) that men trained in mine rescue work very readily accept apparatus which satisfies the maximum allowable breathing resistance proposed by Senneck (1962); these proposals were later used in the formulation of resistance standards for breathing apparatus (British Standard, 1971).

Mine Rescue Breathing Apparatus

Nearly all closed-circuit breathing apparatus are of the compressed oxygen type; the oxygen is stored in one or more cylinders and usually charged to either 12·2 or 20·4 MN/m^2 (120 or 200 atmospheres) pressure. The wearer is provided with oxygen either from a lung-governed demand system or from a constant supply of not less than 2 litres per minute or, more usually, from a constant supply of about 1·5 litres per minute supplemented by a lung-governed mechanism. Although the system most economical in its use of oxygen is the totally lung-governed type, apparatus using this form of oxygen supply are rare because the need to ensure that the oxygen concentration is at all times adequate requires the addition of a venting device to the breathing circuit. The system of constant supply is probably the simpler, but may be very wasteful of oxygen; it has the further disadvantage that the wearer must operate the appropriate valve when, owing to increased exertion, his oxygen demand is greater than the oxygen supply. Whichever method of oxygen supply is used, however, compressed oxygen breathing apparatus require a manually operated by-pass valve as a protection against possible blockage of the usual oxygen supply system.

The most recent designs of compressed oxygen breathing apparatus have concentrated on either (a) reducing the overall size and weight of the apparatus or alternatively (b) reducing the temperature of the air breathed by the wearer. Savings in weight have been achieved by introducing smaller and more elegant oxygen demand systems, lighter frames and improved carrying harness. One such apparatus (Fig. 5a) has a 2 litre cylinder which may be charged to a little more than 15·3 MN/m^2 (150 atm) pressure. When in use oxygen enters the breathing circuit at a constant rate of 1·6 litres per minute and the additional automatic supply mechanism is operated by the pressure in the breathing bag. On expiration, a valve in the circuit directs the carbon dioxide contaminated air through a factory filled purifier containing caustic-soda pellets and into a breathing bag. The relief valve operates automatically when the bag becomes full. On inspiration air is drawn from the breathing bag, through a second circuit valve and then through the breathing tubes into either a facemask or mouthpiece. The working parts of this apparatus, which is not normally supplied with a cooler, are contained in a light alloy case; the ready to use weight is 12·9 kg (28 lb). With only minor changes, this description of a compressed oxygen breathing apparatus is representative of apparatus now in use in many countries, e.g. the U.S.S.R., Germany and the U.S.A. This type of apparatus, however, may provide the user with hot humid air to breathe; at the ventilation rate corresponding to heavy work (40 litres/minute) the air breathed increases the thermal load of the wearer for much of the wearing period (Fig. 3). The potential hazard of breathing air at temperatures much above body temperature is recognized, and the design of some apparatus makes provision for the use of a cooler as an optional accessory; one such cooler consists of a box containing either solid carbon dioxide or ice chippings, which is carried at the waist.

Other designers have paid particular attention to the provision of cool air to breathe. The main components of one such apparatus are contained in a metal shell which has access ports for the purifier, breathing bag, relief valve and coolant. The apparatus is protected by a glass-fibre cover (Fig. 5b) and weighs 16.8 kg (37 lb) when fully charged. The method of working is based on the conventional arrangement of purifier, relief valve, breathing bag, compressed oxygen supply and

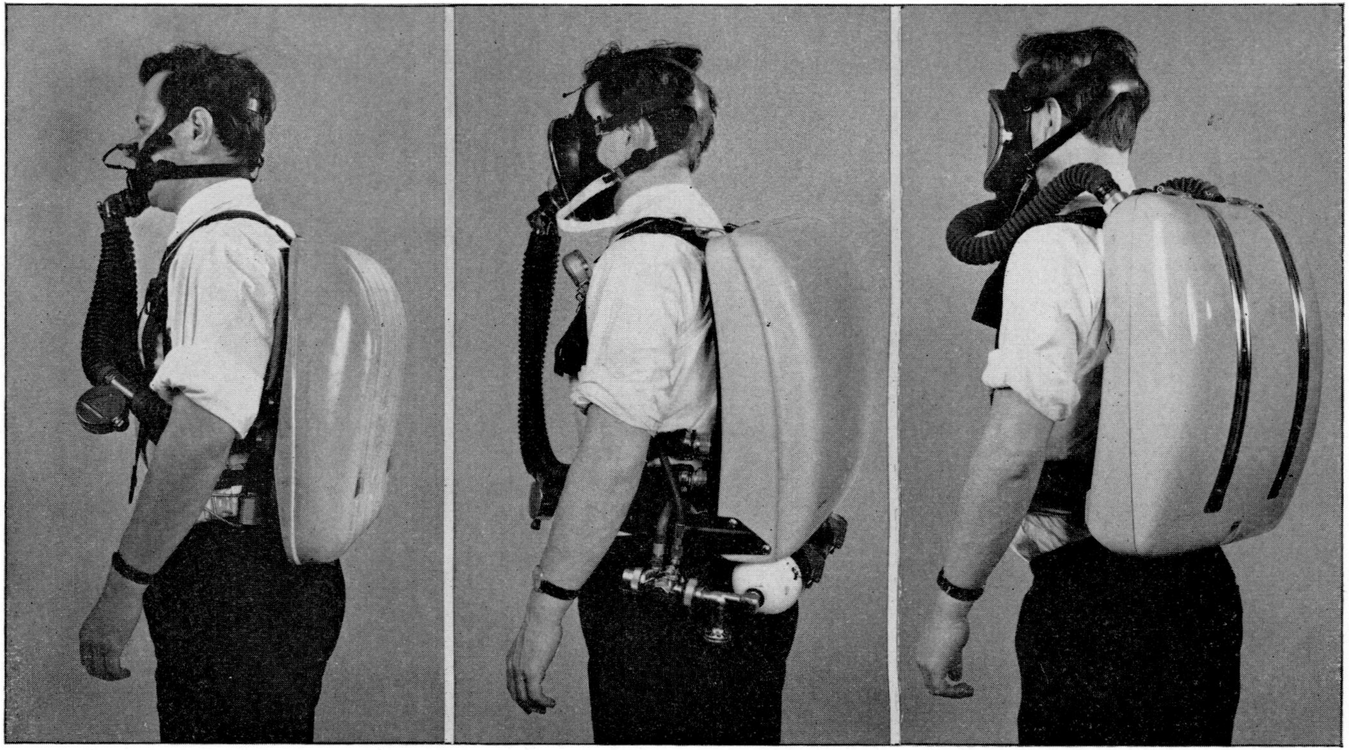

Fig. 5. Modern mines-rescue breathing apparatus.

cooler. The apparatus is supplied with either a mouthpiece or a face-mask; underarm breathing tubes connect the facepiece to the apparatus which is carried on the back.

Soda lime is contained in a rechargeable, radial-flow purifier of low flow resistance. The breathing resistance is low and the chemical efficiency of its purifier is good (Fig. 2).

The breathing bag arrangement in this apparatus is unusual; the bag is reversed, that is to say the changing pressures in the apparatus are applied to the outside of the bag. The inside of the bag is open to atmosphere through a port in the side of the metal case; thus during inspiration the bag inflates. The advantage of such a system is twofold; first, the surface available for heat exchange is large and mainly metallic, and since condensation on this surface is expected, the heat loss from the circuit gas will be greater than from the usual breathing bag arrangement; secondly, the movement of the bag should ensure an effective transfer of heat away from the flexible surface of the breathing bag.

On inspiration, air is drawn from the breathing bag through the cooler and into the breathing tubes. The cooler has a 0·8 kg (1·7 lb) charge of ice; as the ice melts the water is channelled through wicks to an exterior fabric cover, fitted over the metal shell, and around which the mine air circulates. In non-saturated atmospheres evaporation from the wetted surface cools the metal surface of the apparatus (Fig. 3).

A comparatively recent development in closed-circuit breathing apparatus has been the introduction of apparatus using liquid oxygen. This type of apparatus is now standard equipment in Australia, South Africa and the United Kingdom.

An example of this type of apparatus is shown in Fig. 5c. The components are housed in a glass-fibre case suspended from the shoulders and held off the back by a rucksack-type suspension; when fully charged it weighs 13·4 kg (29·5 lb). The method of working can be followed from the block diagram (Fig. 6). Starting at the point A, the

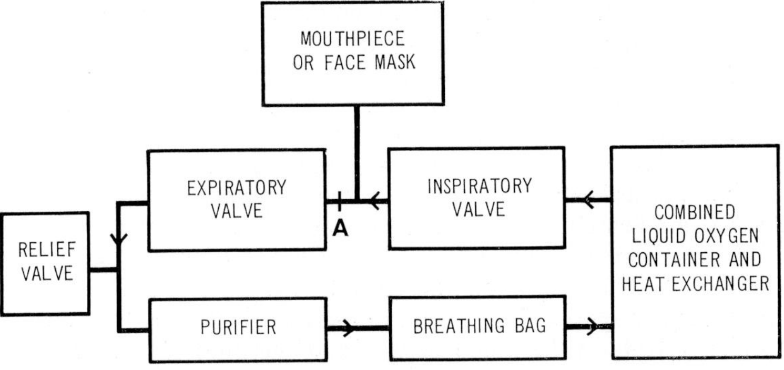

FIG. 6. Circuit of liquid oxygen breathing apparatus.

expired air is returned to the circuit through the expiratory valve. The next component, which is inside the case of the apparatus, is an automatic relief valve, which allows excess gas to escape to atmosphere, and which is necessary because the oxygen supply always exceeds the wearer's normal demands. For maximum efficiency, the relief valve must be placed at this position in the circuit, where the wasted gas is unpurified expired air. If the air is purified before the waste gas is discarded, the weight of purifying agent would be unnecessarily high. The next components in the circuit are the purifier and the breathing bag. Again, for maximum efficiency the bag must follow the purifier, because it is important to make the most efficient use of the heat exchange that occurs between the bag and its surroundings; the air is at its hottest, and the heat exchange is most effective, at the point immediately following the purifier. The remaining components of the circuit are the liquid oxygen container, which cools the purified air and enriches it with oxygen, and the inspiratory valve.

The purifier is of the radial-flow type and is charged with 1·6 kg (3·5 lb) of soda lime; it has a high carbon dioxide absorption efficiency (Fig. 2) and a very low resistance, about 0·10 kN/m² or 1 cm water gauge at a flow rate of 300 litres/minute. Because of the low resistance of the purifier it is possible to use a relief valve with the very low opening pressure of 0·25 kN/m² (2·5 cm water gauge).

The liquid oxygen pack is a key component in the design of the apparatus. Immediately before an apparatus is to be used, it must be charged with 2·5 kg (5·5 lb) of liquid oxygen; the apparatus will then provide the wearer with enough oxygen for a minimum of two and a half hours. The liquid, normally carried in 25 litre dewar flasks, is poured through a funnel into the centre compartment of the liquid oxygen pack. Once the apparatus is charged with oxygen, the useful life of the charge commences; the flow of gas from the evaporator cannot be manually controlled and is only slightly affected by external conditions such as the ambient temperature or the work rate of the wearer. The heat-exchange system consists of concentric cylinders surrounding the liquid oxygen container; the gases flow through the annular spaces separating the cylinders. During inspiration the hot purified air from the breathing bag is drawn through the outermost annular space, and subsequently passes out of the exchanger; there is no communication between the outermost space and the inner spaces. As the hot purified air passes through the outermost annular space a thermal gradient from the outside to the inside of the evaporator is produced; heat flow inwards causes the liquid oxygen to evaporate. The cold freshly evaporated oxygen flows from the container into the inner annular spaces. The freshly evaporated oxygen is thus in close proximity to both the liquid oxygen and the purified air. The inner annular space serves (a) to cool the purified air in the outer annulus,

(b) to warm the gaseous oxygen and (c) to insulate the liquid oxygen so that a satisfactory evaporation rate can be obtained. After passing through the inner spaces, the oxygen flows into the breathing bag, where it is mixed with the purified air.

This type of heat exchanger allows much of the cooling potential of the liquid oxygen to be used to cool the air supplied by the apparatus. As a consequence, the air inspired is noticeably cooler and drier than the air breathed from the more conventional compressed oxygen breathing apparatus (Fig. 3). Work in hot and humid atmospheres can be safely endured for a longer time (Fig. 4) and the wearer obtains in addition the obvious subjective benefits of breathing cool air.

References

Bannister, R. G. and Cunningham, D. J. C. (1954), "The effects on the respiration and performance during exercise of adding oxygen to the inspired air." *Journal of Applied Physiology*, **125**, 118.

Bentley, R. A., Griffin, O. G., Love, R. G., Muir, D. C. F. and Sweetland, K. S. To be published.

British Standard (1971), Specification 4667. Breathing Apparatus. British Standards Institution, London.

Cooper, E. A. (1960), "Suggested methods of testing and standards of resistance for respiratory protective devices." *Journal of Applied Physiology*, **15**, 1053.

Cooper, E. A. (1961), "Behaviour of Respiratory Apparatus". *Med. Res, Memo. No. 2*, National Coal Board, London.

Craig, F. N. (1955) "Pulmonary ventilation during exercise and inhalation of carbon dioxide." *Journal of Applied Physiology*, **7**, 467.

Lind, A. R., Hellon, R. F., Weiner, J. S. and Jones, R. M. (1955), "Tolerance of men to work in hot saturated environments with reference to Mines Rescue Operations." *British Journal of Industrial Medicine*, **12**, 296.

Senneck, C. R. (1962), *Design and Use of Respirators*, p. 143. Pergamon Press, Oxford.

Silverman, L., Lee, G., Yancey, A. R., Amory, L., Barney, L. J. and Lee, R. C. (1945), "Fundamental factors in the design of protective respiratory equipment; a study and an evaluation on inspiratory and expiratory resistance for protective respiratory equipment." *U.S. Office of Scientific Research and Development Report No. 5339*, Washington.

Chapter 20

Personal Protective Equipment

Introduction

Early drawings and paintings of mining subjects make it clear that for many centuries miners have tried to adapt their clothing to offer some protection from the hazards of their work. Only in recent decades however has this subject received serious attention.

Protective clothing, widely interpreted, is usually provided by the employer free, free on loan or at a subsidized price. There are several reasons for this:

(*a*) protective clothing may protect vulnerable parts of the body e.g. head or knee, thus reducing accidents and minimizing production losses;

(*b*) protective clothing may replace manifestly unsuitable clothing which workers otherwise tend to wear at work and which may not only offer no protection but may be a positive hazard e.g. flapping buttonless jackets or torn trouser legs;

(*c*) protective clothing issued by management can be of the standard required and control over the quality of items issued can be exercised;

(*d*) well designed protective clothing can add to rather than detract from the appearance of the worker thus contributing positively to the morale of mining communities.

Before considering in detail the various items available it must be stressed that the issue of protective clothing often presents a subtle problem in industrial relationships. Items of protective clothing or equipment will be worn for substantial periods by miners; understandably they will look critically at new items or issues which should only be made after full consultation with their representatives. In many cases it will be desirable to carry out user trials—these should be carefully organized and evaluated at a preliminary stage. Unless a particular item is manifestly superior to all alternatives the miner should be allowed a choice. The fact that he has been able to choose an article personally is likely to increase its acceptability.

The following subjects will be considered separately:

Helmets	Self Rescuers	Boots
Eye protection	Elbow pads	Stockings
Ear protection	Gloves	Miners' suits
Protection from dust	Knee pads	

Helmets

In selecting a suitable helmet for mining the criteria to be observed are as follows: the helmet must provide adequate protection to the head, it must not be too heavy, it must have a bracket to hold a cap lamp and a clip or fastening at the back to which the trailing cable can be secured and the interior harness should fit comfortably and securely to the skull while providing ventilation.

In Great Britain there is a British Standard for safety helmets (British Standard, 1957). In addition to the specifications laid down in this standard for tests of shock absorption, inflammability and penetration it is possible to devise tests which measure the helmet's resistance to repeated impact, penetration and shrinkage following repeated wetting and drying and resistance to side pressures.

When the head band of the interior harness is made of leather, cases of dermatitis may occur due to the sensitivity of the wearer to the chrome salts used in tanning. Plastic headbands do not produce such lesions. Alternatively disposable paper skull caps can be worn.

Eye Protection

Freeman (1962) suggests that this is the most difficult of all types of protection to enforce. There is a large number of suppliers and a great variety of equipment available. Therefore, before selecting any particular type of goggles, it is desirable to consider how well they meet the following requirements:

(a) they can be worn over ordinary prescription lenses if necessary,
(b) they do not restrict the visual field,
(c) misting of the lenses is unlikely to be a problem,
(d) they are comfortable to wear,
(e) the transparent surfaces do not pit or scratch easily,
(f) the ear pieces and nose bridge are well fitted,
(g) the whole assembly moulds well to the face.

If an underground worker requires to wear corrective lenses for a visual defect while at work these should always be unsplinterable. Suitable arrangements for the supply of such unsplinterable lenses should be made. Any one-eyed, or virtually one-eyed man should wear eye protection all the time at work as a matter of principle.

Ear Protection

With the steady development of mechanization mines are becoming much noiser places. It has been shown that intermittent exposure to noise does not appear to have such a deleterious effect on hearing as continual high intensity noise. Nonetheless certain machines such as compressed air boring machines undoubtedly produce temporary hearing loss which persists after the end of the shift (Spencer, 1971).

The earliest types of ear muffs which were used, chiefly, in the aircraft industry were not suitable for underground use because helmets could not be worn over them. However, presumably in response to the increased awareness of the undesirable effects of excessive industrial noise, considerable progress has been made by the manufacturers in producing either a combined helmet and ear muff or ear muffs which can be worn in conjunction with a helmet. These items of protection must always be regarded as a third line of defence after suppression of noise at source or the removal of workmen from the noisy environment which may, of course, be impracticable in some underground situations. Significant sound attenuation can be expected if well constructed and fitted ear muffs are worn. Another method of protection is the ear plug of which a number of reasonably effective types are available. Care should be taken to ensure that they are properly fitted by a specially designated member of the medical or safety staff. The use of glass wool fibre supplied so that men can make their own plugs has its advocates. A firm container in which they can be kept should be issued to the miner because they should only be used when he is exposed to noise.

The ear muff is the method of choice where the noise hazard is substantial. But there will be many circumstances in which less sophisticated measures will suffice. For these glass wool is probably preferable to ear plugs because it is disposable and a fresh plug can be used on each occasion. Ear plugs have the disadvantage that they may irritate the external ear.

Protection from Dust

In historic times the miner sought to protect himself from dust by putting a handkerchief (often wetted) over his nose and mouth. The first masks commercially produced offered little more protection.

Some modern dust respirators are highly efficient and while dust suppression must remain the basic measure in the control of occupational pulmonary disease the dust mask will often have a significant role. In places where, in spite of all reasonable efforts, dust control measures remain unsatisfactory dust respirators should be used. Individual miners who are showing signs of dust retention in their lungs should also be advised to wear dust respirators.

There have been considerable advances in the design of dust respirators. Most types presently available have both coarse and fine filters. The coarse filters are designed to prevent undue dust loading of the fine filters and make use of an electrostatic effect to assist the normal interception and impaction of particles in the fibrous bed. This results in a high retention efficiency, yet the inspiratory resistance is not so high that work, wearing a respirator, is uncomfortable. With the improvement in filter design the fit between face and facepiece can become the major source of leakage and to overcome this difficulty some manufacturers have incorporated an inflatable or pneumatic rim into the facepiece. This is intended to take care of the considerable variation in facial contours and especially of the hollowed cheeks of miners who leave their dentures on the surface. Without some such device an unmeasured amount of dust is inhaled through the gaps between mask and face. In Great Britain the criteria for construction and performance are set out in a British Standard (1969) while in the United States approval testing is undertaken by the U.S. Bureau of Mines.

The modern mask is undoubtedly much more effective in trapping respirable dust than its primitive predecessors; it is also more complex and requires adequate maintenance.

An effective administrative system is necessary for the smooth working of any issue of dust respirators. In the first place an adequate, and continuous, supply of filters and spare parts must be available. A room should be designated for the issue and storage of masks and spares and should be furnished with adequate facilities for washing, cleaning and drying masks. Depending on the number of masks in use at a mine a full-time or part-time attendant will be needed to carry out daily inspection and servicing. It is important that this should be the responsibility of one individual and that the miner should not be left to devise his own servicing arrangements. A register should be kept to record the daily issue, return and maintenance of the masks in use. Five to six minutes is a reasonable time in which to service a dusty mask and thus an attendant can hope to deal with ten to twelve masks each hour. Mechanical methods of servicing are being developed.

These arrangements should ensure that this costly and relatively sophisticated protective equipment is used most effectively.

Self Rescuers

Underground fires, explosions and ignitions of methane can all produce dangerous atmospheres with potentially lethal concentrations of carbon monoxide. The self rescuer (Fig. 1) is designed to remove carbon monoxide from the air before it is inhaled. A bed of hopcalite (a mixture of the oxides of magnesium and copper together with small amounts of other oxides) converts the carbon monoxide to carbon dioxide. Since mine air is usually moist it is passed through a drying agent before reaching the hopcalite which deteriorates rapidly in the presence of moisture. Dust is also removed by filter. The self rescuer is fitted with a cooler as the hopcalite is heat producing and the higher the concentration of carbon monoxide present the higher the temperature of the inhaled air; the maximum temperature which can be tolerated is about 90°C.

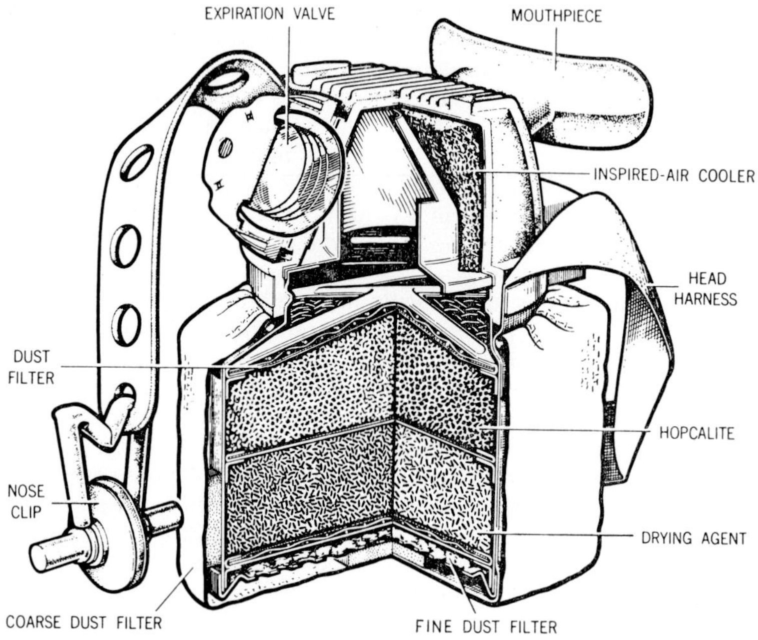

Fig. 1. A typical self rescuer.

High inspiratory resistance is always a problem in canister type respirators and this must be reduced as much as possible by giving attention to the way in which the chemicals are packed, to the design of valves and to the filtering out of coarse dust particles.

The self rescuer should be light, should be readily attached to the miner's clothing or equipment and should have a container stout enough to protect the breathing unit from damage.

As with dust masks it is essential to have an effective checking and replacement system if self rescuers are to be fully effective in an emergency.

Elbow Pads

Where thin seams of less than 0·75 metre in height are worked pressure on the elbows may cause a condition known as beat elbow. This condition is characterized by a tender, painful swelling of the soft tissues over the bony prominence at the back of the elbow joint (see Chapter 12). Movement at the elbow joint is not merely that of a simple hinge but in addition involves rotation of the forearm on the upper arm. Nevertheless protective pads are available which are fairly loose fitting, composed of leather-backed sponge rubber or similar material, held in place by straps above and below the joint; these protect the joint without impeding movement to any material degree (Archibald, Kay and Scott, 1966).

Gloves

Safety gloves inevitably represent a compromise between protection of the hand and fingers and limitation of tactile sensation and fine movement. Heat and dust add to the problems confronting the designer of gloves suitable for mining conditions.

The need for hand protection in mining is clearly illustrated by the findings of a survey in a large mining medical service where it was found that hand and finger injuries accounted for at least one third of all injuries treated (Archibald, 1964).

Gloves of cotton or similar light-weight materials will not stand up to the robust conditions encountered underground. Thus the most popular gloves are made of leather. Much care has to be devoted to the manufacture of leather gloves if rough seams are not to chafe the skin of the finger webs and if the thumb part is not to form a weak area which splits from the rest of the glove. An alternative to leather, indicated for miners whose jobs involve contact with oil, is a polyvinyl chloride coated cotton glove which is impermeable; in hot conditions it may retain sweat and cause maceration of the skin of the hand. Knitted nylon gloves allow free circulation of air although they afford less protection than leather. Elasticized wrists may protect against dust and dirt but may decrease still further the ease of rotation of the hand.

Thus it will be seen that no one glove will suit all conditions. If it is proposed to issue gloves on a large scale carefully controlled user trials should be carried out, the various qualities which it is designed to test having been clearly defined beforehand.

Though it is a commonplace that hands vary in size the fact is sometimes overlooked that gloves must fit well if they are not to add to, rather than protect from, the hazards of mining. One sixth of all men require large size gloves, two thirds medium and one sixth small. Gloves should therefore be stocked in three sizes in these proportions.

Knee Pads

Where mineworkers, particularly coalminers, work in seam heights below 1·5 metres they spend much of the time on their knees; it has been demonstrated that the pressure exerted on the area of contact is very considerable (Sharrard, 1963). In these circumstances they may develop the condition known as Beat Knee which, like Beat Elbow, is characterized by a tender and painful swelling of the soft tissues over or immediately below the kneecap (Roantree, 1957). This condition prevents work in the kneeling position until it has subsided (see Chapter 12).

Traditionally miners have worn knee pads to protect their knees; an investigation by a British working party into all types of knee pads commercially available showed defects of design and construction in almost every pad and some were judged to provide little, if any, protection.

Testing of pads was carried out on machines simulating the kneeling process and attention was paid to the following points:

(*a*) pliability of the outer casing,
(*b*) tear-out strength of the straps,
(*c*) abrasion resistance of the outer casing,
(*d*) cushioning of the inner casing,
(*e*) ventilation property,
(*f*) stability when kneeling.

Pads were then subjected to impregnation with coal dust and water and tested in a conditioning machine.

As a result of this work a specification for knee pads was produced which dealt with design, materials, and dimensions (National Coal Board, 1971). Manufacturers now make knee pads which meet this specification and which have been shown to be satisfactory in user trials, though consistently good straps have yet to be produced.

Boots

Boots for mining should be safe, should support the ankles and should be comfortable to wear (British Standard, 1961; 1966; 1970).

For dry conditions a boot is required with a strong but pliable sole of leather or equivalent synthetic material strongly joined to the upper which should give support to the ankle. A steel toe cap is essential and should preferably be an integral part of the boot. The boot must be light enough to be capable of being worn for a whole shift without discomfort or fatigue.

Leather boots, and sometimes clogs, were traditionally worn by miners. However in the last decade satisfactory man-made materials have become available although leather has not yet been replaced. Advances in production techniques have allowed manufacturers to produce a boot in which the upper and sole are moulded together in a continuous whole, thereby eliminating a source of weakness, namely, the separation of the upper from the sole before the boot was worn out. As slipping is a common cause of injury when walking underground it is important that the design of the sole be such as to counteract this tendency. Certainly the patterning of the synthetic sole is probably more effective in this respect than the studding of the conventional leather sole which was at one time universal. But boots are like car tyres—both are dangerous if worn until smooth and there is a greater tendency to slip in smooth-soled boots. To overcome this problem tungsten carbide studs, added mechanically to the finished boot, show promise.

In wet conditions, which may range from mud patches to shallow water, a different solution is required. Formerly in such conditions miners wore Wellington boots (gum-boots) which protected them only from water. These failed to protect the toes and the soles were too flimsy to prevent damage by sharp objects which might puncture the sole of the foot. However the rubber manufacturers have developed the safety Wellington with in-built steel toe cap and a reinforced, patterned sole—the whole of such stout construction as to be suitable for mining conditions.

Further progress in the design of mining boots is likely to lie in weight reduction if this can be achieved without loss of effectiveness.

Stockings

If stockings are too thin or holed, blistering or chafing of the skin is likely to result, which may lead to incapacitating sores. These are eminently preventable. Woollen socks, properly maintained, have been preferred for many years. However, recently socks made of polyester long-staple fibre have appeared which have the "feel" of wool. They are hard wearing, do not seem to interfere with the natural sweating of the feet and are worth considering as an alternative to wool. There can be no place for thin nylon or nylon-cotton socks in mining conditions. For both boots and socks correct fitting is important; many men are ignorant of the size they require and facilities to try on boots and socks should be available.

Miners Suits

If the employer takes no initiative in the provision of suits, miners are likely to wear a variety of old clothes, often unhygienic and sometimes unsafe. In some mining industries it has long been the practice to provide the miners with uniform clothing—the gain to their morale has already been mentioned. In a time when clothes consciousness is increasing there is no reason why miners' suits should not be well designed and good looking.

The type of suit to be adopted will depend on the working conditions. The overall or boiler suit is probably more widely used than any other— yet it was not designed for mining and is not ideal. In certain circumstances a two-piece outer garment will be the most suitable, in others the one-piece suit. Outside pockets or flaps which can catch in machinery should be avoided. Adequate gussets should be provided behind the shoulders to allow full mobility of the arms. Elastic gathering at wrists and ankles has advantages from the point of view of safety but may cause skin irritation in hot or dusty atmospheres. Suits should be wind-proof and waterproof under wet and cold conditions but, of course, largely impermeable cloth is unsuitable for hot conditions. Indeed, in very hot workings the miner will be most comfortable in boots, socks and helmet.

In mines where there is no risk of ignition of gas, nylon is a very suitable material for suits. When this danger exists nylon can, in dry air, produce electrostatic sparking and it would be prudent to use some such material as a blend of two-thirds terylene and one-third cotton.

It is not enough simply to provide miners' suits. Arrangement should be made for cleaning or laundering and maintenance; if laundry arrangements can also be made for underclothing so much the better.

The Administrative Aspects

It is always good management practice for issues of protective clothing to be controlled and administered so that the ensuing benefit can be related to the outlay. Each separate occupation, both underground and surface, should be reviewed and its requirements in terms of individual items of protective clothing listed.

At all but the smallest mines a protective clothing store should be established, either separately, or as part of the main store. The items available for issue should be displayed in showcases so that both workers and management can see at a glance the full range of protective equipment available and the alternatives within which some degree of personal preference may be exercised. The storekeeper, in addition to controlling the issue of each item should keep a record of all workers together with their current job description. From this and the master list described above he can see what each man is entitled to and, by noting the individual issues, what item he has had and how frequently replacements have been made. A scheme such as this gives management control over the issue of protective clothing and should form an integral part of the general mine safety programme.

References

Archibald, R. McL. (1964), "Men and machines, the medical problems of the sixties." *The Mining Engineer*, **50**, 118.
Archibald, R. McL., Kay, D. G. and Scott, E. (1966), "A study of beat elbow and related conditions at one colliery." *Occupational Health*, **28**, 118.
British Standard (1961, 1966, 1970), Specification 1870 (Pt. 1, 1970, Pt. 2, 1961, Pt. 3, 1966), *Safety Footwear*. British Standards Institution, London.
British Standard (1969), Specification 2091, *Respirators for Protection Against Harmful Dust, Gases and Scheduled Agricultural Chemicals*. British Standards Institution, London.
British Standard (1957), Specification 2826, *Industrial Safety Helmets (Heavy Duty)*. British Standards Institution, London.
Freeman, N. T. (1962), *Protective Clothing and Devices*, p. 20. United Trade Press, London.

National Coal Board (1971), Specification 581, *Knee Pads*. National Coal Board, London.

Roantree, W. B. (1957), "A review of 102 cases of beat conditions of the knee." *British Journal of Industrial Medicine*, **14**, 253.

Sharrard, W. J. W. (1963), "Aetiology and pathology of beat knee." *British Journal of Industrial Medicine*, **20**, 24.

Spencer, T. D. (1971), Personal communication.

Chapter 21
Ergonomics of Mining

Introduction

Ergonomics is the science concerned with the relationship between man and his occupation, equipment and environment. It participates in fitting the job to the man: thus it is concerned with selection and training, with machine design and use, with provision of optimum conditions for the task in question, and with improvements in efficiency and reduction of fatigue. Equally, it is concerned with the problems of men working in large organizations, and is especially concerned with aspects of communications and information flow in such situations (Sell, 1969; Ergonomics Research Society, 1970). Thus in general it is concerned with improving the efficiency of man–machine systems, and with improving individual well-being (Chapanis, 1970).

In mining, the work of the ergonomist clearly overlaps that of a number of other interests. In designing the layout of the mine, the engineer is concerned with the provision of clean air at the right temperature and humidity, adequate lighting, and with safety precautions, as well as with the efficient removal of ore or coal and the design of machinery for this end. Historically the engineer has made mining possible for human beings. Today the proper object is to provide conditions in which the miner is a contented individual operating at maximum efficiency.

This change in emphasis is of relatively recent origin, and ergonomics has yet to be applied fully to the mining situation. The change appears to arise from three new sets of circumstances. The first is the recent wide introduction of mechanization, with its remote control and automatic mechanisms, the second is the change in the social and educational status of mine workers in developed countries, and the third is the increase in knowledge concerning the capabilities and limitations of people and the effects upon productivity of adverse environments.

Mine Mechanization

It is common knowledge that the first phase of industrial development started with the introduction of steam in Britain in the late 18th century. This eliminated the use of human effort as a prime mover in the production process and replaced it by mechanical or electrical power under human control. This changeover, known as the Industrial Revolution, has nearly reached completion in advanced countries, so that from start to finish the Revolution is taking about 200 years. If a graph were made of the proportion of human physical work that has been replaced by mechanical power by a given date, the resulting curve would have roughly a sigmoid shape with a slow onset, a rapid rise and a gradual approach to final completion which will never quite be reached (Crossman, 1964). The mechanical horse-power now in use per head of the population of mine-workers vastly exceeds the single man-power that it has historically replaced.

Since mechanization is characterized by the fact that man ceases to be a source of power and becomes, for the most part, a controller of extraneous power, it might be concluded that the physical strain on man in a mechanized situation must also have been reduced.

The question now arises as to what extent this hypothesis is valid. Is muscle fatigue in mine mechanization really less and by how much relative to other occupations? Amounts of human work are usually expressed in calories since mechanical work is directly related to the amount of heat generated by chemical transformations. In such assessments, the muscular effort can be expressed as the calorie consumption related to a given length of time. Providing that the consumption is equally distributed over the whole mass of muscle the values obtained by this method are directly related to a person's aggregated physical strain. Thus the data concerning the average calorie consumption per minute can be used as a guide to the physical strain imposed by the work whether it is done with hand tools or machines. Table 1 shows a classification of work by Christensen (1953) based on energy expenditure and other body measurements.

Table 1

A Classification of Work Intensities (Christensen, 1953)

Grade of work	Energy expenditure (kcal/min)	Pulse rate (beats/min)	Oxygen consumed (l/min)	Rectal temperature (°C)
Very light	<2·5	<75	<0·25	37·5
Light	2·5– 5·0	75–100	0·5	37·5
Moderate	5·0– 7·5	100–125	1·0	37·5–38·0
Hard	7·5–10·0	125–150	1·5	38·0–38·5
Very hard	10·0–12·5	150–175	2·0	38·5–39·0
Extremely hard	>12·5	>175	>2·0	39·0

Many studies of energy expenditure in mining have been carried out (Durnin and Passmore, 1967). However, conditions of work in mines of developed countries are changing so rapidly that some traditional occupations can no longer be found and new tasks and working environments are in existence. An example in coal mining of the energy expenditure levels of activities measured prior to increases in mechanization and activities which have been created by the introduction of power loaders and powered supports is shown in Table 2.

Table 2

Values of Energy Expenditure of Mining Activities Prior To and Following the Introduction of Mechanization by Power Loading and Powered Supports

	Prior			Following		
		kcal/min				kcal/min	
Activity	*Range*	*Mean*	*Activity*	*Range*	*Mean*
Drilling coal	3·7– 9·5	6·1	Shearer driver	3·2–7·1	4·4
Erecting roof supports	4·2–10·1	6·7	Advanced powered supports and face		
Loading coal with shovel	5·1– 9·4	7·0	conveyor	3·1–5·9	5·1

While the levels of energy expenditure in these examples are lower following mechanization, the comparison is not as simple as it would appear from a straightforward examination of these figures. For instance, the time available for productive work at the coal face varies widely due to differing travelling times and delays. The introduction of the power loader changes the working situation from a self-paced or socially paced task to one paced by the machine. Furthermore, factors in the working situation such as the thickness of the seam, the space available for travelling through the face and the gradient may confound direct comparisons.

Estimates have been made of the total energy expenditure of miners during a shift for the same groups of workers as are represented in Table 2. These levels are shown in Table 3.

Table 3

Average Energy Expenditure per Shift before and after Mechanization

	Before		After	
Activity	kcal/shift	*Activity*	kcal/shift
Hand coal getters on longwall faces	1,990	Mechanized face team men	1,790
		Shearer drivers	1,780

By comparison of the values shown in Tables 2 and 3 with those of Table 1, it can be seen that mechanization appears at present to have reduced the energy expenditure level of miners whose work has been mechanized. But attention must be drawn to the fact that mechanization of individual face operations has in some cases *increased* the work required by groups of face workers, for example the work of ripping and packing for gate roads; moreover, the rate of advance of mechanized faces may be limited by the rate at which men can carry out this manual work. For this reason, considerable effort is now being made to design equipment to mechanize ripping and gate-side packing. With the growing need for increased productivity, higher work rates are being introduced in many types of mining, and these will inevitably raise the energy expenditure of individual workers in proportion to this demand.

Mine Automation

After reducing or dispensing with the need for human muscle power the remaining human activity in the production process (and often the limitation on it) is man's use of the information supplied by the human senses to the brain to guide and control the newly available mechanical power. Technological progress has now enabled this human activity to be replaced by machinery and the resulting 'automation' can be regarded as Phase 2 of the Industrial Revolution. It is the second stage in eliminating human labour and the contraints imposed on the production processes by limited human capacities.

John Diebold (1952), who originally made popular the term 'automation', used it to denote both automatic operation and the process of making things automatic. This role of machinery in replacing human control functions has been made clearer by such workers as Shannon (1948), Weiner (1968) and Von Neumann (1952). Essentially their idea is that information is something which can be measured in the same way as length or energy, that it is capable of being communicated from place to place through arbitrary physical signals forming messages, and that it is subject to such processes as coding, filtering and storage. In their theory, information is an entity which can be manipulated and used to control machinery much as energy can be generated as heat, transformed into chemical or electrical forms, stored and recovered, and finally used as kinetic energy.

With this concept in mind, all human mental processes involved in guidance and control, operating machinery, remembering, calculating, solving problems and planning, are 'information-processes'. These processes can be carried out equally well by mechanisms other than the human brain. To a limited extent machines can now make value judgements, although this aspect of human activity will not be replaced fully for a long time to come. Crossman (1964) has, therefore, proposed as a definition of automation "the replacement of human information processes by mechanical ones". While it may be a highly fallible prediction, if we can draw an historical parallel with the growth of mechanical power and use it to predict the percentage of human information-processes that will have been replaced by a given time in the future, we might expect automation to go to completion in perhaps 100 years from now.

Individual items of automatically controlled machinery have been employed underground for many years, for example, the sequence control of the earth-leakage protection, which automatically cuts off the power if a cable is damaged or equipment is overloaded. On the surface all winding engines should have automatic safety equipment which cuts off power and applies the brakes if the winder exceeds its proper speed, does not decelerate at the prescribed rate at the ends of the shaft, or attempts to overwind. Systems are in use where the control of mine car circuits, airlocks and winders has been centralized to give control from one point. Generally, these automatic operations are initiated by limit switches operating relay controlled electromagnetic contactor boards, but transistorized systems are also available.

The development of automation underground has not been as rapid as was first anticipated. The difficulties have been both economic and technical. The economic problems are related to the high capital cost of items of machinery and supports associated with automatic methods, compared to partial mechanization. This means that the automatic methods must produce higher outputs per shift than the existing partial mechanization methods to offset this extra capital cost. In thin coal seams and narrow workings there is increased likelihood of low utilization of equipment caused by geological conditions and engineering breakdowns which makes the situation especially difficult (Joint C.E.E./C.U.M.M. meeting, 1966). The technical problems are mainly in the development of sensing devices and the co-ordination of control. It appears that the progress which has been made with automatic steering of coal face shearer machines and the batch control of powered supports will continue, but it will be a long time before fully automatic systems are available for the extremely complex range of geological conditions which are met with underground. Therefore, remote control of machinery by men, together with improved communication methods are features of mining which will become more common in the coming century.

The Practical Application of Ergonomics in Mining

Since modern mining is a highly specialized occupation many aspects of ergonomics are included in other sections of this work. Certain aspects not covered in these sections are included here.

Lifting and Handling

While the use of human muscle power as a prime mover is being phased out, it is still employed in ripping, stable work, and much maintenance and recovery activities. The main contributions to these activities so far reported comprise studies of lifting methods, prop handling, and shovel design.

For lifting and handling certain basic principles have emerged and these have been incorporated in a number of training pamphlets and booklets. The principles are:

(i) Ensure that the load is within the miner's capacity (50 kg is a working upper limit).

(ii) Ensure that the ground is as level and clear of obstruction as possible.

(iii) Keep the load as close to the trunk as possible.

(iv) Use a full hand grip.

(v) Avoid stooping by bending the knees and hips.

(vi) Carry out lifts smoothly, avoiding jerks.

(vii) Plan the stacks of supplies so that heavy weights requiring repeated handling are stored at a convenient height, usually about 70 cm (Davis and Troup, 1964, 1966; I.L.O. Report, 1964).

With regard to shovelling, there exists a wide variety of shovel designs, many of these being jealously guarded as part of the mystique of a given mine. In principle the pan should allow the load to rest as near the handle as possible and the haft should be as short as conditions will allow and the handle should be well rounded to allow changes in wrist position (Davis, 1965). These factors ensure that the load exerts least leverage on the operator, and minimize the amount of muscular work involved in handling the shovel.

Machinery and Controls

Where the miner is in continuous control of machinery, every effort should be made to ensure that the seating and control systems match human needs. This has not been true of many machines in the past.

Seating should be designed for the tasks required on the particular machine, and should take account of regional variations in anthropometrical data. Much more knowledge is required before fully satisfactory seats can be designed for mining situations, as any given machine poses different problems from any other.

Controls can be divided generally into knobs and levers (input to the machine) and dials (feedback from the machine, or information displays). The relationships between these two divisions are subject to the stereotyped reactions of the operators: for instance, turning a rotary control clockwise is normally considered to increase the magnitude of the output, except in the case of liquid flow controls where the opposite is the case. In general, pointers on dials should move in the same direction as the controls, and a given control should be placed in clear association with its dial. Optimal sizes and shapes and required torques of knobs and levers, and the preferred layouts for information displays, are well described by Grandjean (1969).

Ergonomic Assessment of Working Situations

It would be impossible here to summarize fully the knowledge required for proper ergonomic appraisal of any given task. References should

22

be made to one or more of a number of text books giving general treatments of the subject (Fogel, 1963; McCormick, 1964; Murrell, 1965; Edholm, 1967; Sherrer, 1967 and Grandjean, 1969). The ergonomics of lighting has been described by Hopkinson and Collins (1970), and Burns (1968) has described noise and its effects on man. However, much research has been carried out on these and other topics which can be traced through the journal *Ergonomics*, *Human Factors*, *Ergonomics Abstracts* and its associated information services, and the new journal *Applied Ergonomics*.

Another approach to the application of ergonomics has been the production of handbooks and guide books which interpret research results so that industry can apply the findings without knowing the reasoning behind the recommendations (Woodson, 1964; Murrell, 1957; Kellerman, Van Wely and Willems, 1963; Morgan, Cook, Chapanis and Lund, 1963; Damon, Stoudt and McFarland, 1966). A few years ago a study was made of how engineers, provided with human factor hand-books, analysed design problems demanding consideration of human operator and other factors (Meister and Farr, 1967). While only ten designers were studied the results startled many people—it was concluded that the designers had little or no interest in human factor information or in the incorporation of human criteria in their designs. Meister and Farr considered that the situation was not one of unrelieved gloom and suggested that a way of improving the situation is to place emphasis on human factors not only in the training of design engineers, but also of those concerned with higher levels of management. In other industries the proper application of ergonomics has achieved startling increases in productivity and worker satisfaction, and both of these matters are of considerable concern to modern mining management.

A third approach has been the use of check lists (Burger and de Jong, 1962; 1967, and Krasucki, Cwirko, Kliks and Bajorek, 1969). A check list takes the form of a systematic list of queries about the human aspects of a work task. The check list may be used to examine a machine in being, or at the drawing office or prototype stage, or to study a work station in a system. This assessment normally covers both the physical and the mental requirements of the task. At the Second International Congress on Ergonomics in Dortmund (1964) an ergonomics system check list was published by an expert committee. This list was a basic attempt to evaluate work tasks and work environments and from it a number of more specialized lists have been compiled. There have also been a number of attempts to improve on this and other check lists which are in existence (Dirken, 1969). Examples of specialized subjects for which lists have been compiled from the Dortmund Committee's work include work design, traffic accidents, occupational health surveys, and machine tools. It is difficult to determine how widely check lists are in use but they do appear to be used commonly in the Netherlands; certainly great value should be attached to their increased use throughout the mining world.

The Human Factor

The view is often expressed that one of the reasons why scientific investigation into human performance waned during the 1930s was that machines were, on the whole, the limiting factor in performance. Today, there is evidence in mining that in some instances human performance is the limiting factor. Robens (1970) quotes the situation where, with identical geology, with identical organization and with groups of men identical in terms of age and physical fitness, the productivity of different units varies by a factor of 5. Of equal importance to productivity, although much more difficult to evaluate from a financial point of view, are the effects of the machine on man. Accordingly the qualities of machines and tools must be evaluated in terms not only of productivity but also of the physiological changes in people and the changes in health occurring at work as a result of physical or mental tension, or worsening of environmental conditions produced by a machine or by the technology of a process (Roscin, Mojkin, Razumov and Livcak, 1969). However, modern mining machinery manufacturers are still far from such an assessment of their products. Therefore, it is necessary to make provision for consideration of the physiological and health demands of miners in machinery and system design.

It has often been stated that the majority of industrial accidents can be attributed to human error. Many believe, therefore, that the greatest promise in the control of accidents lies in the elimination of the human element by complete mechanization. Although this has been accomplished in some fields the fact remains that a large percentage of the persons who are gainfully employed in mining operate or are exposed to some type of equipment or machine. It is necessary to think of men working with mining machines of all types, with conveyors, support systems, underground and surface locomotives, tractors, forklift trucks, tippers, vans, cranes, winding machines and so forth, as well as the small but important number of men still employing tools such as hammers and shovels. In some cases men are exposed to extremes of lighting, noise and vibration, or to harmful dusts, fumes and gas. Human error or failure may occur in any of these situations and environmental conditions or operating practices may increase the stress of work sufficiently to cause accidents. Where in the past a miner has had one simple job to do, his accident liability was low. With the need for each man to possess and use an increasing number of skills his accident liability is increased proportionally. As automation increases, the stresses on those working in control rooms will also increase and must be combated by careful design of control systems.

In addition to the established methods of mining accident prevention such as safety-education programmes, competitions and special safety equipment, accidents can be reduced in frequency by relating the mechanical design of the equipment to the biological and psychological characteristics of the operator. It seems reasonable to require that machines be designed from the man outwards, with the instruments and controls considered as extensions of his nervous system and body appendages. This implies that machines and working areas must be built around the operators rather than placing the workers in a setting without due regard for their requirements and capacities. Unless machines are so constructed it is foolish to attribute so many accidents to human failure.

In the introduction to this chapter it was emphasized that ergonomics has not yet been applied widely to mining. There is great scope for its application both in terms of the design of existing and new equipment and to the investigation of human performance, health and safety and of the work place. In France, ergonomics is being used to design controls of heading machines (Pternitis, Pean, Quinot and Rameau, 1967a and b) while in Poland, selection tests are being carried out on a wide scale for certain mining occupations (Spiewak, 1967).

Trends and Prospects

In conclusion the trends and prospects of the further development of the application of ergonomics in mining are:

(1) The increased use of ergonomic knowledge to aid in the design of new mining machinery and systems.

(2) The assessment of existing machinery by checklists and measurements and the modification or rejection of this machinery in relation, not only to productivity factors, but also to health and safety considerations.

(3) Increasingly, individual machines created to achieve one function are being used in combination. These combinations are becoming more complex. Their control is more than a management problem in terms of the relative cycle times of the component operations and of the relative capacities and maintenance requirements of the individual machines. Men will be required to work in these systems. Therefore, new techniques of ergonomics must be evolved to deal with such systems, in which the critical factors are likely to be the inspecting, sensing, monitoring, control and maintenance aspects of human performance.

(4) The use of anthropometry in mining machinery design is not satisfactory. It is well known that age, race and occupation affect body dimensions and capabilities. The designer must make

informed guesses from available data and must sometimes measure small groups himself, but such information is generally inadequate as a basis for determining dimensions for equipment which is to be mass produced for operation by miners. This problem is liable to become more acute with the introduction of larger and heavier equipment of all types.

(5) With changes in mine mechanization and automation it is obvious that the tasks that miners are required to perform are changing. New training methods are required. These training methods must be soundly based on job analysis and must include education in occupational health, safety, and ergonomic efficiency at all levels from mining apprentice to top management.

References

Burger, G. C. E. and De Jong, J. R. (1962), "Aspects of ergonomics. Job analysis." *Ergonomics*, **5**, 185.

Burger, G. C. E. and De Jong, J. R. (1967), "The ergonomic system analysis checklist (Dortmund 1964). Some critical remarks on further developments and results." *Ergonomics*, **10**, 717.

Burns, W. (1968), *Noise and Man*. John Murray, London.

C.E.E./C.U.M.M. (1966), Fourth Mining Engineering Conference "Read-in" on Thin Seam Mining. National Coal Board, London.

Chapanis, A. (1970), "Relevance of physiological and psychological criteria to man-machine systems." *Ergonomics*, **13**, 337–346.

Christensen, E. H. (1953), "Physiological valuation of work in Nykroppa iron works." In *Ergonomics Society Symposium on Fatigue*, ed. W. F. Floyd and A. T. Welford, pp. 93–108. Lewis, London.

Crossman, E. R. F. W. (1964),"European experience with the changing nature of jobs due to automation." Paper delivered at Conference of the Manpower Implication of Automation, Dec. 3–10, 1964. Organization for Economics Cooperation and Development, Manpower and Social Affairs Directorate.

Damon, A., Stoudt, H. W. and McFarland, R. A. (1966), *The Human Body in Equipment Design*. Harvard University Press, Cambridge (Massachusetts).

Davis, P. R. (1965), Report to the Medical Service, National Coal Board.

Davis, P. R. and Troup, J. D. G. (1964), "Pressures in the trunk cavities when pulling, pushing and lifting." *Ergonomics*, **7**, 465–474.

Davis, P. R. and Troup, J. D. G. (1966), "Effects on the trunk of erecting pit props at different working heights." *Ergonomics*, **9**, 475–484.

Diebold, J. (1952), *Automation: the Advent of the Automatic Factory*. Van Nostrand, New York.

Dirken, J. M. (1969), "Ergonomic checklist analysis of printing machines." In International Labour Office. *Ergonomics in Machine Design*, Vol. II, pp. 903–913. I.L.O., Geneva.

Durnin, J. V. G. A. and Passmore, R. (1967), *Energy Work and Leisure*. Heinemann, London.

Edholm, O. G. (1967), *Biology of Work*. Weidenfeld and Nicolson, London.

Ergonomics Research Society (1970), "The present position of the society." A report prepared by the Policy Committee.

Fogel, L. J. (1963), *Biotechnology: Concepts and Applications*. Prentice-Hall, New York.

Grandjean, E. (1969), *Fitting the Task to the Man*. Taylor and Francis, London.

Hopkinson, R. G. and Collins, J. B. (1970), *The Ergonomics of Lighting*. Macdonald Technical and Scientific, London.

International Labour Organization: Report on maximum permissible weight to be carried by one worker. Geneva, 1964.

Kellerman, F. T., Van Wely, P. A. and Willems, P. J. (1963), *Vademecum Ergonomics in Industry*. Cleaver Hum (Phillips Technical Library), London.

Krasucki, P., Cwirko, J., Kliks, I. and Bajorek, E. (1969), "Application of the ergonomic checklist to the evaluation of machine tasks." In: International Labour Office. *Ergonomics in Machine Design*, Vol. II, pp. 915–918. I.L.O., Geneva.

McCormick (1964), *Human Factors—Engineering*, 2nd ed. McGraw-Hill, New York.

Meister, D. and Farr, D. E. (1967), "The utilisation of human factors information by designers." *Human Factors*, **9**, 71–87.

Morgan, C. T., Cook, J. S., Chapanis, A. and Lund, M. W. (1963), *Human Engineering Guide to Equipment Design*. McGraw-Hill, New York.

Murrell, K. F. H. (1957), "Data on human performance for engineering designers." *Engineering*, London.

Murrell, K. F. H. (1965), *Ergonomics*. Chapman and Hall, London.

Pternitis, C., Pean, J., Quinot, E. and Rameau, R. (1967a), "Ergonomics research on a coal cutting machine for inclined formations." Abstract of paper contributed to 3rd I.E.A. Congress. *Ergonomics*, **10**, 721.

Pternitis, C., Pean, J., Quinot, E. and Rameau, R. (1967b), "Ergonomic study of a coal cutting machine for driving rooms in an inclined seam." In: International Labour Office. *Ergonomics in Machine Design*, Vol. II, pp. 619–832. I.L.O., Geneva.

Robens, Lord of Woldingham (1970), Opening address to the Conference on "Performance under Sub-optimal Conditions." *Ergonomics*, **13**, 531–534.

Roscin, A. V., Mojkin, Y. V., Razumov, I. K. and Livcak, I. F. (1969), "Hygiene and the physiology of work in the man-machine problem." In: International Labour Office. *Ergonomics in Machine Design*, Vol. II, pp. 619–631. I.L.O., Geneva.

Second International Ergonomics Association Congress, Dortmund (1964), Proceedings. Taylor and Francis, London.

Sell, R. G. (1969), "Ergonomics around the world." *Applied Ergonomics*, **1**, 42–44.

Shannon, C. E. (1948), "A mathematical theory of communication." *Bell system Tech. J.*, **27**, 379–423 and 623–656.

Sherrer, J. (Ed.) (1967), *Physiologie du Travail*. Masson, Paris.

Spiewak, F. (1967), "Application of psychology in the Polish coal-mining industry." In: International Labour Office. *Ergonomics in Machine Design*, Vol. II, pp. 1071–1076. I.L.O., Geneva.

Von Neumann, J. (1952), *Probabilistic Logics*. California Institute of Technology.

Weiner, N. (1968), *Cybernetics*. John Wiley and Sons, New York.

Woodson, W. E. (1964), *Human Engineering Guide for Equipment Designers*. University of California Press, Berkeley (California).

Chapter 22

Hygiene in Mines

Introduction

The importance of good hygiene in mines needs no emphasis. Yet the more obstinate hygienic problems are seldom discussed and are all too often solved in traditional and primitive ways.

In most mining countries laws and regulations relating to hygiene are few and the wording is brief. In theory there is no reason why the standards of hygiene in mines should not conform to those in other industries and should not be the same underground as above ground. In practice ingenuity may be required to achieve this, particularly in some underground conditions.

This chapter will be concerned with the provision of food and water, bathing facilities, the cleanliness of mine water, conservancy and the consequences of indifferent hygiene.

The solutions to problems of hygiene may vary considerably according to the geographical location and the type of mining.

Thus in metalliferous mining the structure of the surrounding rock is very solid facilitating the construction of spacious tunnels and rooms underground, whereas in coalmines the surrounding strata tend to be brittle and do not permit the construction of spaces without substantial support.

The Hygienic Provision of Food and Drink

Canteens and Meals

Canteens or dining halls where the workers can eat their own food or be served with meals are now established at most working places above ground. It is important for the general wellbeing that there should be a pleasant, clean room adjacent to the working area where meals can be enjoyed. The room should be well lighted and the ventilation adequate. Consideration should be given to lining the ceiling with acoustic tiles and the walls with noise absorbent materials.

This provision should be made both for surface and underground workers and for office staff. In some of the larger Scandinavian mines a hall is provided adjacent to the canteen in which the miners can lie down and rest for a short while after their meal.

As an alternative to the surface canteen the miners may bring their own food for consumption underground or they may be served with meals in suitable localities there. In either case there should be facilities for washing hands and face before eating. In some mines it may be practicable to establish underground canteens. Serving meals underground, however, creates special problems. The most convenient arrangement is for the food to be prepared above ground and transported underground while it is still hot. Otherwise the food can be vacuum-packed and frozen immediately after preparation and reheated underground before being served. To minimize washing up underground, the dishes can be brought to the surface after meals or disposable utensils may be used throughout. As will be discussed in more detail later it is important that water used in rest rooms for washing or in the canteens should not be mixed with the water which is going to be used in mining operations.

Drinking Water

An adequate supply of wholesome drinking water should be provided and maintained at suitable points, reasonably accessible to most work places in the mine. Where access is difficult water bottles may have to be used. Mine water seldom satisfies the requirements for drinking water. Generally speaking the water must be led underground from safe surface sources. The supply of drinking water is, of course, particularly important in hot deep mines where in dry heat a miner may require as much as 12 litres per day (MacFarlane, 1966). In these conditions the loss of salt in sweat has to be made good and it should be supplied, either added to the water in a concentration of 0·1 to 0·25 per cent or as salt tablets.

Bathing Facilities

Facilities for bathing after work should be available above ground. Communal shower baths have been established since the beginning of this century and are now to be found at virtually all mines. The baths should consist of two separate sections with clothes-lockers, one for home clothes and one for working clothes. The lockers should be well ventilated by mechanical means and heated if necessary to dry the clothes. The two sections should be separated by the bathing area with shower baths, approximately one to every fifteen lockers. In very wet mines it is common, and probably just as effective, to dry the working clothes by leaving them hanging on hooks suspended from the ceiling.

Epidermophytosis

Fungus infection of the feet ("athletes foot", epidermophytosis) is always a problem when many persons bathe together. Surveys carried out during 1953 and 1954 by the Medical Research Council in different British coalfields (Gentles and Holmes, 1957) showed conclusively that pit-head baths are primarily responsible for the prevalence of this disease. About one-third of the men using baths had epidermophytosis whereas less than 5 per cent of those bathing at home were found to be infected. In mines where nearly everybody wears rubber boots during working hours this is a troublesome condition and it is worth making considerable efforts to control it. The floors of the baths should be swept over with a mycostatic disinfectant daily. Wooden gratings and wooden floors should be avoided since they are very difficult to disinfect.

Everyone with fungus infection should be encouraged to seek medical treatment as soon as possible. Frequently miners do not recognize it as a fungus infection and try to cure it with soap and water or different home remedies. Epidermophytosis should therefore be included in regular health education.

The daily bath does much to prevent infection of small wounds and of the skin in general. At the same time the high standard of cleanliness which it entails is an important factor in the general wellbeing of the workers.

Cleanliness of General Mine Water

Pollution with Excreta

The usage of water in mines is high, in particular in connection with wet-drilling and water-spraying which are employed to suppress dust. In addition there is a variable flow of ground water in mine shafts and galleries. Water from these sources collects in the reservoirs which always exist in a mine in the form of old sumps.

It is common practice in mining to pump water from these reservoirs back into the system and in this way a continuous circulation of much the same water is maintained. On its way to the reservoir the water can become contaminated in different ways, particularly with human excreta, but also with excreta from animals, especially rats. In addition water from underground canteens may be led into the system and further contaminate the mine water. Contaminated water from above ground may also drain into the mine.

In this way the water in the mine becomes a medium in which pathogens from different sources may be augmented continuously and disseminated to all working places.

Pollution with Oil and Radon

Pollution of mine water may also be caused by oil and radon. Oil may leak from drilling equipment, from oil tanks underground or from diesel vehicles. It is not a health risk in this context. It may, however, create a serious nuisance if oil-polluted mine water is evacuated into water reservoirs above ground which are in communication with the public water supplies.

The important subject of radon in mines is dealt with in another chapter. Suffice it to say that radon pollution in the mine air may sometimes originate from radon dissolved in mine water (White, 1968). In that case it is very important to try to isolate the source of the radon polluted water so as to prevent the radon from contaminating all the water in the mine.

Separation of Polluted Water and Clean Water

In order to prevent bacterial pollution of the general mine water, all water discharged from floor washings in the underground canteens and rest rooms or from washing up should be sterilized by suitable methods (e.g. sodium hypochlorite) and not mixed in with the water used for mining operations.

Bacteriological Examination of Water

In spite of every effort it is often difficult or impossible to prevent contamination of the water in the mine. Regular bacteriological examinations should be carried out to obtain information on the situation. It is reasonable to set the same standards for the mine water as for water for washing and bathing (not as for swimming pools). The following limits apply:

			Presumptive coliform count per 100 ml water (in lactose bile-salt medium at 37°C)
Class	I	Excellent	<10
Class	II	Satisfactory	10–100
Class	III	Suspicious	100–1,000
Class	IV	Unsatisfactory	$>1,000$

From both aesthetic and hygienic points of view it is highly desirable to keep the mine water reasonably free from faecal contamination, as indicated by a presumptive coliform count of less than 100 bacilli per 100 ml water.

Purification of Water

If mine water for recirculation cannot be kept sufficiently clean by preventive methods it is necessary to consider either carrying out secondary purification of the water or abandoning underground reservoir water altogether and using clean water instead. In some cases this can be found within the mine (ground water); if not it must be led in from surface sources. Secondary purification of the water may entail filtration as well as sterilization. The best method of sterilization is probably chlorination with gas or sodium hypochlorite. Mechanical sandfilters should be considered as a supplement. They are relatively cheap to install and give a rapid delivery of water. Moreover, they occupy much less space than slow sandfilter beds though the running costs are high.

Conservancy: Disposal of Excreta

Most regulations concerning sanitation in mines assume that it is the duty of the manager of every mine to secure the provision of sufficient and suitable sanitary conveniences for the use of persons employed there. The word "suitable" has to be interpreted in the light of the contemporary sanitary standard of the community and of the technical problems of the mine.

In larger mines it is important that the toilets be placed at strategic points in the vicinity of the work places. Since mining is a dynamic process in which the miners are moved about a great deal it is most convenient for their toilets to be mobile and easily transportable.

All workers must be repeatedly informed about the need to use the proper toilets. It need hardly be said that they will not do so unless the toilets are properly maintained. Good sanitary discipline is, of course, of great assistance in preventing contamination of the mine water.

Technical Problems

The main problem when attempting to provide modern sanitation in mines is the difficulty of procuring satisfactory discharge conditions. The conventional sewage system which is used at the surface is based on the law of gravity and cannot be used in a mine. A traditional sewage system would also be too inflexible and expensive in relation to the time during which it would be used.

Alternative Types of Sanitation in Mines

In a small mine it is often sufficient to have the sanitary arrangements above ground and there are seldom problems in installing ordinary water closets there. In addition, urinals with collecting vessels should be provided within easy reach underground, and particularly at shaft bottom if transport delays are likely there. In larger mines toilet facilities must be available under ground. It is seldom practicable and often impossible to construct a common sewage system for ordinary water closets for reasons mentioned above. Large collecting tanks are required for the amount of flushing water used and the piping system is easily damaged and difficult to alter as work progresses.

In the majority of mines old-fashioned non-flush closets are still in use where the excreta are sterilized by chemical means (e.g. lime or disinfectant solutions). This is of course an acceptable, but by no means ideal, solution. It is difficult to keep the closets in good condition and they require continuous attention with regular emptying of the containers. The cost of this is high. The larger the mine the greater are the problems associated with any attempt to modernize the sanitary installation. In some mines, especially coalmines, it may be difficult or impossible to install any permanent toilets and the restricted space may permit only a very compact type. The chemical type used in caravans can nearly always be fitted in at strategic points even in coalmines.

The Vacuum-Sewage System

A possible solution to the sanitation problem, in larger mines at least, seems to be a new type of water closet which has been introduced in Sweden in the last decade. The system is called the vacuum-sewage system or the Liljendahl system, after its inventor (Essunger, 1962).

It has been employed in, among others, the large iron-ore mines at Kiruna in northern Lapland. In principle the vacuum-sewage system consists of a specially constructed water closet which is connected by a plastic pipe with a collecting tank in which a negative pressure is maintained. The sewage is propelled through the pipe by suction and the amount of water which is needed is only about one tenth of what is used in conventional flushing systems. The pipes are of plastic material, 50 or 63 mm in diameter, and are suspended from the roof of the passageways by wires. They are easily accessible so that removal and rearrangement can easily be carried out.

The actual vacuum closet resembles an ordinary water closet but there is no water tank and no conventional flushing takes place. The pressure in the pipe which connects the closet with the collecting tank is always negative. When the mechanism is operated by pulling a lever powerful suction is applied to the bowl and the contents—about 1·2 litres of water plus excreta—are rapidly evacuated and led directly to the collecting tank. The tank is emptied by a sewage vehicle every 10 or 12 days.

In the Kiruna mines 800 men are employed under ground on each shift and some 70 vacuum toilets are in use at three levels underground. Each level has its own pipeline system and a collecting tank. The most remote vacuum closet has a pipeline 2,700 metres long. About 25 closets are connected to each main collecting pipe but the number can be increased to 80. The majority of the vacuum closets are situated in the vicinity of underground canteens where there are also facilities for hand-washing and rest rooms. As yet no experiments have been made with more permanent installations in the immediate vicinity of the rock face where the risk of structural damage is considerable. It is thus not possible to avoid the use of dry closets at these exposed places in the mine.

The vacuum sewage system not only offers an attractive and hygienically satisfactory solution to the problem of sanitation underground; it is also more economical as the maintenance costs in connection with dry closets far exceed those of the vacuum sewage system.

Diseases Associated with Defective Sanitation

Most underground workers come in close contact with mine water and if the water is contaminated with faeces it carries an obvious health risk. The pathogenic organisms derived therefrom may infect the skin. The wrists and neck, where wet working clothes rub against the skin, are especially at risk.

The development of abscesses is a problem in many African mines. In one investigation among Bantu mine workers Staphylococcus aureus was isolated from 80 per cent of skin infections and Streptococcus faecalis from the skin of as many as 72 per cent of the workers examined (Sonnenfeld, 1969).

Contamination of mine water used for dust suppression would seem to be a possible vehicle of disease transmission—bacteria and viruses could be inhaled and ingested with the water aerosols.

The two diseases which are clearly associated with defective sanitation in mines are leptospirosis (Weil's disease) and ankylostomiasis.

Leptospirosis

This disease is caused by the species of spirochaete, leptospira. World-wide in distribution it is endemic in rodents and is transmitted to man by their urine, or by mud or stagnant water which have been contaminated.

Infection may occur through the intestinal tract or the spirochaete may penetrate apparently unbroken skin. Where miners are at risk they should be safeguarded by protective clothing, boots and gloves. Washing facilities should be provided adjoining the canteens and a good standard of food hygiene should be maintained.

Leptospirosis is now uncommon in mines in Europe and the United States, but it is a constant potential risk. The last serious outbreak in Great Britain occurred in 1951–1952. A total of twenty-three miners were affected and of these, nine died (Roberts, 1952, 1953).

Because leptospirosis is so closely associated with the presence of rats their extermination is the key to prevention. It is difficult to prevent rats from entering mines and if they find something to eat there it is nearly impossible to avoid infestation. All too often rats in mines are accepted as an inevitable nuisance. Indeed in some places they are protected as they may give warning in case of an inrush of water.

To prevent leptospirosis all parts of the mine below ground must be kept free from rats and mice. Food scraps and rubbish should not be left about. The mines in Kiruna were infested with rats up to 1946. Since then all mineworkers have had their meals served daily in underground dining halls and the mines have remained uninfested. When horses were used for transport careless storage of their fodder underground encouraged invasion by rats. Drifts opening onto the surface near habitations can increase the risk of infestation by rats and should be protected accordingly. Rats will eat filth of any sort, including human faeces, and can adapt themselves to extremes of temperature. Usually it is Rattus norvegicus (the brown rat) that is found in mines. It is the larger and clumsier of the two rat species and can be recognized by its small ears.

The most effective method of killing rats is by poisoned bait. Prebaiting to accustom them to the food is usually recommended. Otherwise the best results are obtained by keeping the amount of bait to a minimum because the food is then eaten more quickly. Rats that survive poisoned bait will not take the same bait again and it is therefore necessary to change both the bait and the poison. The annihilation of rats must be systematically and continuously carried out. Rat destruction both underground and on the surface in the vicinity of the mine should always be coordinated.

Ankylostomiasis

Hookworm disease is also known as miners' anaemia or tunnel-workers' anaemia. The cause was traced to the hookworm by Perroncito (1880).

There are two types of hookworm, Ankylostoma duodenale and Necator americanus. The eggs are passed in the faeces from an individual suffering from the disease. Moist warm soil or mud is the ideal medium for development of the ovum. The optimum temperature is 25°C; the larva will not hatch below 15°C. The larva passes from the soil or from contaminated water and penetrates the human skin. After being transported in the blood stream to the heart and lungs it finally reaches the small intestine where it remains. Each female then starts to produce about 6,000 eggs a day.

The disease is prevalent within a belt 35 degrees north and south of the equator. It is not uncommon, however, in the warm conditions of deep mines and tunnels in temperate climates and it is still said to be found in the collieries of Northern France, Belgium and Hungary. It is also found in mines in Spain, Russia, Southern United States and Central America. It is common in mines in Africa, India, and Malaysia.

Hookworm disease may spread in a mine when the water is polluted with faeces from a hookworm sufferer. The important thing, of course, is to avoid such pollution by good sanitation. Prevention starts with the medical examination of all applicants for employment. The stools should be examined for ova at this time and, in endemic areas, also at regular intervals as part of general health examinations. Rubber boots must always be worn in the mine. Most important of all, but at the same time most difficult to enforce, is strict sanitary discipline.

Mycotic Infection

An important fungal infection associated with mining is sporotrichosis (Bengtsson, 1971). This is one of the deep mycoses and is a chronic subcutaneous infection with little tendency to suppurate caused by the sporotrichum schenckii. The usual presenting lesion is an indolent papule which may ulcerate. The disease is found in most tropical regions with a high humidity and a median temperature around 16–20°C, particularly in the south and west of Africa. In Brazil and Mexico epizootics are quite common among domestic animals and rodents. Cases are found mainly among people whose occupation brings them in contact with soil or decaying wood as in mining, especially coal mining. Infection takes place when the organism is introduced by trauma into the skin, the hand, arm or foot being often involved. Sporotrichosis is not uncommon among miners. There was an extensive epidemic of about 3,000 cases in 1941–1943 among gold miners in the Transvaal. Prevention consists in treatment of the woodwork in the mine with copper salts to prevent decay caused by moisture and fungus infection.

Insect Infestations

In recent years several unusual insect infestations of British coal mines have been noted (Evans, Roantree and Thomas, 1971). In each case the infestation seems to have originated in timber props. Several varieties of insect were involved. The most troublesome was the flying black ant, Ponera punctissima Roger, which both bites and stings. Sawflies of the species Urocerus auger auger, though apparently incapable of stinging or biting, were suspect of causing skin irritation. In one mine, house flies were found breeding in rotting wood underground—they settled on the miners' food during meal breaks.

Such infestations can be effectively terminated by appropriate insecticides.

References

Bengtsson, E. (1971), Personal communication.

Essunger, G. (1962), "Sewage system consuming very little water." *Proceedings of United Nations Conference on the Application of Science and Technology for the benefit of the less developed areas.* United Nations, New York.

Evans, D. L., Roantree, W. B. and Thomas, D. J. (1971), Personal communication.

Gentles, J. C. and Holmes, J. G. (1967), "Foot ringworm in coal-miners." *British Journal of Industrial Medicine,* **14,** 22.

MacFarlane, W. (1966), "Content and turnover of water in Bantu miners acclimatizing to humid heat." *Journal of Applied Physiology,* **21,** 978.

Perroncito, E. (1880), "Observations helmintuologiques et recherches experimentales sur la maladie des ouvriers de St. Gothard." *C. r. hebd. Seanc. Acad. Sci., Paris,* **XL,** 1373.

Roberts, H. W. C. (1952), Report of H.M. Inspector of Mines for 1951. H.M.S.O. London.

Roberts, H. W. C. (1953), Report of H.M. Inspector of Mines for 1952. H.M.S.O., London.

Sonnenfeld, E. D. (1969), "An investigation into wound infection and abscess formation in a mine." *South African Medical Journal*, **43,** 705.

White, F. T. (1968), "The total environment of mining." *Occupational Health Review*, **20,** 21.

Chapter 23

Attendance and Absence

Introduction

This chapter is about performance at work in general as well as about attendance and absence which are the first measures of it. The point is important because improvements in one aspect of performance can be offset by deterioration in another. If men are persuaded by incentives or by punishment to attend more than should properly be asked of them, the increased attendance will sooner or later be offset by lower productivity, by disputes or strikes or by miners leaving, or leaving the more arduous occupations at an earlier age.

The practical effects of absence must also be assessed with caution. They are likely to be less serious where trained men are in plentiful supply. The cost of absence will be lower where no allowances are paid for injury or sickness or where men are engaged for work from day to day. When attendance fluctuates greatly the disturbance to production may be more than the absolute amount of absence may suggest; conversely, when periods of much absence can be anticipated, such as before or after public holidays or in association with other strongly established customs, the practical effects will be less serious.

Absence may be the result of fatigue arising from the nature of the work or from its physical environment, the hours spent at it, inadequate training, poor supervision or inappropriate incentives. It may reflect differences in the customs, expectations and attitudes to work of miners and their employers. It may be the result of underlying sickness whether or not the absence is ascribed to sickness. This chapter discusses first, the broad nature of the problem as a whole, secondly, the chief factors known or suspected to contribute to it, thirdly, the essentials for its measurement and for statistical analysis.

The Broad Nature of the Problem

The Theoretical Dilemma

In England the problem of miners' absence from work has been a subject of controversy probably for as long as coal or other minerals have been mined. Early references appear in writings of the 16th century; more formal evidence about its extent, and argument about its causes, appear regularly in reports of Royal Commissions and other public inquiries from the beginning of the 18th century onwards;

organized research has produced a large body of literature on the subject.

One reason for the controversy lies in the failure on the part of most investigators to take account of the full range of factors that need to be considered in the diagnosis of an absence problem. But reports of past inquiries, including organized research, show another persistent cause to lie in the confusion between the moral and the physiological aspects of the problem. The question why people do not come to work as often as a mine is open for it has in the past often been treated as a purely moral one: that they could if they would. It has usually been asked without due regard to the physiological limitations to continuous hard work: whether they would if they could. The moral approach finds typical expression in the belief that people only work as much as they need in order to maintain the standard of living to which they are accustomed. The physiological limitations have been becoming clearer as a result of a long series of researches represented in the United Kingdom by those of the Health of Munition Workers Committee from 1915 to 1918, the Medical Research Council's Industrial Fatigue Research Board, later the Industrial Health Research Board, between 1919 and 1946, the National Coal Board's study of miners' attendance and absence from 1952 to 1958 and in the implications of many laboratory studies.

Statistical Illustration of the Dilemma

Confusion over the moral and physiological aspects of the problem has been encouraged by the widespread convention of expressing the days men spend away from work as a percentage of the days the mine was open to them. The use of such a single measure is misleading (Buzzard and Liddell, 1963a). If a mine is open four days in the week and a man attends all four, he has no absence. But if it is open for five days a week and he stays away one day every four weeks, his average attendance will have risen to four and three quarter days a week but he will have had $\dfrac{1 \times 100}{20}$ or five per cent lost time. If the mine is open for six days in the week and he stays away two days every four weeks his attendance will have risen to five and a half days a week on average but he will have had $\dfrac{2 \times 100}{24}$ or eight and a third per cent lost time.

The time men spend at work is increased by overtime and this distorts the measure further. Some miners, not in the most arduous occupations, have thus been found to have attended the equivalent of eight days a week if the actual hours they spent in the mine are expressed in terms of the seven and a half hour day prevailing at the time. Expressing hours lost as a percentage of the hours available for work does not overcome the distortion. Absence and attendance normally rise and fall together if not in the same ratio. No single index of the ratio of days or time lost to days or time available for work provides an adequate measure of absence unless the time available is constant. If it is constant, the ratio, as a measure, is unnecessary.

Since the medical officer's first concern is with the miners' health and safety, the physiological limitations to attendance should be the first focus of his inquiry. His investigation of an absence problem should begin with the question: how much work should reasonably be expected on average of men in that occupation working in that environment and what individual variations should be expected from the average?

The Factors that Affect Performance

Attendance and absence are influenced by a wide range of factors which may operate directly, indirectly, separately or in combination. Since space is limited these are discussed briefly under the headings most likely to be helpful in guiding a medical officer in his investigations

The Effort Spent at Work

The series of researches mentioned earlier shows the importance of the effort spent at work in causing absence. For some purposes this is best assessed by direct physiological measurement but this is seldom practicable and can be misleading.

The work itself. Work by hand where the mineral is extracted is normally more strenuous than most work elsewhere underground and this in turn is normally more strenuous than work on the surface of a mine (Buzzard and Liddell, 1963b). Particular forms of work vary in the effort they entail within these categories. The effects of mechanization need to be examined carefully since mechanization may only reduce the number of people needed to do the work without lessening the effort of those who remain to do it. For example, the energy spent in handling certain machines used for cutting and loading coal has been found equal to that expended in hand filling.

Posture. Lying, kneeling, crouching and standing while at work are postures commonly found in mining and involve the use of different sets of muscles both in maintaining static posture and in doing the work. Posture has particular importance whenever new men are brought into a mine or are transferred from one work place to another. For example, a man used to working lying down is at a serious disadvantage if transferred to less cramped conditions to work with new colleagues used to working upright or in some other posture. He gets more tired, he loses face among his colleagues and he loses face at home through loss of earnings. Training, graduated introduction to full work loads and protection of earnings until that stage is reached are among the remedies to be considered.

Travelling underground. Posture also increases the effort of travelling underground; oxygen consumption may be doubled or trebled by walking in stooping postures and effort is similarly increased by walking on rough surfaces including sleepers laid for car rails (Bedford and Warner, 1955). Walking distances in British mines can vary from a few hundred yards to three or four miles.

Travelling home from work adds to the time spent at work in the sense that it is not recuperative. Such journeys may amount to more than two hours a day.

Temperature affects effort and performance and work can be shown to be affected over and below a quite narrow range of temperature. Thus accidents in factories in one study were found to be more frequent above 21°C dry bulb and below 18°C and in another to be so above 23°C and below 21°C (Vernon, 1936). Miners' accidents were more frequent and increased in severity above 23°C (Vernon and Bedford, 1927). Laboratory studies have shown deterioration in perception in warm and cold environments (Mackworth, 1950). Temperature must be taken into account for its effects on travelling underground as well as on the work itself. Humidity and air velocities alter the physiological effects of temperature and the reader is referred to other chapters and the sources quoted in the bibliography for discussion of the measurement of temperature as it affects performance.

Pace and rhythm of working affect the effort that a man expends and is related to age, training, experience and custom (Lehmann, 1950; Clark and Dunne, 1955; Welford *et al.*, 1951). For example, where custom gives older people priority in entering the better paid and usually more arduous occupations, a slower pace and steadier rhythm of working is likely to be found compared with a situation where no such priority is given. Rhythm is especially disturbed by the frequent interruptions which are common in working underground. Since their incidence and duration are usually unpredictable, unrecorded short interruptions can be as disturbing in this way as longer ones.

Hours worked. The time spent in different forms of work in different physical environments has already been noted as a factor influencing absence.

Cumulative effects. Factors contributing to increased effort are inter-related and cumulative. The investigator should take account of the total effect of all the factors he can identify as well as the effects of each one individually.

Individual differences in men's physical capacity whether innate, or due to training, habituation, age or disability are clearly important in assessing the effort spent at work.

Comfort

Although there is little evidence that discomfort directly causes absence, its indirect effects may be considerable, especially where the sources of discomfort appear to miners to be remediable but are not attended to. Of the factors already mentioned as affecting effort, *posture* affects comfort and *temperatures* can be uncomfortably hot or cold.

Water falling from roofs or lying in pools is a source of discomfort especially where men lie or kneel to work.

Dust as a cause of pneumoconiosis is dealt with in another chapter; measures of dust in this connection concern small particles only (less than 10 microns). It is the large dust particles not routinely measured in pneumoconiosis surveys which are important causes of discomfort by irritating eyes and mucous membranes. Dust can be intensified where explosives are frequently in use and discomfort is worse where air velocities are high. There is usually less dust in the atmosphere in wet environments but it may then form a coating on skin which may increase body temperatures.

Air velocities can feel like high winds and cause discomfort, especially at low temperatures and, as seen above, where there is much dust.

Toxic fumes from firing explosives underground can cause discomfort and headaches to the men who fire them and to others present in the vicinity. More severe discomfort with marked headaches can be caused by absorption of some kinds of explosives through the skin and is more prominent in warm environments when men are sweating (Powell and Lomax, 1960).

Visibility in mines is seldom good and can be made worse by dust, fumes, water vapour and water falling from roofs.

Noise is not a common feature in most forms of mining but can be considerable near conveyor transfer points and other machinery. Compressed air motors and pneumatic borers are a special source of noise which may cause transient deafness at least. Noise also needs to be considered for the way in which it can hide warning sounds of the movements of roofs and supports.

Clothing as protection. Even in quite warm environments extra clothing may be worn to prevent chilling where air velocities are high; waterproof clothing may be worn in wet environments; trousers may be worn instead of shorts to protect legs from falling debris especially where men work standing; extra clothing may be worn to protect backs and shoulders when working in low seams. While a protection rather than a cause of discomfort, extra clothing worn for such reasons needs to be considered because it affects the interpretation of measurements of temperature.

Training and Experience
Inadequate training can lead miners to fail when transferred to new forms of work or new environments. As noted earlier, good training and graduated introduction to new forms of work can prevent fatigue and social stigma, both of which may be a cause of absence.

Age
While physical capacity declines with age the relationship to absence is complex partly because of the different style of working noted earlier and partly from other inter-related factors including differences in financial responsibilities and leisure needs discussed below. On average, older men tend to take fewer but longer absences (Buzzard and Shaw, 1953; London Transport Executive, 1956).

Incentives and Pay
It is difficult to substantiate the theory that men work only as much as they need to support the standard of living to which they are accustomed. In the first place, men attend more when more work is available and failure to attend as much as is possible can equally be explained in terms of fatigue. Similarly, although there is usually more absence in the better paid occupations these are usually the most arduous as well. Neither incentives to increase attendance nor fines to discourage absence have been found to have more than short-term effects (Buzzard and Liddell, 1963c). But financial considerations may alter the amount and pattern of attendance for different people in other ways.

Financial responsibilities. Younger men with few financial responsibilities tend to be away from work more often than older men with growing families but care is needed before ascribing this to financial considerations alone (Buzzard and Liddell, 1963d). Older men are more settled in their style of working and well habituated to its conditions while their social life is apt to be more settled too. Younger and unmarried men have more need for leisure.

Allowances for injury or sickness may be expected to increase the total amount of absence from all causes and also to change the reasons given for it. Studies in mining and in other industries do not suggest that malingering is an important cause. In the first place, allowances for sickness or for injury enable men to afford the convalescence they may need for full recovery; in the long term this may enable them to remain at work and in the more arduous forms of it to a later age (Buzzard and Shaw, 1952; Denerley, 1952). Secondly, an increase in the absences ascribed to sickness or to injury is as likely to be due to the greater care taken by the recording clerk as to the claims men make themselves (Buzzard, 1968).

Pay day. The day and shift on which wages are paid is an important consideration in determining the days on which absence will be greatest.

Deterrents. Many attempts have been made throughout the history of mining to reduce absence by fines and punishments but there is no evidence that they have had any substantial or permanent effect. They can, however, alter the incidence and duration of absences. It was shown in one study (Buzzard, 1968) that men who were reprimanded and threatened with suspension subsequently took the same amount of absence as before but in less frequent absences of longer duration.

Holidays and Length of Working Year

The effects of daily or weekly hours of work in causing absence have been noted earlier. The length of the working year must also be considered in interpreting historical evidence about absence and in comparing different countries. In England, the holidays that miners took were usually more frequent than they are today even until well into the 19th century; periods of sustained full employment in mining never exceeded five years at a stretch until after the beginning of the second World War and were not equally spread throughout the country. Technological advances in engineering, ventilation and transport have enabled mines to stay open longer than in the past. The differences in the amount of holidays customarily taken in different countries in Europe are substantial.

Shift Cycles and Starting Times

The influence of shift work on diurnal rhythm, on fatigue and on social life is too large a subject to be entered into here except to note that different patterns of shift working affect absence. The starting and finishing times of shifts also need to be considered, especially in their relation to transport arrangements (Walker and de la Mare, 1971).

Selection of the Working Group

Although people differ in their individual attendance, one person is normally consistent in the attendance he maintains over long periods (Buzzard and Liddell, 1963e). The average attendance of a group of people will therefore be affected by the composition of the group. Thus one group may tolerate the presence of bad workmen which another would reject; custom may reserve some forms of work for older and experienced men or may allow the less experienced to do it. Management may deliberately influence the selection of men working in different occupations. Inter-relations with other factors are complex. For example, better selected teams tend to be found in the most productive places in a mine and less well selected teams to be found in the less popular ones.

Supervision

The quality of supervision influences attendance and is closely related to other factors such as the pace of work and safety. Where access is easy a supervisor can attend to more people at a time than in difficult conditions when it will take longer to see each man. The supervisor's other duties, such as inspecting roadways, affect the time he can give to the men under his charge. Well selected and experienced teams need little or no attention while poorly selected ones need much. The personality and training of the supervisor are important.

Illness

Illness is sometimes underestimated as a cause of absence. Even when the apparent reasons for absence are carefully recorded, much absence not ascribed to illness may have been due to it in some degree. Increasing amounts of absence by one man should be investigated carefully lest they prove a symptom of approaching illness, of illness in the family or other difficulties for which he might be given help. Similarly, marked increases in absence of any category among a mine population as a whole may be the first sign of epidemic illness.

Customs and Attitudes of Miners

Despite attempts to relate absence and other measures of performance to the social histories of particular mines, there is little evidence that custom is an important factor influencing the amount of absence as a whole. It may, however, do so and needs to be considered especially in defining absence problems in industrially underdeveloped countries. For example, where miners are engaged to work at a mine far distant from their homes, their visits to their tribes and families may be conceived as absence or as resignation from that mine followed by later re-engagement. As noted earlier, custom can influence the times at which absence is likely to be greatest.

Size of Mine, Morale and Other Factors

Researches in mining and in other industries have suggested many other factors contributing to absence. They include poor morale associated with the size of an organization, mine or working group (Revans, 1960) and various assumptions about unconscious desires to withdraw from unattractive work and even to sustain injuries to do so (Hill and Trist, 1953). The distribution of absence on different days of the week has similarly been treated as a measure of morale (Behrend, 1951). As guides to the practical investigation of an absence problem theories of these kinds need to be treated with discretion. In the first place, the statistical evidence is capable of alternative interpretations: deep mines, for example, tend to be large but tend also to be hot and to have difficult geological conditions; large working groups are more likely to tolerate poor workmen. Secondly, the effects of size are assumed to be due to greater difficulties of communication and of supervision leading to poor morale, while any theories about desires to stay away from work raise the question of what makes work unattractive. For practical purposes, the theories are as yet of little help and the investigator would be well advised to look for underlying causes directly on the lines suggested.

Essentials for Statistical Investigation

Problems of absence arise because too many people are away from work, some people are away too long, the daily fluctuations are too great, or the direct cost of absence appears to be too high. The search for causes has accordingly been dominated by statistical comparisons between mines, occupations, groups of people and individual men in relation to factors of the kind discussed above. The medical officer can go a long way in identifying and alleviating causes of absence by their systematic study without recourse to statistical analysis. But, if he is to persuade others of his diagnosis or evaluate the remedies suggested, he will need some acquaintance with the main essentials for statistical analysis of absence problems.

Taking Account of Effort

Since effort is one factor influencing attendance comparisons of groups of men must take account of their occupations and of the physical environments in which they are pursued. Since men may change their occupations and work places often, account must also be taken of the time each man spends in each.

Individual Differences

Since absence has been shown to be influenced by age, experience, physical capacity and individual financial responsibilities, comparisons must take account of the way these things are distributed among the members of the groups compared. The investigator also needs to know whether a high absence rate can be ascribed to all the members of the group or to a few with unusual amounts of absence.

Statistical Definitions

Statistical measures of performance at work are easily and often markedly distorted by differences in the way that definitions are applied, however carefully the instructions have been drafted. They include the way that overtime is treated, the way that part time or seasonal workers are treated in the populations compared, the length of time men are treated as absent before being taken off the records as having left the mine. In a study made in 1931 (Vernon, 1931) the much lower absence rates of Scottish compared with English miners were found to be due to the shorter time that men absent from work remained on the statistical records in Scottish mines compared with English ones and by the exclusion in most Scottish mines of absence due to injury and the frequent exclusion of absence due to illness. Large differences in the absence in collieries and coalfields in Britain in 1952 could often be explained as due to differences in statistical definitions and in calculations which are difficult to discover from superficial examination (Buzzard and Liddell, 1963f).

Daily Variations

Unless there is a good reserve of trained men in occupations of low priority daily variations in attendance can be especially disturbing to the efficient running of a mine but great care is needed in their measurement. In Europe, for example, Monday is commonly the day on which there is most absence on average if large populations are studied (Behrend, 1951). But any daily patterns can be found in particular mines, occupations, work places or on different shifts, while averages can conceal marked differences between the patterns of individual men. The days when wages are paid, transport systems, occupation, local custom and age are among the many factors that affect such distributions. Remedies suggested from the study of large populations can be ineffective or do harm when applied in particular instances.

The Records Needed for Statistical Analysis

The following information is needed about each man if statistical analyses are to take account of the factors which have been discussed in this chapter (Buzzard and Radforth, 1964).

Age;
An indication of domestic responsibilities—tax codes can sometimes be a useful index;
Address, from which can be derived length of journey from home to work and possible differences in custom;
Occupation, place of work and time spent in each;
Number of days worked, overtime, date of start and finish of an absence;
Occupation and place of work at the time the absence started;
The ostensible cause of absence;
The date of leaving the mine and, if possible, the reason for it.

The information should be on a separate record for each man whether on manuscript cards, punched cards or computer tape. Often the wages record, or copies of it, with a few additions can provide all the information that is needed, but the recording clerk must be trained to do the work and must be supervised. Accuracy and consistency in the use of statistical definitions should be checked by careful examination of sample records.

This minimum information for each man can then be supplemented by the records the medical officer has compiled of the health of individual men, his knowledge of the operation of the mine, and the work and its conditions.

Analysis

The records or copies of them must be sent to some central point for analysis. Statistics which have been compiled locally will not be comparable and will not allow adequate account to be taken of factors that need to be considered when examining specific questions. Some of the statistical techniques to enable those making comparisons to take account of the factors which have been discussed are described in the sources quoted in the bibliography (Buzzard and Liddell, 1963g; Martin, 1971).

Conclusion

So much has been written about absence from work in general and miners' absence in particular that the subject has acquired a spurious identity as some "disease" for which there must be a cure. But the opinions about its nature and its real importance remain so varied and contradictory as to make so simple a concept entirely inadequate.

Two things especially emerge from the controversy. First, attendance at work and absence are exceptionally difficult to describe and measure satisfactorily and this increases the difficulty of identifying underlying causes of differences in attendance. Secondly, so far as they can be identified, the underlying causes are numerous.

This chapter has stressed the physiological factors limiting attendance rather than the psychological or sociological factors contributing to absence. This is partly because they also affect health and partly because, where work and the physical environments are arduous, these causes will be proportionately more important. Accordingly, before considering other remedies for absence, the medical officer should consider whether effort could be reduced by improving the working methods and the physical environment, by more careful selection of men for particular occupations or by better training for them. If warranted, these should be the first remedies to suggest to the manager of a mine.

Recommendations for increasing men's attendance through psychological or sociological approaches rest on less sure ground and also vary greatly in importance from one mine and one working group within it to another. Certain general suggestions can, however, be put forward on the basis of the accumulation of studies in mining and other industries over many years.

(i) The physiological limitations discussed in this paper and sources of discomfort have a separate psychological importance. Failure to attend to things a man believes to be remediable increases frustration and dislike of the work he has to do. If, therefore, they cannot be remedied every effort should be made to ensure that the reason is understood.

(ii) Training, as well as improving physical ability to perform a job, can increase interest and pride in its performance. So can the encouragement and help provided by efficient and interested supervision. Initial training, training on the job and supervision should always be examined from this standpoint.

(iii) People work better if they know where they stand. For example, although it may not be possible to guarantee security of employment, men should be given the fullest information possible about the mine they work in and the matters which affect employment in it to enable them to plan their own lives properly. Failure to keep people properly informed is a major factor in deteriorating morale.

(iv) One way of helping to ensure both the above types of communication is to encourage senior managers to spend much time visiting work places underground to answer questions and to be seen to be involved.

Other things which can often be brought to the attention of management in particular instances include alternating strenuous with lighter work (where payment systems permit it), adjusting shift times to suit men's preferences and the transport systems and improving the transport of men from home to work.

References

Bedford, T. and Warner, C. G. (1955), "The energy expended while walking in stooping postures." *Brit. J. Industr. Med.*, **12**, 290.

Behrend, H. (1951), *Absence under Full Employment*. University of Birmingham, Studies in Economics and Society. Monograph A.3.

Buzzard, R. B. and Shaw, W. W. J. (1952), "An analysis of absence under a scheme of paid sick leave." *Brit. J. industr. Med.*, **9**, 282.

Buzzard, R. B. and Liddell, F. D. K. (1963a), "Coalminers Attendance at Work," p. 7, *Med. Res. Mem. No. 3*, National Coal Board, London.

Buzzard, R. B. and Liddell, F. D. K. (1963b), "Coalminers Attendance at Work," p. 92, *Med. Res. Mem. No. 3*, National Coal Board, London.

Buzzard, R. B. and Liddell, F. D. K. (1963c), "Coalminers Attendance at Work," pp. 85 and 95, *Med. Res. Mem. No. 3*, National Coal Board, London.

Buzzard, R. B. and Liddell, F. D. K. (1963d), "Coalminers Attendance at Work," p. 85, *Med. Res. Mem. No. 3*, National Coal Board, London.

Buzzard, R. B. and Liddell, F. D. K. (1963e), "Coalminers Attendance at Work," p. 55, *Med. Res. Mem. No. 3*, National Coal Board, London.

Buzzard, R. B. and Liddell, F. D. K. (1963f), "Coalminers Attendance at Work," p. 15, *Med. Res. Mem. No. 3*, National Coal Board, London.

Buzzard, R. B. and Liddell, F. D. K. (1963g), "Coalminers Attendance at Work," pp. 130–160, *Med. Res. Mem. No. 3*, National Coal Board, London.

Buzzard, R. B. and Radforth, J. L. (1964), *Statistical Records about People at Work*. NIIP Report No. 16. National Institute of Industrial Psychology, London.

Buzzard, R. B. (1968), *Proceedings of the Symposium on Absence from Work Attributed to Sickness*, pp. 91–97. (Ed. A. Ward Gardner.) Society of Occupational Medicine, London.

Clark, F. L. and Dunne, A. C. (1955), *Ageing in Industry*. The Nuffield Foundation, London.

Denerley, R. A. (1952), "Some effects of paid sick leave on sickness absence." *Brit. J. industr. Med.*, **9**, 275.

Hill, J. M. M. and Trist, E. L. (1953), "A consideration of industrial accidents as a means of withdrawal from the work situation: a study of their relation to other absences in an iron and steel works." *Human Relations*, **6**, 357–380.

Lehmann, G. (1950), "Notes on the physiology of work performed in mining." *Bergbau Rundschau*, **2**, 162 and 251.

Linden, V. (1969), "Absence from work and physical fitness." *Brit. J. industr. Med.*, **26**, 47–53.

London Transport Executive (1956), *Health in Industry*. Butterworth, London.

Mackworth, N. H. (1950), *Researches on the Measurement of Human Performance*. Medical Research Council Special Report Series, No. 268. H.M.S.O., London.

Martin, J. (1971), "Some aspects of absence in a light engineering factory." *Occup. Psychol.*, **45** (2).

Ministry of Munitions. Health of Munition Workers' Committee (1918), *Final Report. Industrial Health and Efficiency* (Cd. 9065). H.M.S.O., London.

Powell, M. and Lomax, M. A. (1960), "The toxic effects of handling and firing explosives in coal-mines." *Ann. Occup. Hyg.*, **2**, 141.

Revans, R. N. (1960), "Morale and size of working group." *Modern Trends in Occupational Health.* (Ed. R. S. F. Schilling.) Butterworth, London.

Shepherd, R. D. and Walker, J. (1958), "Absence from work in relation to wage level and family responsibility." *Brit. J. industr. Med.,* **15,** 52–61.

Shepherd, R. D. and Walker, J. (1957), "Absence and the physical conditions of work." *Brit. J. industr. Med.,* **14,** 266–274.

Vernon, H. M. (1936), *Accidents and their Prevention.* Cambridge University Press, London.

Vernon, H. M., Bedford, T. and Warner, C. G. (1931), *Two Studies of Absenteeism in Coal-mines.* IHRB Report No. 62. H.M.S.O., London.

Walker, J. and de la Made, G. (1971), "Absence from work in relation to length and distribution of shift hours." *Brit. J. industr. Med.,* **28,** 36–44.

Welford, A. T. (1951), *Skill and Age: an Experimental Approach.* Oxford University Press, London.

Chapter 24
Rehabilitation of Mineworkers

Introduction

The medical approach to this complex subject has been defined thus: "Broadly speaking, the aim of rehabilitation is not only to reintegrate the worker into the economic system, but, beyond the material interests of the individual and of society, beyond medical healing, we must aim at social healing" (Ruyssen, 1962). This very general definition should be kept in mind. This concept involves not only the restoration of organic function, but also the treatment of the psychological consequences of the accident or illness. In other words, the injured man needs help to overcome his handicap, his sense of purpose must be restored, his *joie de vivre* has to be restored.

It is a tradition in the industry that the handicapped worker is re-employed in the mine if at all possible. The large size of many mining undertakings makes resettlement easier, because a relatively wide range of jobs is available.

It is desirable to bear in mind certain characteristics of the miner's job. It is a hard job, or, more precisely, "semi-hard" according to Lehmann's definition (1955), with relatively little light work. It is performed in very unusual conditions, poor lighting, an atmosphere which is dusty in varying degree, awkward working positions which produce static fatigue. It also has its own peculiar occupational hazards, particularly pneumoconiosis, and accidents—mining is one of the most accident-prone occupations.

The miner's job has economic and sociological characteristics which must be briefly mentioned. Mines are usually situated in rural areas and form closed communities, away from urban and other industrial centres. Their men take a traditional pride in their job and are often disinclined to learn a new one once they are in their thirties. In some countries mines may be affected by economic recession; as a result, men are no longer being recruited, and this alters the age structure.

The resettlement of handicapped workers may be obstructed by psychological difficulties which are inherent in the mining job. It may thus be very difficult to integrate the man into a team if he is likely to slow down the rhythm of production. The creation of "protected workshops", at least underground, is not a reasonable proposition. Resettlement in surface work may involve permanent reduction in earnings. Finally, there is a marked, even conflicting, difference in character between the communities of underground and surface workers respectively; the underground miner re-employed on the surface is inclined to resent the change of milieu.

Such are the main obstacles to resettlement. Unless they are largely overcome, the aim of rehabilitation, to place as many men as possible in their former jobs, will not be realized.

The following table shows not only the phases of rehabilitation and resettlement but also the phase of accident prevention which naturally precedes the other two.

Prevention
$\begin{cases} \text{Organization} \\ \text{Ergonomics and human engineering} \end{cases}$

ACCIDENT

Rehabilitation
$\begin{cases} \text{First aid} \\ \text{Surgical treatment} \\ \text{Rehabilitation centre} \end{cases}$

CONSOLIDATION

Resettlement
$\begin{cases} \text{Assessment by the company doctor in collaboration with} \\ \text{Personnel Department} \\ \text{Production Department} \\ \text{Trade Union} \end{cases}$

Prevention

The need for accident prevention is obvious. Prevention includes not only good general organization of the work by the mining engineer but also more specialized studies, e.g. surveys involving ergonomics and human engineering. Ergonomics and human engineering should play their part in prevention, but should also assist in the process of re-settlement. Thus the aim of job study in this context is to make jobs physically accessible to a greater number of workers. It is in this field that the future of resettlement and job allocation in general lies. And it is in this direction that the mining industry can still make considerable progress. The company doctor must collaborate with the engineers and ergonomists in the analysis of specific occupations. He will be concerned with those aspects of industrial physiology which determine the maximum work load for a clearly defined job. For healthy subjects, energy expenditure during normal work must not exceed 50 per cent of the maximum load. This load should be less than 50 per cent for handicapped men until their recovery is complete. (The company doctor should therefore be capable of carrying out or supervising studies in industrial physiology, a subject which must form part of his training.)

Rehabilitation

As we have seen, rehabilitation in the general sense comprehends the following three post-accident phases: First aid, surgical treatment, the physical and psychological process of rehabilitation; the last two may be carried out simultaneously in most cases.

First aid is most important. The National Coal Board's system is a good prototype. This consists of well-equipped first-aid posts at colliery or plant level, manned by qualified and competent nursing staff, and very well-equipped underground first-aid supplies depots containing, e.g. sterilized sheets for severe burn cases. Provision must be made for major accidents with multiple casualties; these are often due to firedamp or dust explosions which result in a large number of severe burn cases whose evacuation calls for a specialized technique. A few ampoules of morphine are held underground and are available to the qualified first-aid man who reaches the site of the accident before the doctor in charge of the medical services at the mine. In Western Europe, where hospitals are usually within easy reach of the mines, there is seldom need for ambulances to be manned and equipped for the treatment of shock. In countries where the distances are greater such provision may be necessary.

The surgical services will sometimes be provided by the company (as in the case of Charbonnages de France) and sometimes (as in Great Britain), they form an integral part of the National Health Service. The same applies to rehabilitation centres.

These administrative considerations in no way affect the standard procedures guiding the work of surgical teams. The work of these teams should have one constant aim: functional restoration which is as near perfect as possible. Thus surgeons who work in hospitals where injured miners are treated must have adequate training in accident surgery and orthopaedics. The services of a physiotherapist are essential from the commencement of hospitalisation. To take one example: a miner has had a blow on the spine involving fractures of the transverse processes (without a cord lesion). It is essential to get the man to move his lower limbs as soon as the plaster cast is in place; this will prevent the joints from stiffening and also prevent atrophy of the muscle masses.

Rehabilitation centres were developed in their modern form in Great Britain and the United States during the last war.

The Charbonnages de France established the centre at Oignies after an exhaustive survey of the layout and organization of various British centres. It may serve as an example of the large centre which can be maintained by a substantial mining organization. The Oignies centre

24—24 pp.

was opened in 1950, the first in France to have in-patients. It is run by a specialist physician, assisted by a consultant neuro-psychiatrist. It is situated in the centre of the Nord Pas-de-Calais coalfield, on an estate consisting of 15 hectares of woods, coppices and pastures, interspersed with ponds. The château, which dates from the last century, has been modernized and equipped to accommodate, feed and entertain residents; it can take 100 miners. The building, although not excessively luxurious, is very comfortable and has a capacious living room, an assembly hall also used for games, a library and two dining rooms where the men have their meals at small tables. The upper floors contain dormitories and wash-rooms.

The miners spend their day in a relaxed and cheerful atmosphere. The supervisors pay great attention to the men's recreation, because they know that the psychological factor plays a very big part in successful rehabilitation. The treatment rooms have been constructed in annexes near the château. They include a large gymnasium—this is the focus of the treatment wing and is equipped for standard gymnastics as well as for medical and corrective gymnastics. The latter includes a system of ropes and pulleys (pulley therapy) with sandbags of different weights which call for graduated effort from each patient. Next to the gymnasium there are dressing rooms, showers and lavatories. The physiotherapy rooms provide a full range of treatments.

The prosthetics room, for the repair of plaster casts, is next to the surgery. Three very large occupational therapy workshops are adjacent to the gymnasium; one for weaving (this is equipped with special looms), one for carpentry and one for basket-making and wicker work.

A sports ground has been laid out in the park which is also available for long walks and for cycling.

The staff includes six specialized supervisors and a (female) physiotherapist. There are also three ladies who act as medical secretary, administrative secretary and social-activities supervisor, respectively; they, and the domestic staff, are answerable to the matron. It should be stressed that the purpose of the rehabilitation which is practised at Oignies is to re-adapt the worker for his subsequent job, once he has recovered his physical capacities and moral fibre.

An incomplete picture would be given of this centre if nothing were said of the importance of the rehabilitation which must occur at the injured man's bedside in the hospital, from the very first days which follow the accident, the operation or the placing of a plaster cast. It is organized at each of the colliery hospitals in the Pas-de-Calais coalfield. It makes only slender demands on resources and can be concentrated in a relatively small room; it must be practised by a qualified physiotherapist under the supervision of the surgeon. This centre, which might be called the first-stage centre, also deals with minor injuries; a miner with, say, a fracture of the radius or of a finger does not require residential rehabilitation at a centre such as Oignies, but he will benefit from treatment carried out at the local centre whilst living at home with his family. The average stay at Oignies lasts approximately ten weeks, and this does not allow a rapid turnover. The miner spends each weekend with his family, from mid-day on Saturday to Monday morning. This does much to sustain the injured man's equanimity.

The results recorded are most encouraging; of 3,000 patients who stayed at the Centre over a recent ten-year period, 60 per cent were able to resume their former jobs, 39 per cent had to be resettled in lighter work and only 1 per cent had to be invalided out. It should be noted that the 60 per cent mentioned above includes men who return to their previous jobs or to a job requiring the same physical capacities, either when they leave the centre or after a temporary period of light work lasting 8–9 months on average. Of course, this result varies in relation to the nature of the injury.

A qualitative analysis of these results is illuminating, particularly from the psychological point of view. Subjects who readapted either well or normally constituted 87·5 per cent of the total whereas 12·5 per cent readapted badly. The latter presented a variety of psychological problems. After a major accident or illness it is not at all surprising that a proportion of miners will show signs of severe anxiety. It may be manifest in a variety of syndromes, such as paranoia, hysteria or depression. Pre-existing constitutional inadequacies may be intensified. All such cases present a challenge which can be met much more effectively if the services of a capable psychiatrist are available during rehabilitation.

In many cases a proper and satisfactory rehabilitation is only possible if we regard the patient as having been injured, not only somatically and psychologically, but also socially, professionally and in his family life. In this connection it must be appreciated that the main thing is to act quickly. Good work means quick work. In the rebuilding and maintenance of morale, group psychotherapy is of particular value. It must have a play element, but only up to a certain point. The British concept of giving it a sporting (or even competitive) character is worthy of emulation. Another promising concept is the introduction of workshops into rehabilitation centres so that as the patient recovers his fitness he is re-introduced to work discipline and routine. During the whole period of treatment, whether at the hospital or at the rehabilitation centre, the company must keep in touch with the injured man through its specialist services—i.e. Personnel Department, the company doctor, the medico-social workers, and the Trade Unions must not be overlooked. This is essential for the future resettlement of the handicapped man, whether he goes back to his old job or is given another job within the company.

The organization which we have just described is only applicable in very big undertakings where special establishments and equipment can be justified. In all other cases (and these are the general rule) reliance will have to be placed on the regional or national organizations which, it is to be hoped, would share the ideas expressed above. Artificial-limb centres are likely to be available only on a national basis. Considerable progress has been made during the last few years in prosthetic techniques. The importance of the quality of an artificial limb to an amputated man, both for his leisure and for his work needs no emphasis.

So far only the orthopaedic rehabilitation of injured miners has been discussed. Clearly the rehabilitation of miners after illness must also be considered. Individuals in the following three major groups may well benefit from systematic rehabilitation:

Early respiratory insufficiency;
Gastro-intestinal conditions, particularly partial gastrectomy;
Myocardial infarction.

Before rehabilitation is effectively employed during convalescence an entirely new attitude of mind will have to be created within the medical profession, and, particularly, among hospital physicians. With a little imagination, the methodology should fall into place. Admission to rehabilitation centres must depend on the three-fold condition that the patient can genuinely benefit in the sense that he can be retrained for physical exertion, that a full (or nearly full) recovery may reasonably be expected and, finally, that his stay in such a centre will not exceed several months.

In passing it may be noted that these criteria apply equally to injured men.

Once rehabilitation is completed, resettlement is effected. (In French law the accident period ends with what is known as consolidation—the patient is classified as either normal or having partial permanent incapacity.)

Resettlement

As comprehensive a report as possible on the miner's condition at this stage will be drawn up by the company doctor, perhaps with the assistance of the industrial psychologist. Then, if necessary, the case will be considered by a committee consisting of representatives from the Medical, Personnel, Production and Training Departments, and the Trade Union.

If it is found impossible to re-employ the miner within the company and it is decided, with his agreement, that he should change his occupation, he will be admitted to a vocational training centre; it would not, of course, generally be possible for a mine to run such a centre.

The difficulties which are inherent in the miner's job and which make resettlement difficult have already been alluded to at the beginning of this chapter. However, this survey would not be complete without mentioning certain other inhibiting psychological factors.

In the first place, there is legislation covering compensation for industrial injuries and occupational diseases. In most countries this sector enjoys preferential treatment. In France, the "accident on the journey" (road accidents on the journey from the home to the place of work or vice versa) is compensated as an industrial accident, whereas a leisure-time accident will receive far less compensation. In Great Britain the "accident on the journey" is not compensated as an industrial accident. It is difficult to see the natural justice of these distinctions. Holland is the only country where compensation is now the same in either case. These legal distinctions and provisos may well induce neuroses which are far from helpful in retraining the patient to exert himself.

It should be added that the family background often has an adverse influence. Psychiatrists are well aware of these frequent situations where the injured man, suffering from emotional shock, subconsciously turns to his wife for additional protection, the wife being only too pleased to take over as effective head of the family. This state of affairs does nothing to help the rehabilitation of the man concerned.

Finally, the family background is not the only potential source of trouble. The hospital staff, doctors and, above all, supervisors (at rehabilitation centres in particular) sometimes display an over-paternalistic attitude towards the patients. There are many female supervisors whose work nearly always deserves nothing but praise; but, on occasion, their tendency towards "maternalism" may emerge with the worst possible results.

When the patient has been resettled it is particularly important that his further progress should be regularly reviewed until it is judged that he has made the maximum recovery possible. Without a review system men may settle down indefinitely in light jobs when they are capable of better performance.

To summarize: the problem of rehabilitation is, above all, psychological. It should be remembered that the time during which a man will stay away from work because of a given handicap is in inverse proportion to his own idea of his status and usefulness within the Company. There is a minority which has no need of rehabilitation centres. The spirit which reigns in these centres, the idea of doing as well as (or better than) the next man, is far more important than the techniques which are practised. Most human beings require emotional support and help after a serious accident, and miners are no exception.

References

Lehmann, G. (1955), *Physiologie Pratique du Travail*, p. 137. Editions d'Organisation, Paris.

Ruyssen, L. (1962), *C. r. des Journées Francaises de Pathologie Minière*, p. 111. Paris.

24A

Chapter 25

Epidemiology

Introduction

An important question for the mining industries is what kind of environment should be maintained to minimize the occurrence of disease and injury in the employed population. To answer this, it is necessary to know whether factors in the environment are related to the incidence of disease and injury, how changes in the environment will affect the incidence of disease and injury, and finally what changes in the environment are economically and technically possible. The first two questions are ones that can be answered by epidemiologic studies; the last is a question that must be answered by engineers and by the conscience of management and government.

Seldom is it possible to prevent all disease and injury associated with productive labour, not only because engineering changes frequently cannot make environments totally safe but also because as total safety is approached costs of control become prohibitive. A generally accepted philosophy is to create a working environment in which adverse effects will occur only rarely. "Rarely" is variously defined. For example, the Threshold Limit Values published by the American Congress of Governmental Industrial Hygienists refer to time weighted concentrations of substances for a seven or eight hour work day and a 40 hour work week. This report states that at these concentrations "nearly all workers may be repeatedly exposed day after day without adverse effect" (American Congress of Governmental Industrial Hygienists, 1970). On the other hand, in dealing with a single substance, asbestos, the British Occupational Hygiene Society has been more specific and recommends a dust standard that permits asbestosis to develop in only 1 per cent of persons over a 50 year period (British Occupational Hygiene Society, 1968).

The Nature of Epidemiology

Whether a "safe" environment should allow 1 per cent, or 5 per cent, or 10 per cent of a population to develop a disease is not a question that can be answered by the application of epidemiologic methods. Rather, epidemiology can only reveal the relationship between the environment and the occurrence of some disease or injury. This is a definition of epidemiology and is similar to one proposed by Payne (1969). It is intended to embody the notion of various physical, biological, and behavioural factors interacting to produce health or disease. As Terris (1962) points out, a variety of methods can be employed drawn from a variety of disciplines. While these methods will be referred to here as epidemiologic methods, it is recognized that they are employed in other fields and are not the exclusive property of epidemiology. Primary emphasis here will be on disease since this traditionally has been of interest to the field of medicine. Also important, however, has been the use of epidemiology for the identification and elimination of causes of accidental injuries (Iskrant and Joliet, 1968).

The inference drawn from epidemiologic studies is that an environmental cause has a medical effect. The ability to make this inference is an essential part of epidemiology. By cause and effect is meant that substance A causes disease X, and that a reduction in substance A will be accompanied by a reduction in disease X. In some instances it can also be inferred that disease X will only occur in the presence of substance A. The pneumoconioses, for example, are presumed to occur only in the presence of dust in amounts which exceed that in the general environment, so that for workers in the mining industries elimination of dust would result in the virtual elimination of pneumoconiosis. This notion is firmly embedded in occupational medicine and evidence of exposure is often one of the requirements for the diagnosis of certain diseases. On the other hand, for diseases widespread in the general population, such as lung cancer, while it might be demonstrated that workers in certain occupations are at increased risk and that changes in their work environment will modify this risk, it cannot be inferred that changes in the work environment will eliminate these diseases.

Epidemiologic studies rarely prove the existence of a causal relationship but usually provide sufficient evidence to serve as the basis for action. The strength of this evidence will depend both on the nature of the disease and upon the nature of the evidence. Diseases with multiple causes are more difficult to relate to a single set of environmental factors than diseases with only a single cause. As noted above, the pneumoconioses are easily related to environmental agents whereas many other diseases, and in particular the chronic diseases where many causative or predisposing factors are operative, are usually more difficult to associate with the work environment.

The nature of epidemiologic evidence may vary from simply showing that the presence or absence of a substance is related to the presence or absence of a disease in some defined population, to showing that there is a quantitive relationship between the substance and the disease, to showing that removal of the substance results in disappearance or decline in the disease. The first two types of evidence arise from studies usually referred to as *descriptive* epidemiology and are based on observations of populations in some natural setting undisturbed by the investigator. The third type of evidence arises from studies called

experimental epidemiology and usually requires some deliberate intervention by the investigator.

Descriptive Epidemiology

Sometimes the effects of occupational exposure are so overwhelming
and so unique that only very crude observations are necessary to
establish a probable cause and effect relationship. Nevertheless, these
qualify as descriptive epidemiology. During the years 1932–1934 at
Gauley Bridge in West Virginia, for example, 476 workers died from
silicosis and 1,500 others contracted the disease while digging out a
rock tunnel. The cause-effect relationship here was unmistakable and
initiated widespread efforts by both industry and government to control
quartz dust in the working environment (Subcommittee of the Committee of Labour, 1936).

More often occupational effects are less dramatic or environments
less easily describable requiring somewhat more sophisticated types of
information before action can be taken. Higgins, Cochrane, Gilson and
Wood (1959) compared the prevalence of chronic bronchitis in miners
and ex-miners in Staveley, Derbyshire, aged 55 to 64 with the prevalence
in men of the same age who worked at non-dusty occupations in the
same area with the following results:

	Number in sample	Number with chronic bronchitis	Per cent with chronic bronchitis
Miners and Ex-miners	191	40	20·9
Non-Dusty Workers	81	12	14·8

Similarly, Oettle (1963) provides data which allow comparison of
the frequency of lung cancer in South African white miners with that
of non-miners as seen at autopsy during the period 1935–1945:

	Number of necropsies	Number with lung cancer	Per cent with lung cancer
Miners	550	20	3·6
Non-Miners	750	30	4·0

Somewhat stronger evidence of the presence or absence of a causal
relationship in descriptive epidemiology is provided by studies which
show quantitative relationships between exposure to some substance
and the occurrence of a disease. For example, Lainhart (1969) reported
on chest X-ray examinations of a random sample of 449 coal miners
aged 55 to 64 working in the Appalachian region of the United States.
His data show the following relationship between years spent underground in coal mining and definite roentgenographic evidence of
pneumoconiosis:

Years underground	Number of miners examined	Number with pneumoconiosis	Per cent with pneumoconiosis
0–9	60	4⎫	6·7
10–19	14	1⎭	
20–29	76	8	10·5
30–39	213	56	26·3
40 or more	136	34	25·0

Wagoner, Archer, Lundin, Holaday, and Lloyd (1965), studying the relationship between the amount of airborne radiation to which 1,200 uranium miners had been exposed and the incidence of respiratory cancer, reported the following:

Cumulative radiation exposure (*working level months*)	Number of person-years at risk after exposure	Number of respiratory cancers	Incidence of respiratory cancer per 10,000 miners-years
Under 120	7,437	2	2·7
120–359	6,296	6⎫	6·3
360–839	4,762	1⎭	
840–1,799	3,299	6	18·2
1,800–3,719	1,601	8	50·0
3,720 and over	467	8	171·3

Evidence provided by the last two studies is considerably more convincing than that provided where comparisons were made with some non-exposed population. For one thing, it is difficult to develop evidence that the non-exposed workers are truly comparable to exposed workers in terms of predisposition to disease or in terms of exposure to other environmental factors that might influence the development of disease. For another, the underlying assumption in relating disease incidence to some environmental agent usually involves the notion of a dose-response relationship. That is, if causality really exists increased dose should be related to increased response. The last two study examples provide this type of evidence.

The problem of separating the effects of exposure to agents outside the working environment from agents in the work environment has been approached by comparing disease in wives of exposed workers with disease in wives of non-exposed workers. Enterline (1969), for example, compared the prevalence of symptoms of chronic bronchitis in age matched groups of miners, non-miners, and their wives in Mullens, West Virginia:

	Number examined	Number with symptoms of chronic bronchitis	Per cent with symptoms of chronic bronchitis
Miners	185	26	14·1
Non-Miners	194	17	8·8
Wives of Miners	163	10	6·1
Wives of Non-Miners	163	7	4·3

Here, the fact that wives of coal miners had a greater prevalence than wives of non-miners suggests that something outside the work environment may be partly responsible for the greater frequency of symptoms of chronic bronchitis among miners as compared with non-miners.

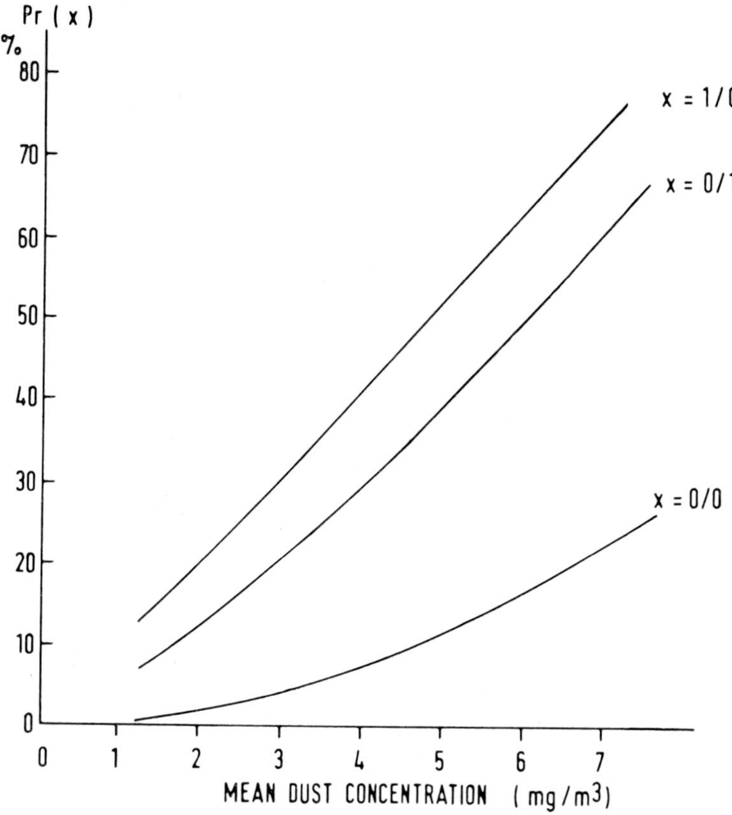

FIG. 1. $Pr(x)$ = percentage of men whose radiographs show some sign of progression of simple pneumoconiosis over ten years starting from point (x) on the extended (1968) I.L.O. classification of pneumoconioses. (Statistically fitted curves.)

(Reproduced by permission of Unwin Bros. Ltd., Surrey, England, from "The relation between pneumoconiosis and dust-exposure in British coal mines" in *Inhaled Particles, III*, edited by W. H. Walton.)

One of the most sophisticated descriptive epidemiological investigations in the mining industry to date is that conducted by the British National Coal Board. This involves follow-up by X-ray and other tests of men working in 25 collieries and relating the development of pneumoconiosis to dust dosage (Fay, 1957). An interim analysis of results from this investigation produced estimates of the probability of developing simple coal workers' pneumoconiosis given a 35-year exposure to different mean concentrations of respirable dust. Although the observed radiological changes were over a ten year period, the extrapolation to 35 years utilized a statistical argument which allowed for substantial variations in the probability of the disease progressing depending on the radiological state at the start of a ten-year period. Figure 1 illustrates this variation. 0/0 represents men with completely negative chest X-rays while 1/0 reflects some evidence of pneumoconiosis. Jacobsen, Rae, Walton and Rogan (1970) have reported how these results were used as a basis for recommendations on permissible dust levels. While the data were derived from observations of a particular population over a specified time period and thus are entirely unique, the applications of the results are intended to be fairly general. That is, in order to use these observations based on coal miners in Great Britain for setting dust standards in other countries, for example, it must be assumed that they reflect some underlying truth about coal mine dust and coal miners and therefore the results are applicable in other settings. This is, in fact, the nature and use of scientific data and not peculiar to epidemiologic observations. It does, however, occasionally pose a problem for users of epidemiologic data due to possible qualitative differences in some substance or differences in the susceptibility of the subjects exposed to this substance. For this reason epidemiologic studies are often duplicated in a variety of settings and results compared. Thus, Reisner (1971) reports probabilities of developing pneumoconiosis based on a ten-year study of miners in the Ruhr coalfield. Quantitative comparison with the British results is difficult because different scales and instruments were used to measure radiological change and dust exposure respectively. (The need for international agreement on measuring scales and instrumentation is discussed in a later section of this chapter.) Nevertheless, it is evident that both studies reflect the same basic relationship between the disease and the industrial environment.

Experimental Epidemiology

Instances in the mining industries where it has been well documented that the removal of a substance or agent has resulted in the decline or disappearance of a disease qualify as examples of experimental epidemiology and provide the strongest type of evidence that a cause-effect relationship exists. Cochrane (1962) discusses results from an ingenious attempt at experimental epidemiology in the coal mining industry. In order to investigate the suggestion that the occurrence of progressive massive fibrosis (P.M.F.) might be related to the presence of exogenous tuberculous infection, the attack rate of P.M.F. was studied in two similar Welsh mining valleys. An abnormally intensive campaign for tuberculosis eradication in one of these valleys was introduced to reduce exogenous tuberculous infectivity there at an accelerated rate. The positive evidence on the "tuberculosis" hypothesis which was sought from this experiment was not forthcoming because at the end of the eight-year period there appeared to be little difference in tuberculosis attack rates between the two valleys despite eradication efforts in one of them. Thus, no direct conclusion could be drawn from the similar P.M.F. attack rates in the two valleys. However, Cochrane noted the continuous fall in tuberculous attack rates over the eight years in both valleys, and argued *a posteriori* that under the hypothesis, the higher infectivity in the earlier part of the period should be associated with a higher attack rate of P.M.F. No such difference in attack rate occurred, and this provided weaker descriptive "absence of evidence in support of the hypothesis". In the metal mining industry the prevalence of silicosis has been studied before and after the introduction of extensive dust control measures (Flinn, Brinton, Doyle, Cralley and Harris, 1963). Silicosis is reported to have fallen from a prevalence of 30 to 80 per cent among workers in the early 1900s to less than 4 per cent in 1954.

Sometimes it is difficult to document relationships between dust concentrations and improvements in the health of workers due possibly to changes in techniques for dust sampling, changes in techniques for the diagnosis of disease, or a changing population of workers. For example, Flinn, Seifert, Brinton, Jones and Frank (1942) described X-ray examinations of 507 coal miners in Utah and reported 16 cases of pneumoconiosis (3·2 per cent). Lainhart (1969) reports on 567 chest X-ray examinations of coal miners in Utah conducted in 1964 with almost identical results. While it was generally felt that working conditions improved during this 22 year period this is difficult to document. Moreover it is not clear that there is much comparability between the definition of pneumoconiosis used in 1942 and 1964.

Epidemiologic Methods

There are three principal methods used in epidemiologic investigations: cross-sectional studies, retrospective studies, and prospective studies. Each method has advantages and disadvantages and its appropriateness will be dependent on the population available for study, the disease under investigation, the use to which the data will be put and the time and resources available. Among the studies discussed so far some were cross sectional (Higgins *et al.*, 1959; Oettle, 1963; Lainhart, 1969; Enterline, 1967) and others used the prospective approach (Wagoner *et al.*, 1965; Jacobsen *et al.*, 1970; Reisner, 1971; Cochrane, 1962).

Cross-sectional studies are probably the weakest but most frequently used epidemiologic method. They consist of a single examination conducted on persons who have a common occupation or potential exposure. This might be compared with examinations on persons outside the occupation or without the potential exposure. Examinations might proceed rapidly, as where a special survey of a group of workers is conducted, or be extended over a considerable period of time, as might be the case in giving periodic physical examinations. Cross-sectional surveys are most effective in detecting conditions which last for a long period of time and are not severely disabling. Things like dermatitis, allergies, pneumoconiosis, residual effects of illnesses or injuries, high blood pressure and chronic bronchitis fit this category. For surveys confined to employed populations it is important that the condition to be detected be not so severe, at least in its early stage, as to cause a person to leave his job. Where a condition may be involved in job separation, it is important to obtain some information on persons who have left employment. Higgins *et al.* (1959) examined both coal miners and ex-coal miners in Staveley to obtain an estimate of the prevalence of chronic bronchitis both among men still in the industry and among those who had left. In the coal miners in the Appalachian region of the United States, Lainhart *et al.* (1969) report on the prevalence of pneumoconiosis both among a sample of coal miners and a sample of ex-miners.

Stating that cross-sectional studies are particularly useful in studying diseases which last for a long time is saying, in effect, that such studies are useful where the prevalence of the disease is large in relation to its incidence. In discussing cross-sectional studies, therefore, it is important to define prevalence and incidence and how these measures are related. Prevalence, expressed as a percentage, is defined as:

$$\frac{\text{Number of cases at one moment in time}}{\text{Population at risk at that moment}} \times 100$$

Since it is never possible to make all observations in a single moment, the concept is usually approximated by:

$$\frac{\text{Number of cases found during a given period}}{\text{Population examined during that period}} \times 100$$

Thus, if it took a week or a month to conduct examinations of a group of workers the prevalence rate would simply be the percentage of workers examined who were found to have a particular disease or condition.

Incidence, expressed as a percentage, is:

$$\frac{\text{Number of cases beginning during a period of time}}{\text{Population observed during the period of time}} \times 100$$

The incidence of pneumoconiosis in a working population, say during the past year, would ordinarily be much lower than the prevalence, since pneumoconiosis is usually not severely disabling and men with evidence of the disease might stay at their jobs for many years. Suppose in a working population the prevalence of pneumoconiosis as revealed by X-ray is 10 per cent and workers remain on the job an average of five years after the first X-ray changes take place. An annual incidence of only 2 per cent would be required to maintain the 10 per cent prevalence rate under these conditions. The relationship between prevalence, incidence, and duration of disease is therefore:

$$\text{Prevalence} = \text{Incidence} \times \text{Duration of disease}$$

$$\text{Incidence} = \frac{\text{Prevalence}}{\text{Duration of disease}}$$

$$\text{Duration of disease} = \frac{\text{Prevalence}}{\text{Incidence}}$$

As stated at the outset, the important question for epidemiologic investigation is the relationship between the environment and the *incidence* of disease since the ultimate object of epidemiology as applied to industrial populations is to point to measures which will minimize or prevent the occurrence or incidence of disease. Prevalence is only an indirect way of measuring incidence and is useful only if some assumptions about duration of disease in the population under study can be made.

For acute events or diseases cross-sectional studies are not very effective. For example, examinations of workers would be of little or no use in learning about deaths or accidents. These kinds of events have no meaningful prevalence but rather are related only to the concept of incidence. There are also many important diseases with high fatality rates or which have a relatively short duration for which cross-sectional studies are unsuitable. Cross-sectional studies involving chest X-rays of uranium miners in the United States were not useful in detecting an excess in lung cancer (Flinn *et al.*, 1963) while from prospective studies it is now known that a serious hazard exists (Lundin, Lloyd, Smith, Archer and Holaday, 1969).

Retrospective and prospective studies differ from cross-sectional studies in that rather than dealing with the prevalence of disease they deal with the incidence. Thus, the kinds of disease appropriate for retrospective studies are also suitable for prospective studies, although from a practical standpoint these two types of studies are not necessarily interchangeable. Moreover, the methodology employed for retrospective studies is very different from that employed for prospective studies.

Retrospective studies start with a series of cases of a particular disease and attempt to discover what these cases have in common. This is done by contrasting the series with a parallel series of controls without the disease and is sometimes referred to as the case-control approach. They are relatively inexpensive, excellent for rare disease, and can often be carried out entirely within some clinical setting, such as a hospital. Newhouse and Thompson (1965), for example, established occupational histories for all cases of mesothelioma (an extremely rare disease) seen at the London Hospital over a 50 year period and compared these histories with those of a control series without mesothelioma of the same sex and age distribution selected from records of the same hospital. The results were as follows:

	Cases	*Controls*
Total	76	76
History of exposure to asbestos dust	40	9
No history of exposure to asbestos dust	36	67

This is evidence of an association between asbestos dust and mesothelioma and supports other data on this subject. For a disease as rare and fatal as mesothelioma probably no other epidemiologic method would be suitable. Unfortunately this type of study does not permit estimates of the incidence of mesothelioma in persons exposed to asbestos dust as compared with those not exposed and thus provides no measure of risk. Moreover, it offers many opportunities for bias. If, for example, the investigator believes that mesothelioma and asbestos dust are associated he may try harder to elicit a history of exposure in cases than in controls. Also, there is no assurance that the proper control group was used or that it was drawn from the same population as the cases. For these reasons and where the disease being investigated is not rare, most epidemiological investigations dealing with incidence are prospective rather than retrospective.

Prospective studies start with persons without disease, rather than those with disease, and determine the incidence of disease in relation to selected characteristics of the people and of their environment. Often this is referred to as the cohort approach—meaning a cohort or band of people traced through time. The starting point for this tracing is purely a matter of convenience. The starting point might be a cross-sectional survey. In the studies of coal miners by the British National Coal Board and of uranium miners by the U.S. Public Health Service the starting point was an X-ray survey at which time certain demographic and health data were gathered and persons without pneumoconiosis were identified. In these studies a long waiting period has been required for the production of a sufficient number of cases to draw inferences. Given the time, the resources, and much patience this is by a considerable margin the most productive type of descriptive epidemiologic investigation. The investigator can control the information initially used to describe the cohort, he can control environmental information collected during the follow-up period, and he can define disease in advance in any manner he feels would be most useful.

Given a lack of time, money, and/or patience prospective studies can be conducted retrospectively. That is, a population can be identified at some point in the past and observations brought up to the present. A recent example of this is the study of lung cancer among chrysotile asbestos mills and mines in Quebec (McDonald, McDonald, Gibbs, Siemiatycki and Rossiter, 1971). In this study a cohort of 11,788 persons born between 1891 and 1920 employed in mines or mills for one month or more prior to November 1, 1966 was identified. For each person a work history was obtained and an estimate of total dust exposure made. Deaths and causes of death were determined as of November 1, 1966. Death rates for lung cancer were as follows:

Dust Index	*Number of deaths*	*Death rate per 1,000*
Under 10	25	7·6
10–99	26	8·6
100–199	10	11·2
200–399	8	8·9
400–799	11	15·8
800 and over	14	24·2

Another example of a prospective study done retrospectively is that reported by Beadle (1971) relating the development of radiological signs of silicosis to dust exposure. Twelve hundred underground workers who started work between 1934 and 1938 are involved and results are being updated at regular intervals until all men in the cohort will have died. Interim analyses have been made and an equation has been derived expressing the probability of developing silicosis in terms of the number of shifts worked and the average dust level.

The use of official mortality statistics may also be considered as a prospective study. Where official counts of death for particular occupations are related to persons at risk in those occupations the rates can be viewed as reflecting the incidence of death in a cohort followed for a fairly short period of time—usually one year.

Measurement in Epidemiology

The value of any scientific study depends upon the clarity with which the aims are defined and upon the ability of the investigator to make measurements related to the defined objects. This general principle is as valid for epidemiology as for other branches of science, but it merits special emphasis in the present context because of a common misunderstanding concerning the way in which conclusions are drawn from epidemiologic data. Inferences of a statistical nature are frequently necessary in order to complete an epidemiologic study, but contrary to a belief held by some no mathematical or statistical technique can extract useful information from ill-conceived projects or irrelevant observations.

One type of measurement used in epidemiology is the re-assembly and supplementation of existing information in such a way that it is relevant to the defined objects although originally the information may have been recorded for some other reason. The hospital records of mesotheliomas collected by Newhouse and Thompson (1965) and cited above are of this kind. Frequently public records and reports of morbidity and mortality are used. In the United States a valuable source is information published by the National Center for Health Statistics. In Great Britain mortality data by geographic area and for various occupations are published regularly by the Registrars-General. The force of mortality is summarized in these reports as the ratio of the observed number of deaths in an occupation or area to the number that would have been expected had the death rates for the general population (usually the death rates for persons of the same age and sex distribution in the country in which the observation is being made) prevailed. The resulting ratios are multiplied by 100 and the result is called a standardized mortality ratio. A ratio of 100 means that there is no excess or deficit of deaths. Ratios above 100 reflect an excess and below 100 a deficit. Examples of the use of official mortality data are studies by Ashley and Davies, and Ashley (1966, 1967). Ashley (1967) examined published death rates due to lung cancer in England and Wales and noted a deficiency in mining areas. This work stimulated Crofton (1969) to compare the deficiency of lung cancer deaths in coal-mining areas in England and Wales with the experience in the coal-mining areas of Scotland. Among men in Scotland, there was excess mortality due to lung cancer and bronchitis in areas concerned with coal mining. In her discussion of these results, Crofton suggests that they may be connected with the lower prevalence of pneumoconiosis in Scotland noted in other studies.

Observations of this kind often suggest hypotheses for further research. Rarely do they permit definitive conclusions, and this is usually because it is difficult to ensure that the measurements are indeed strictly relevant to the objects of the study. The data will have been collected with a variety of purposes in mind. None of them are likely to coincide precisely with the specific aims of a particular study. Moreover, it may be difficult or impossible to identify retrospectively sources of bias in the way the data were collected. Liddell (1961) reported on an investigation which revealed such a bias. The British Registrars-General classify deaths according to last occupation of the deceased as reported by a survivor. A high standardized mortality ratio for coal miners working at the coal face was apparently due to incorrect reporting of the last occupation before death. It appeared that in mining communities the social status associated with face-work had resulted in posthumous "promotion" of surface mineworkers, as is shown by the standardized mortality ratios in the following table:

	Official data	*Independent investigation of true last occupation*
Face workers	142	81
Surface mineworkers	109	135

Accumulated information from periodic medical examinations may also provide useful measurements. More than 90 per cent of British coal miners take advantage of the National Coal Board's Periodic X-ray Scheme. McLintock, Rae and Jacobsen (1971) have used results from the first five years of the scheme to specify the attack rate of progressive massive fibrosis in British coal miners. In doing so they were able to confirm for Great Britain as a whole Cochrane's (1962) earlier findings from South Wales, which showed that the chance of developing progressive massive fibrosis increases with increasing degree of simple coalworkers' pneumoconiosis (Figure 2).

A second type of measurements used in epidemiology are those acquired specifically for the purposes of the investigation. All the normal criteria for sound scientific measurement apply: internal consistency of technique, comparability with recognized standards, reproducibility over time and between observers. Reproducibility should be quantified so that the conclusions may be assessed by other workers. In the case of measurement by chest X-rays, for example, this would mean more than one reading of each X-ray with comparisons of results by various readers.

Reproducibility is particularly important where measurements are in the form of classifications based on subjective judgments, such as the radiological diagnosis of pneumoconioses. The International Labour Office's (1970) Classification of Radiographs of Pneumoconioses is an important advance towards generally recognized criteria in radiology concerned with mining industries. In addition to adequate training of film readers, quality and consistency in radiographic technique, certainly of interest in any clinical situation, assume great significance in epidemiologic work where findings may result in decisions affecting large numbers of workers. Investigations by Pearson, Ashford, Morgan, Pasqual and Rae (1965) demonstrated a tendency for less pneumoconiosis to be read on films with unsatisfactory technique. Clearly, differences in film quality between two series of films could affect assessments of radiological progression of lung disease. This consideration affects, in turn, the question of how measurements of radiological change should be made in epidemiologic studies. Should serial films from the same subject be assessed side-by-side on the viewing box, or should they be read singly in random order? Liddell and May (1966) describe trials from which they concluded that the side-by-side method resulted in less observer variation, but Oldham (1968) points to a number of reasons why independent and randomized readings of serial films are desirable in research.

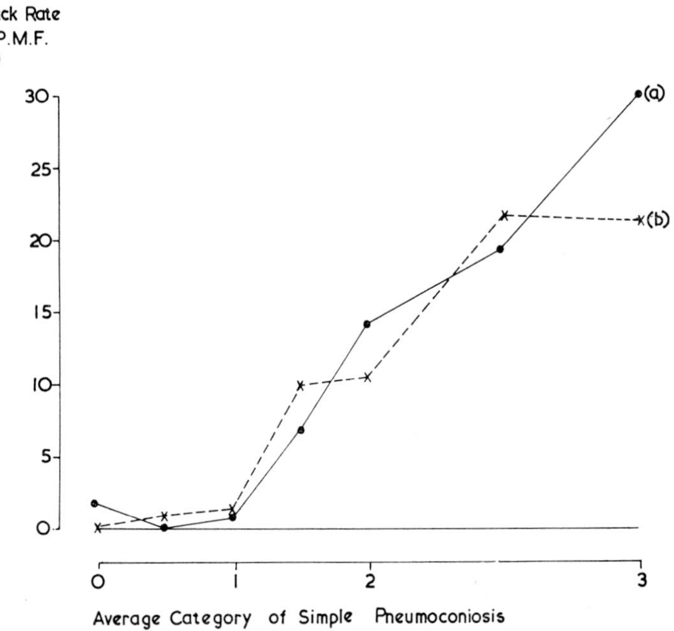

FIG. 2. Attack rate (%) of progressive massive fibrosis in coal miners over eight years in relation to average category of simple pneumoconiosis as defined by Cochrane (1962).

(Reproduced by permission of Unwin Bros. Ltd., Surrey, England, from "The attack rate of PMF in British coal miners" in *Inhaled Particles, III*, edited by W. H. Walton.)

Where measurements are dependent on the response of subjects to questions relating to symptomatology, rigour in methods and definitions can determine whether a study concludes with an objective analysis of subjective data or whether it ends with unjustifiable inferences from anecdotal reports. The British Medical Research Council's (1966) questionnaire concerning bronchitis is an example of a measuring technique designed to measure subjective responses in an objective manner, so that results from one study can be compared with results from another. When such a measuring tool is used for epidemiologic purposes suitable safeguards must be employed to ensure that possible biases arising from the manner in which questions are asked are reduced to a minimum. Careful instruction of interviewers on the aims and methods of epidemiology are essential in order to avoid negating the purpose of the questionnaire by unscheduled, well-meant, but impermissible qualifying questions and leading formulations. Tape-recorders may be used intermittently in order to monitor compliance with the strict research protocol and to identify possible sources of bias.

Measurements characterizing the environment surrounding a working population require the same precautions as the medical assessments, since results from both will affect the validity and reproducibility of the estimated relationships between the disease and its hypothesized antecedents. Validity refers here to the underlying truth of an apparent relationship, and it implies an absence of bias. It is distinguished from reproducibility, which is a measure of the repeatability of a set of observations.

Chapter 9 is devoted to what is by far the most important environmental measurement in mining epidemiology: the recording of airborne dust concentration and composition. Temperature, humidity, noise levels, air composition and head-room are examples of variables which the epidemiologist may wish to measure in mining situations.

References

American Conference of Governmental Industrial Hygienists (1970), "Threshold limit values of airborne contaminants and intended changes." Industrial Health Foundation, Pittsburgh.

Ashley, D. J. B. (1967), "The distribution of lung cancer and bronchitis in England and Wales." *British Journal of Cancer*, **21**, 243.

Ashley, D. J. B. and Davies, H. D. (1966), "Lung cancer and chronic bronchitis in Wales." *British Journal of Preventive and Social Medicine*, **20**, 148.

Beadle, D. G. (1971), "The relationship between the amount of dust breathed and the development of radiological signs of silicosis: an epidemiological study in South African gold miners." *Inhaled Particles, III*, ed. W. H. Walton. Unwin, London.

British Occupational Hygiene Society (1968), "Hygiene standards for chrysotile asbestos dust." *Annals of Occupational Health*, **11**, 47.

Cochrane, A. L. (9162), "The attack rate of progressive massive fibrosis." *British Journal of Industrial Medicine*, **19**, 52.

Crofton, E. C. (1969), "A study of lung cancer and bronchitis mortality in relation to coal-mining in Scotland." *British Journal of Preventive and Social Medicine*, **23**, 141.

Enterline, P. E. (1967), "The effects of occupation on chronic respiratory disease." *Archives of Environmental Health*, **14**, 189.

Fay, J. W. J. (1957), "The National Coal Board's Pneumoconiosis Field Research." *Nature*, **180**, 309.

Flinn, R. H., Brinton, H. P., Doyle, H. N., Cralley, L. F., Harris, R. L. (1963), *Silicosis in the Metal Mining Industry: a Revaluation—1958–1961*. Public Health Service Publication No. 1076, Washington, D.C.

Flinn, R. H., Seifert, H. E., Brinton, H. E., Jones, J. L. and Frank, R. W. (1942), "Soft coal miners' health and working environment." *U.S. Public Health Bulletin*, **270**, Washington, D.C.

Higgins, I. T. T., Cochrane, A. L., Gilson, J. C. and Wood, C. H. (1959), "Population studies of chronic respiratory disease—a comparison of miners, foundry workers, and others in Staveley, Derbyshire." *British Journal of Industrial Medicine*, **16**, 255.

International Labour Office (1970), International Classification of Radiographs of Pneumoconioses (revised, 1968). International Labour Office, Geneva.

Iskrant, A. P. and Joliet, P. V. (1968), *Accidents and Homicide*. Harvard University Press, Cambridge.

Jacobsen, M., Rae, S., Walton, W. H., Rogan, J. M. (1970), "New dust standards for British coal mines." *Nature*, **227**, 445.

Lainhart, W. S. (1969), "Prevalence of coal miners' pneumoconiosis in Appalachian bituminous coal miners." Taken from *Pneumoconiosis in Appalachian Bituminous Coal Miners*, Lainhart, W. S., Doyle, H. N., Enterline, P. E., Henschel, A. and Kendrick, J. A. (1969). Bureau of Occupational Safety and Health, Cincinnati.

Lainhart, W. S. (1969), "Roentgenographic evidence of coal workers' pneumoconiosis in three geographic areas in the United States." *Journal of Occupational Medicine*, **11**, 399.

Liddell, F. D. K. (1961), "Miners' mortality." *Incorporated Statistician*, **11**, 103.

Liddell, F. D. K. and May, J. D. (1966), "Assessing the Radiological Progression of Simple Pneumoconiosis', p. 36. *Med. Res. Memo*. No. 4. National Coal Board, London.

Lundin, F. E., Lloyd, J. W., Smith, E. M., Archer, V. E. and Holaday, D. A. (1969), "Mortality of uranium miners in relation to radiation exposure, hard-rock mining and cigarette smoking—1950 through September, 1967." *Health Physics*, **16**, 571.

McDonald, J. C., McDonald, A. D., Gibbs, G. W., Siemiatycki, J., Rossiter, C. E. (1971), "Mortality from lung cancer and other causes in the chrysotile asbestos mines and mills of Quebec." *Archives of Environmental Health*. (In press.)

McLintock, J. S., Rae, S. and Jacobsen, M. (1971), "The attack rate of progressive massive fibrosis in British coalminers." *Inhaled Particles, III*, ed. W. H. Walton. Unwin, London.

Medical Research Council (1966), *Instructions for the Use of the Questionnaire on Respiratory Symptoms*. W. J. Holman, Dawlish, Devon.

Newhouse, M. L. and Thompson, H. (1965), "Mesothelioma of pleura and peritoneum following exposure to asbestos in the London area." *British Journal of Industrial Medicine*, **22**, 261.

Oettle, A. G. (1963), "Cigarette smoking as the major cause of lung cancer." *South African Medical Journal*, **37**, 983.

Oldham, P. D. (1968), "Assessing the radiological progression of simple pneumoconiosis." *British Journal of Industrial Medicine*, **25**, 150.

Payne, A. M. (1969), "The scope and methods of epidemiology" (editorial). *The Bulletin of the International Epidemiological Association*, **18**, 54.

Pearson, N. G., Ashford, J. R., Morgan, D. C., Pasqual, R. S. H. and Rae, S. (1965), "Effect of quality of chest radiographs on the categorisation of coalworkers' pneumoconiosis." *British Journal of Industrial Medicine*, **22**, 81.

Reisner, M. T. R. (1971), "Results of epidemiological studies on pneumoconiosis in West German coal mines." *Inhaled Particles, III*, ed. W. H. Walton. Unwin, London.

Subcommittee of the Committee of Labor, House of Representatives (1936), "An investigation relating to health conditions of workers employed in construction and maintenance of public utilities." *74th Congress. H. J. Res*. 449, 2603.

Terris, M. (1962), "The scope and methods of epidemiology." *American Journal of Public Health*, **52**, 1371.

Wagoner, J. K., Archer, V. E., Lundin, F. E., Holaday, D. A. and Lloyd, J. W. (1965), "Radiation as the cause of lung cancer among uranium miners." *New England Journal of Medicine*, **273**, 181.

Chapter 26

Administration

The aim of this chapter is to describe the principal areas in occupational medicine in which good administration is essential. It does not purport to set out the various administrative techniques which may be used; several textbooks have been written on this subject and these are readily obtainable.

General

The health problems of an industry coupled with the broad corporate or company policy should be the major factors in determining the shape of the medical programme within that organisation, but the particular interests of the doctor in charge cannot be neglected. His personality and interests play a considerable part in the administration of the programme. Of at least equal importance are the executive level to which he reports and the relationship between the doctor and the executive. To implement a medical programme successfully the status of the doctor is important; he must have sufficient standing within the organisation to be accepted as one of the senior management team. His title, whether it be Chief Physician, Medical Director or other apposite term, does not in itself make much difference to the success or failure of the programme, but what does is the level to which he reports; the nearer this be to the chief executive officer the better. Not only is high status likely to attract the more able medical administrator, but the degree of freedom of action and the ability to carry out a programme effectively are commonly related to reporting level and status, It is of course implicit that there must be mutual respect between physician and executive; without this the likelihood of success decreases sharply.

Programme Planning

Each occupational health service should have a clear programme of duties. This programme will vary from time to time as change occurs in work processes and in consequence the measures necessary for the health protection of the operatives, or as company policy alters in response to, *inter alia*, governmental regulations. The major responsibilities will naturally vary from organisation to organisation but the basic elements are as follows:

(*a*) Preventive and Constructive Medicine . . . for proper job placement and health maintenance, through pre-employment physical examination (and psychological in some cases) and possibly also on re-engagement or transfer; periodic examinations of employees in certain critical occupations where the safety of fellow operatives is dependent on physical and mental fitness, or of those men who run the risk of exposure to toxic substances or otherwise harmful materials; for employees following sickness or injury absence or in relation to retirement; and a management health examination programme.

(*b*) Curative Medicine and Rehabilitation . . . for the application of modern principles of medical treatment and rehabilitation to restore the individual to maximum usefulness to himself and his organisation. Where a comprehensive treatment service is provided by the government or is in some other way readily available to each member of the community, this aspect of the service may be limited. But in those parts of the world where an efficient treatment service is not available, a company may make itself responsible for such treatment for all its employees and perhaps for dependants also. Naturally in circumstances between these extremes intermediate arrangements require to be made.

The minimum provision in any occupational health programme should be for the primary treatment of any person injured or falling sick at work. It is also essential that close liaison be maintained with the doctors responsible for treatment and rehabilitation who will wish to know about the type of work to which the patient can return; equally the industrial physician will wish sufficient clinical information to ensure that he has not missed any environmental hazard at work.

(*c*) Industrial Hygiene . . . wherein the special knowledge of the profession of environmental health engineering is applied through the anticipation, identification, measurement and recommendation for control of health hazards presented by chemical, physical and biological factors in the work or community environment.

(*d*) Health Education . . . for medical guidance of employees and management toward improved health and thus work effectiveness, through health counselling and health education, and assistance to management in handling personnel, plant and community programmes having medical or industrial hygiene aspects.

(*e*) Medical Research . . . on occupational health problems. The engineering (chemical or mechanical) development of new industrial processes may lead to new health problems. Attention must be devoted to this possibility; indeed, as a member of the management team the industrial physician should be involved at the earliest stage of development. In complex health problems it may be appropriate to seek the assistance of an outside research agency. Nevertheless the control of the research should remain within the industrial medical department.

(*f*) Adequate record keeping . . . to permit good clinical case-handling, to assist in making good judgments in personnel and labour

relations matters, to provide clinical data for industrial medical research activities, to furnish statistical and epidemiological data, and to
meet legal and financial responsibilities.

In some circumstances the medical department may be called upon
for sick pay scheme purposes to certify inability to work because of
sickness or injury. This is a function to be avoided if possible. It is
virtually impossible to arbitrate on financial matters between employer
and employee and still be regarded by both as expert and unbiassed in
comment on occupational health matters such as those concerned with
the environment at work.

The needs of the organisation will determine the size of the basic
programme. Requirements of governmental regulations in the safety
and health field will influence and may determine the relative size of
these various elements. In addition, the related programmes on Safety,
Water and Air Pollution Control and Solid Waste Disposal (sanitation)
will make their contribution. Operations change, as do processes, each
with different hazards and exposures; regulations change and the needs
of the organisation also. Because of these changes, so too must a
medical programme, oftentimes in anticipation of such events so that
a smooth service to the employees can be maintained and a healthy
environment continued. Research projects may and often are a major
contributor to the needed changes in order to keep small problems from
becoming large ones, or for that matter from even occurring.

Budgeting

A programme and a budget go hand in hand. Management will
certainly wish to know and approve the estimated cost of its medical
service. The budgeting system is mainly determined by the financial
accounting system of the organisation. The medical department can
operate successfully within a realistic and approved budget; in this
respect it is no different from other departments.

Yearly budget estimates are usually required. This necessitates
administrative procedures within the medical department to ensure
adequate preparation within the time limit set out. Anticipated expenditure for medical supplies and equipment, both new and replacement, and capital expenditures for major alterations to the department
or erection of new facilities must be estimated with considerable
accuracy if budget deficits are to be avoided. In some organisations the
capital expenditure items are in a separate budget and are considered
with other capital items. Salaries are usually altered by specific review
procedures. When all items specified in the accounting procedure have
been included, the total expenditure on medical activities can be
calculated. In some instances estimates are not required on a periodic
basis, but comparison is made with expenditure during the previous

year. Justification is often demanded for variation above or below certain percentage levels of earlier expenditure.

Whatever the company's accounting system, it is to be expected that in the event of unforeseen circumstances, where additional unbudgeted monies are called for and can be justified, there will be provision to seek approval for this extra expenditure.

Average costs per employee can be calculated, but because of different accounting procedures it is unwise to attach too much significance to comparison of such costs between different industries or organisations. Indeed, accountancy changes may make for difficulties in comparing annual costs within the same medical department.

Staffing

Manpower requirements for physicians, nurses, technical, clerical and other administrative personnel will depend in large measure on the scope of the programme and the budgetary levels available and to a lesser degree on the availability of personnel.

Great care must be exercised in the selection of personnel, especially those in direct contact with employees. The medical department must be responsive to the health needs of the employees, and all departmental staff contribute in some measure to the general feeling of confidence (or lack of it) in the medical services among the company personnel. There is a direct relationship between the level of such confidence and the usage of the facilities provided.

Ideally a balance should be struck between highly detailed instructions on the performance of each task in the medical department and the opposite extreme of "laissez-faire." The purposes and functions of the post should be defined and the limits of responsibility clearly set out. It is desirable to try to match the talents of each member of the staff to the needs of specific jobs; where appropriate staff should be encouraged to utilise skills not fully developed. To attract talented staff, individual initiative must be encouraged wherever possible.

In ever increasing numbers, paramedical personnel are being utilised to relieve the physician and, in some instances, nurses of routine tasks. Thus, the highly skilled have more time to spend dealing with the more difficult problems.

In a medical department employing several doctors and nurses, a non-medical administrative assistant can be of considerable help to the chief medical officer in the administrative field. He should normally be selected from the administrative ranks within the organisation, to ensure that he is well conversant with company policy and practice.

Automation is also contributing to the solution of staffing problems. Automated biological tests are one example. Another is the use of computers to store and analyse medical records of individual patients;

25

here care must be taken to maintain the confidentiality of these personal records. Although automation should help the same number of medical and nursing staff to deal with more patients, it must be used with discretion; a patient must not feel that automation has in any way reduced the personal interest of the doctor or nurse.

Evaluation

The medical programme should be a dynamic operation, changing with the needs of the organisation. It is particularly important that these changes should keep pace with the needs, so that the programme is forward looking, not only meeting current requirements but so far as possible anticipating those of the future. There is neither point nor pleasure in carrying out a programme designed for the problems encountered ten years earlier. Effectiveness can be measured by setting objectives to be fulfilled within a particular period and then by determining at appropriate intervals progress towards these goals. Research projects are often fruitful in giving direction to a programme; they may well point to the need to develop a new aspect of work or to terminate an old one.

The relationship between the work of the medical and that of other departments must be reviewed from time to time. Common interest with the safety programme, with personnel and industrial relations policies is obvious, but new developments in the field of production can well raise problems of a medical nature (e.g. noise from more powerful machinery, laser beams in tunnelling). The medical department must not work in isolation but in continual contact and co-operation with other departments.

The performance of individual members of the staff must also be assessed regularly. Periodic work reviews and face to face discussion assist them to improve their contribution to the overall medical programme. Such reviews can be formalised (e.g. by making a record for that individual's personal file) or not, depending on the pattern of the organisation. Opportunities for additional training, either of an in-service nature or through outside courses, can provide staff with the initiative to improve their performance and can prepare them for future promotion. In the main, the standard of work is in proportion to the individual's understanding of the objectives of the programme, of his part in it and of his inter-relationship with the work of his colleagues.

Finally, sufficient and accurate financial records should be maintained to ensure that regular reviews of expenditure in relation to budget can be carried out and that opportunities for cost reductions can be assessed.

Reporting

A certain amount of reporting is necessary but it should be kept to a minimum; there is no value in recording data or preparing reports which serve no clear purpose.

Reports may be prepared for a number of purposes; e.g.

(*a*) as a record of work done;
(*b*) for financial reasons as a measure of expenditure against budget;
(*c*) to inform management of new findings from research studies;
(*d*) to propose to senior management changes in company policy or practice when the chief physician considers that he cannot himself authorise the change.

Such changes may concern departments other than medical, e.g. an alteration in the medical examination practice for new staff might involve the personnel department, or a proposal to issue protective equipment to workmen at special risk might involve the production and safety departments.

When other departments are involved they should be given the opportunity to comment on the report before it is presented.

The burden of reading which chief executives have to bear is normally very considerable. Medical reports should therefore be simple, clear and concise. Many a good medical case has been lost through obscure, vague, lengthy presentation.

Records of work done may require to be detailed, but it should always be possible to start with a summary highlighting the salient points which need to be brought to the attention of the chief executive —or to the chief physician if the report is within the medical department.

Financial reports too may have to be lengthy and detailed, but once again the main items can be summarised.

Research studies may be particularly difficult to present because of the highly technical, and possibly statistical, material which must be introduced if the report is to be valid in the scientific sense. But it is not to be expected that the chief executive is deeply versed in biological or epidemiological matters. Again it should be possible to present the main core of the work and the recommendations arising concisely in everyday language with, if it seems appropriate, the full report as an appendix. Publication of medical research data can add to the bank of health information and should be encouraged, whether the results reveal the presence or absence of a health hazard.

When changes in company policy are proposed, the executive's main interests will lie in the reasons for the proposals, the methods to be adopted, the financial costs and the likely benefit to the organisation both in human and in financial terms.

Good administration requires considerable effort and thought devoted to:

(*a*) defining the health problems of the industry and the medical needs of the personnel;

(*b*) the optimum programme to meet these problems and needs in the light of the finance available and its co-ordination with other departments;

(*c*) the selection, training, supervision and encouragement of staff;

(*d*) the control of financial expenditure;

(*e*) evaluating the success of the medical programme and defining those areas in which research is warranted to improve the health care of the work force; and

(*f*) reporting on all aspects of the performance of the medical department.

Index

3.28 × 3000

= 9840
  164
10004

9.28
  50
16400